Lasers in Ophthalmic Surgery

To my wife Adrienne, who has encouraged, supported and
inspired me to seek a life in research and teaching, as well as
in clinical ophthalmology.

To my two daughters, Linda Beth and Diane Beth, who have
followed through in the family concept of "there are worlds to
be conquered."

To my late father, Doctor Isaac William, and my late
mother, Bertha Eva, who taught me the meaning of honesty, integrity,
dedication and complete application to the field of ophthalmology.

Lasers in Ophthalmic Surgery

David B. Karlin, AB, M.D., M.Sc. (Ophth.)
Clinical Associate Professor of Ophthalmology
Cornell University Medical College;
Assistant Clinical Professor of Ophthalmology, Mount Sinai School of Medicine
Attending Ophthalmic Surgeon and Director of Vitreoretinal Service II
Manhattan Eye, Ear and Throat Hospital;
Vitreoretinal Consultant
National Heart, Lung, and Blood Institute
National Institutes of Health
Assistant Attending Ophthalmic Surgeon, Lenox Hill Hospital
New York, New York

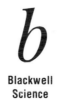

Blackwell
Science

EDITORIAL OFFICES:
238 Main Street, Cambridge, Massachusetts 02142, USA
Osney Mead, Oxford OX2 0EL, England
25 John Street, London WC1N 2BL, England
23 Ainslie Place, Edinburgh EH3 6AJ, Scotland
54 University Street, Carlton, Victoria 3053, Australia
Arnette SA, 1 rue de Lille, 75007 Paris, France
Blackwell Wissenschafts-Verlag GmbH, Kurfürstendamm 57
    10707 Berlin, Germany
Blackwell MZV, Feldgasse 13, A-1238 Vienna, Austria

Acquisitions: Michael Snider
Development: Gail S. Segal
Production: Michelle Choate
Manufacturing: Paul Lansdowne

Typeset by BookMasters, Ashland, Ohio

Printed and bound by Printer S.A., Bilbao, Spain

95 96 97 98 5 4 3 2 1

DISTRIBUTORS:

North America
Blackwell Science, Inc.
238 Main Street
Cambridge, Massachusetts 02142
(Telephone orders: 800-215-1000 or 617-876-7000)

Australia
Blackwell Science (Australia) Pty Ltd
54 University Street
Carlton, Victoria 3053
(Telephone orders: 03-347-5552)

Outside North America and Australia
Blackwell Science, Ltd.
c/o Marston Book Services, Ltd.
P. O. Box 87
Oxford OX2 0DT
England
(Telephone orders: 44-865-791155)

Notice: The indications and dosages of all drugs in this book have been recommended in the medical literature and conform to the practices of the general medical community. The medications described do not necessarily have specific approval by the Food and Drug Administration for use in the diseases and dosages for which they are recommended. The package insert for each drug should be consulted for use and dosage as approved by the FDA. Because standards of usage change, it is advisable to keep abreast of revised recommendations, particularly those concerning new drugs.

Library of Congress Cataloging in Publication Data

Lasers in ophthalmic surgery / edited by David B. Karlin.
    p.   cm.
    Includes bibliographical references and index.
    ISBN 0-86542-260-5
    1. Lasers in ophthalmology. 2. Eye—Surgery. I. Karlin,
David B.
    [DNLM: 1. Eye Diseases—surgery. 2. Eye—surgery.
3. Laser Surgery,—methods.   WW 168 L344 1995]
RE86.L374 1995
617.7'1—dc20
DNLM/DLC
for Library of Congress   94-33489
                                                       CIP

Contents

Contributors, vi

Foreword by Lawrence A. Yannuzzi, MD, viii

Preface, ix

Acknowledgements, x

1. Fundamentals of Lasers, 1
   C. K. N. Patel and O. R. Wood, II

2. Laser Surgery of the Cornea—The Excimer Laser, 30
   Francis A. L'Esperance, Jr. and Olivia N. Serdarevic

3. Laser Surgery in Glaucoma, 67
   Maurice H. Luntz, Raymond Harrison and Andrea F. Katz

4. Lasers in Cataract Surgery, 80
   Stephen A. Obstbaum, King W. To and Ezra L. Galler

5. Laser Surgery in Diabetic Retinopathy, 92
   David B. Karlin

6. Laser Treatment of Choroidal Neovascularization, 112
   Lawrence J. Singerman, Jeffrey C. Lamkin, Rafael Addiego and Hernando Zegarra

7. Laser Treatment of Retinal Vein Occlusions, 140
   Hernando Zegarra, Z. Nicholas Zakov, Lawrence J. Singerman and Jeffrey C. Lamkin

8. Laser Treatment of Less Common Macular Diseases, 152
   Lawrence J. Singerman, Rafael Addiego, Jeffrey C. Lamkin and Hernando Zegarra

9. Laser Surgery for Retinal Tears, Retinal Detachment, Vitrectomy, and Posterior Segment Tumors, 179
   David B. Karlin

10. Recent Laser Techniques in Vitreoretinal Surgery, 197
    David B. Karlin

11. Lasers in Ophthalmic Plastic and Orbital Surgery, 214
    Albert Hornblass and Daniel J. Coden

12. Medicolegal and Safety Aspects of Laser Surgery, 227
    Alfred E. Mamelok and David B. Karlin

Index, 231

Contributors

Rafael Addiego, M.D.
Attending Ophthalmologist, Sparrow Hospital, Lansing, Michigan; Former Vitreoretinal Fellow, Retina Associates of Cleveland and Mt. Sinai Medical Center, Cleveland, Ohio.

Daniel J. Coden, M.D.
Co-Chief, Division of Orbital, Oculoplastic and Reconstructive Surgery, Department of Ophthalmology, University of California School of Medicine, San Diego, California; Co-Chief, Division of Orbital, Oculoplastic and Reconstructive Surgery, Veterans Administration Hospital, La Jolla, California; Civilian Consultant, Balboa U. S. Naval Hospital, San Diego, California.

Ezra Galler, M.D.
Chief Resident, Department of Ophthalmology, Lenox Hill Hospital, an affiliate of New York University School of Medicine, New York, New York.

Raymond Harrison, M.D.
Surgeon Director Emeritus and Co-Chief of Glaucoma Service, Manhattan Eye, Ear and Throat Hospital, New York, New York.

Albert Hornblass, M.D.
Clinical Professor of Ophthalmology, State University of New York, Downstate Medical Center, Brooklyn, New York; Director of Ophthalmic Plastic and Reconstructive Surgery, Manhattan Eye, Ear and Throat Hospital and Lenox Hill Hospital, New York, New York; President, American Society of Ophthalmic Plastic and Reconstructive Surgery and American Israeli Ophthalmological Society.

David B. Karlin, M.D., M.Sc. (Ophth.)
Clinical Associate Professor of Ophthalmology, Cornell University Medical College; Assistant Clinical Professor of Ophthamology, Mount Sinai, Attending Ophthalmic Surgeon and Director of Vitreoretinal Service II, Manhattan Eye, Ear and Throat Hospital; Vitreoretinal Consultant, National Heart, Lung, and Blood Institute, National Institutes of Health, Assistant Attending Ophthalmic Surgeon, Lenox Hill Hospital.

Andrea F. Katz, M.D.
Assistant Attending Ophthalmic Surgeon and Chief of Glaucoma Clinic, Manhattan Eye, Ear and Throat Hospital, New York, New York.

Francis A. L'Esperance, Jr., M.D.
Professor of Clinical Ophthalmology, Columbia University College of Physicians and Surgeons; Attending Ophthalmologist, Columbia-Presbyterian Medical Center, New York, New York; Attending Ophthalmic Surgeon, Manhattan Eye, Ear and Throat Hospital.

Jeffrey C. Lamkin, M.D.
Retinal Specialists of Western Michigan, Grand Rapids, Michigan; Staff Ophthalmologist, Blodgett Memorial Medical Center, Butterworth and St. Mary's Hospitals, Grand Rapids, Michigan.

Maurice H. Luntz, M.D.
Clinical Professor of Ophthalmology, Mount Sinai School of Medicine; President, Board of Surgeon Directors and Surgeon Director, Manhattan Eye, Ear and Throat Hospital; Co-Director, Glaucoma Service, Manhattan Eye, Ear and Throat Hospital, New York, New York.

Alfred E. Mamelok, M.D.
Clinical Associate Professor of Ophthalmology, Cornell University Medical College; Director, Uveitis Clinic, Manhattan Eye, Ear and Throat Hospital; Section Chief of Ophthalmology, Beth Israel North Hospital, New York, New York.

Stephen A. Obstbaum, M.D.
Professor of Clinical Ophthalmology, Cornell University Medical College; Director, Department of Ophthalmology, Lenox Hill Hospital; President Emeritus, American Society of Cataract and Refractive Surgery; Board of Trustees, American Academy of Ophthalmology.

C. K. N. Patel, Ph.D.
Vice Chancellor-Research, University of California, Los Angeles, California; Former Executive Director, Research, Materials, Science & Engineering, Academic Affairs Division, AT&T Bell Labs, New Jersey.

Olivia N. Serdarevic, M.D.
Professor of Ophthalmology, Hotel-Dieu, University of Paris, Paris, France; Attending Ophthalmologist, The New York

Hospital-Cornell University Medical College and The Manhattan Eye, Ear and Throat Hospital, New York, New York.

Lawrence J. Singerman, M.D.
Clinical Professor of Ophthalmology, Case Western Reserve University, Cleveland, Ohio; Director, Retinal Service and Retinal Institute, Mt. Sinai Medical Center, Cleveland, Ohio; Founder and Executive Secretary, Macula Society.

King W. To, M.D.
Assistant Clinical Professor of Ophthalmology and Pathology, Brown University School of Medicine, Providence, Rhode Island; Director of Ophthalmic Pathology and Director of Ophthalmic Residency Program, Rhode Island Hospital.

Obert R. Wood, II, Ph.D.
Distinguished Member, Technical Staff, AT&T Bell Laboratories, Holmdel, New Jersey.

Z. Nicholas Zakov, M.D.
Assistant Clinical Professor of Ophthalmology, Case Western Reserve University, Cleveland, Ohio; Chief, Section of Retina Surgery, Meridia Hillcrest Hospital.

Hernando Zegarra, M.D.
Attending Ophthalmic Surgeon, Mt. Sinai Hospital, Cleveland, Ohio; Retina Associates of Cleveland, Ohio.

Foreword

It has been more than a third of a century since Meyer-Schwickerath first presented his classic monograph on *Licht Koagulation.* Utilizing his recently constructed Zeiss Xenon Photocoagulator, he introduced numerous potential applications and techniques for the treatment of anterior as well as posterior segment ocular diseases with photocoagulation. In spite of his creative genius and his remarkable insight, I doubt that he could have possibly envisioned the explosive technological breakthroughs offered by photobiological scientists and the innovative applications introduced by ophthalmic clinicians since his pioneering work. One of the most important contributions to the widespread use of photocoagulation treatment of the posterior segment, occurred fifteen years after Schwickerath's publication with the introduction of fluorescein angiography. This diagnostic adjunct for the patho-physiological study of macular diseases singularly documented the nature of exudative and angio-proliferative diseases and served as a guide to photocoagulation therapy. Nearly coinciding with the development and use of fluorescein angiography was the discovery of laser light with excellent delivery mechanisms and superb binocular and well-illuminated viewing systems.

The most recent stage in the evolution of light (now laser photocoagulation) was catalyzed by a series of national, collaborative clinical trials, funded by the National Institutes of Health (NIH), on the treatment of diseases of the macula. Based on initial impressions by experienced retinal specialists, these NIH clinical trials were exquisitely designed, and their results were stringently evaluated within a very strict and disciplined environment. Recommendations for laser treatment of common disorders of the macula associated with severe vision loss (such as diabetic retinopathy, age-related macular degeneration, and retinal branch vein occlusion) were disseminated to the ophthalmic public for better patient management.

The development in the use of lasers in ophthalmic surgery was not limited to the posterior segment of the eye. In the past quarter of a century, there have also been discoveries which have favorably influenced the treatment of anterior segment eye diseases as well. Today, laser treatment has expanded as a therapeutic option for disorders involving almost every segment of the eye, including the ocular adnexa.

Dr. David Karlin, a well-known clinical authority in the field of laser surgery, has recruited and actively collaborated with career scientists and clinicians in assembling an ocular laser text under his guidance. Beginning with the fundamental elements to laser light and its use in therapeutic systems, and ending with treatment guidelines suggested by contributing authors for the management of numerous ocular disorders, Dr. Karlin and his co-authors have written an excellent book on laser applications in the entire field of ophthalmic surgery. The text as a whole represents the experience and recommendations of a distinguished panel of clinical and research investigators who have contributed in innovative ways to the applications of laser treatment in various subspecialties in ophthalmology. Many of the authors have been pioneers in the development of these laser techniques in their respective fields.

Finally, one of the purposes of this book was to provide a reference source for ophthalmologists who have not had the opportunity to have formal training. It was also particularly designed for residents in training and for ophthalmologists from developing countries where subspeciality consultations are not always readily available. Each chapter is likely to improve a clinician's judgement in making decisions for patient management, and to enhance his skills in the actual techniques of laser photocoagulation.

Dr. Karlin and his contributors are to be congratulated in providing a timely, well-organized and informative text concerning the present and potential future applications of laser treatment in the field of ophthalmology.

Lawrence A. Yannuzzi, M.D.
Professor of Clinical Ophthalmology,
Columbia University College of
Physicians and Surgeons;
Surgeon Director and Chief of
Retinal Services,
Manhattan Eye, Ear, and Throat Hospital
New York, New York

Preface

The specialty of ophthalmology was the first field in medicine to apply lasers as a surgical tool. Starting with its use in the treatment of retinal diseases in the 1960s, lasers have become the accepted treatment over the past thirty years in almost every subspecialty in ophthalmology, starting with the eyelids and cornea anteriorly and progressing through the angle, iris, ciliary body, lens, retina, and ending with the retro-orbital structures posteriorly.

The book *Lasers in Ophthalmic Surgery* has been written to attract the interest of practicing physicians, fellows, residents, and paramedical personnel in the field of ophthalmology. Each chapter is authored by an expert in that particular discipline. The chapters are divided in a logical progression and present not only the current laser treatments, but also future possible laser applications. The text and figures are presented in a logical manner to enhance the reader's comprehension of each of the many diseases discussed. The first chapter entitled "Fundamentals of Lasers," provides an overview of the subject matter. It has been written by former colleagues of the author who have worked with him on laser projects sponsored by the National Eye Institute in collaboration with Cornell University Medical College and Bell Telephone Laboratories.

David B. Karlin

Acknowledgments

I wish to acknowledge the influence of Dr. Harvey Lincoff who first kindled my interest in vitreoretinal surgery when I was a resident at New York University-Bellevue Medical Center. Dr. Charles Schepens provided the opportunity to study vitreoretinal surgery under his excellent tutelage when I was a Fellow at The Retina Foundation, Massachusetts Eye and Ear Infirmary, and The Harvard Medical School. I also wish to thank Dr. Donald Shafer, who appointed me to the staffs of The Manhattan Eye, Ear & Throat Hospital and The New York Hospital–Cornell University Medical College. His warm personality and expertise during my early career have served me well, as I have gone through life dealing with patients and medical colleagues. Lastly, I have enjoyed teaching, research, and the interchange of ideas with my own Fellows and Residents at The Manhattan Eye, Ear & Throat Hospital, The New York Hospital–Cornell University Medical College, and The Mount Sinai Hos-pital and School of Medicine. It is to this younger gen-eration of Ophthalmic physicians, that I would like to dedicate this book. If I can add in some small measure to their knowledge of lasers in ophthalmic surgery, then I know that this book will prove to be a great success.

Special thanks are given to Sharyn Crichton-Budnetz, my office manager, who provided helpful suggestions in the organization of the material in this book. Rob Wolfson provided most of the illustrations for my chapters. Ms. Janet Kennaugh and Ms. Shellie Silberger did most of the typing of the manuscript dealing with my three chapters on Lasers in Vitreoretinal Surgery. Thanks are also given to my Ophthalmic Technicians, Felicia Kamel and Ms. Beth Soulé.

1

Fundamentals of Lasers

C. K. N. Patel
O. R. Wood, II

The word LASER is an acronym for Light Amplification by Stimulated Emission of Radiation and refers to a device that produces a powerful beam of highly coherent electromagnetic radiation. Although when first developed the laser seemed to be an invention with little immediate use, it has rapidly become quite ubiquitous. It is used in reading the compact discs in home stereo systems, in reading bar codes at supermarket checkout counters, and in transmitting voices in long distance telephone calls. In addition to these prosaic applications, lasers have countless uses in research laboratories, factories, hospitals, and the construction industry and as time goes by there is every reason to expect their uses to continue to proliferate.

The era of lasers began in 1958 with the publication of the seminal theoretical paper of Schawlow and Townes (1), which extended the principles of microwave masers to optical frequencies. The first experimental demonstration of laser oscillation was made by Maiman (2) in 1960, using a ruby crystal pumped with light from a flashlamp. Since then, scientists and physicians have explored hundreds of potential medical applications for lasers. Today, lasers are the tool of choice for sight-saving procedures in ophthalmology, for the removal of various skin lesions in dermatology, as well as for the removal of specific tissue structures in neurosurgery, gynecology, urology, gastroenterology, and orthopedics.

The eye, with its optical accessibility in the visible region, is especially receptive to laser treatment. The iris can be quickly and painlessly perforated with the output from an argon-ion laser to relieve the pressure of fluid in the eye of a glaucoma patient (3). The retina of a diabetic patient can be selectively photocoagulated with light from an argon-ion or semiconductor diode laser to slow or stop the overproduction of new blood vessels (4). The posterior capsule of a lens that has become cloudy after cataract surgery can be cleared using the Q-switched output from a neodymium: yttrium-aluminum-garnet (Nd:YAG) laser (5,6). The cornea can be reshaped to correct for nearsightedness using pulses from an argon-fluoride laser in a procedure called photorefractive keratectomy (7). As exciting as these applications are, in the future it could be that laser systems incorporating feedback to guide the treatment (8)

will find new applications that are even more important. For most surgical and medical applications today, the operating physician is the feedback and control element.

In this chapter, we review the fundamental physics of lasers, especially as it relates to the field of medicine. We begin by briefly reviewing the nature of light and describing the physical processes that lead to laser action. We then describe various population inversion mechanisms and the operational characteristics of a number of lasers of practical importance in medicine and surgery. Next, we discuss three applications of lasers in ophthalmology that show why lasers have become the standard of care in the treatment of many eye diseases. Finally, we comment on the directions laser technology is likely to take in the future that will have an impact on the fields of medicine and surgery.

The Nature of Light

Visible light, x-rays, infrared radiation, and radio waves are all forms of electromagnetic radiation. A graph illustrating the incredible breadth of the electromagnetic spectrum is shown in Fig. 1.1. Electromagnetic radiation consists of time-varying electric and magnetic fields that propagate at the velocity of light. As shown in Fig. 1.2, both electric and magnetic fields oscillate perpendicularly to the direction the light is traveling and perpendicular to each other. Electromagnetic radiation is characterized by the frequency of oscillation of the electric and magnetic fields and the wavelength or distance between successive field peaks. The frequency, f, and the wavelength, λ, are related by the equation $c = f\lambda$, where c is the velocity of light in vacuum, 3×10^8 m/sec (9).

Electromagnetic radiation sometimes exhibits wavelike behavior, for example, when it gives rise to various interference phenomena as in the formation of light and dark bands on reflection from thin films and diffraction of light around obstacles. An example of such an interference effect, the formation of Airy diffraction rings when light waves pass through a small circular hole, is shown in Fig. 1.3 (10). Because of interference, the light transmitted through the hole consists of a central bright spot

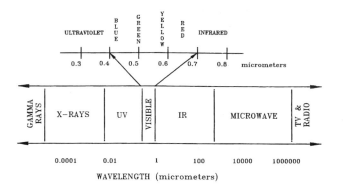

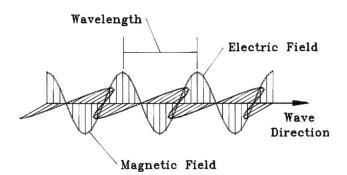

Fig. 1.1 The electromagnetic spectrum.

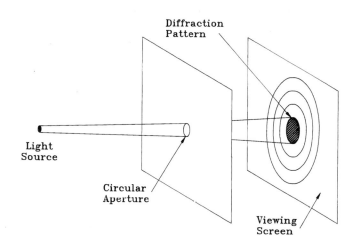

Fig. 1.2 Structure of an electromagnetic wave traveling from left to right, viewed at a particular instant of time.

Fig. 1.3 The production of Airy diffraction rings. (Adapted from Hecht [10]; reproduced by permission from the IEEE.)

surrounded by a series of increasingly faint rings. Electromagnetic radiation sometimes acts as if it consists of particle-like quanta of energy called photons. Each photon possesses a discrete amount of energy given by $E = hf$, where E is the photon energy in joules, and h is Planck's constant, 6.63×10^{-34} joule-seconds (9). This particle-like behavior is important in applications that involve the interaction of light with matter. For example, absorption of

radiation by atoms or molecules occurs at various discrete frequencies, which are characteristic of the particular atom or molecule, and each absorbed photon results in a discrete change in the excitation of the atom. The absorption spectrum of most atoms can be complex. However, the absorption spectrum of some elements like sodium (Fig. 1.4) consists of an easily recognizable series of discrete lines converging toward a limit. Because the behavior of electromagnetic radiation contains elements of both waves and particles, it is sometimes said to have a dual nature.

Laser light is a highly coherent form of electromagnetic radiation falling in the spectral range between the x-rays and the far infrared. Long before the advent of the laser, light possessing various degrees of coherence could be obtained by filtering ordinary light. However, the filtering process resulted in an output beam of such low intensity as to render such beams useless in most practical applications. The usefulness of laser light in medicine stems from its high intensity and coherence that it derives from its unique combination of monochromaticity, directionality, and brightness.

Monochromaticity

The word *monochromatic* applied to electromagnetic radiation means single frequency or single wavelength. In practice, no radiation source, not even the laser, is absolutely monochromatic. Conventional light sources tend to emit a broad spectrum of light, sometimes called blackbody radiation, in all directions. For an ideal blackbody source, the amount of light emitted per unit area of radiator per unit spectral width is given by Planck's law (12) a graph of which is shown at the top of Fig. 1.5. As can be seen from these curves, the emissive properties of an ideal blackbody are a strong function of the temperature of the radiator. The total amount of radiation intensity over all wavelengths, I (W/cm^2), is given by the Stefan-Boltzmann equation, $I = \sigma T^4$, where $\sigma = 5.673 \times 10^{-12}$ W/cm^2 per degree Kelvin (4). Of course, no real light source looks like a perfect blackbody. Instead it radiates somewhat less by a factor ϵ than that predicted by the Planck curves. The factor ϵ is known as the emissivity and is usually a function of wavelength. Lasers,

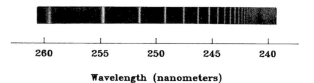

Fig. 1.4 Photograph of the absorption spectrum of sodium, showing some of the lines in the ultraviolet region. (From Herzberg [11]); reproduced by permission from Dover Publications.)

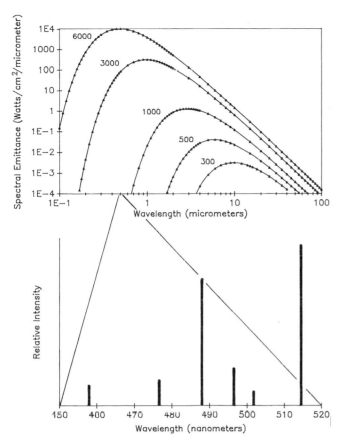

Fig. 1.5 The spectral emittance of a blackbody (*top*) and the emission spectrum of an argon-ion laser (*bottom*).

on the other hand, tend to emit in a narrow spectrum and are, thus, highly monochromatic. For comparison, the spectral output from a multiline argon-ion laser is shown at the bottom of Fig. 1.5. In medicine, high spectral purity or monochromaticity is important because it allows for the possibility of highly specific reactions. In other words, only those specific cells or tissues that absorb the light are modified. It should be emphasized, however, that the absorption features of biologic materials can be quite broad compared to those of the sodium atoms discussed earlier. Therefore, the monochromaticity needed to affect specific cells while leaving others unaffected is not quite as stringent as in atomic or molecular spectroscopy.

Directionality

Laser light possesses a high degree of spatial coherence, which means that at any given time there is nearly constant phase across the wavefront. A conventional (i.e., incoherent) light source will typically have a coherence length, l_c (the distance over which the phase is constant), of at most a few wavelengths, whereas a laser will generally have a coherence length of the order of its beam di-

ameter. Because the angular spread of a light source, θ (in radians), is given by

$$\theta \sim \lambda/l_c \qquad \text{(Eq. 1)}$$

and the coherence length of laser light is much larger than that of incoherent light, laser light is much more directional, as illustrated in Fig. 1.6. For example, a CO_2 laser with a 1-mm diameter beam has an angular spread of only 10 milliradians (about 0.5°). Because laser light is so directional, a lens can collect all of the laser energy. In addition, a laser beam can be focused with a lens to a very small spot. In contrast, it is not possible to focus efficiently incoherent light to a small spot. The best that can be done is to image and demagnify the source. As one moves the lens further and further away from a conventional source, the spot size can be made smaller, but only at the expense of having the lens collect less and less light. In surgery, high directionality and a small focal spot are important because they allow high intensities needed for tissue to be cut precisely and coagulated with little harm to surrounding tissue.

Brightness

Although an incoherent light source can emit as much power as a laser and with greater efficiency, this power is generally broad-band spectrally and in addition is omnidirectional, as shown in Figs. 1.5 and 1.6. Some xenon arc lamps, for example, can deliver more than 100 W of power; however, their brightness (defined in units of power per unit area of radiation emitted per unit solid angle) is actually much less than that of even a low-power laser. For

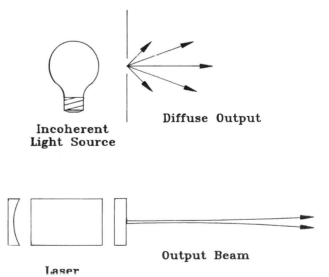

Fig. 1.6 Schematic diagram of an incoherent source and a laser illustrating the differences in their output.

example, the brightness of a 100-W xenon lamp with a radiating area of 2 mm² is approximately 500 W/cm²/steradian. A 1-W diffraction-limited CO_2 laser, on the other hand, has a brightness of approximately 1,000,000 W/cm²/steradian. Hence, the brightness of a 1-W CO_2 laser is more than 2000 times greater than a 100-W xenon lamp! In surgery, high brightness is important because it allows tissue to be coagulated or cut rapidly.

The Physics of Lasers

A laser, then, is a device that produces a highly directional beam of light with high spectral purity that can be focused to a very small spot. Lasers make available intensities many orders of magnitude higher than that possible with conventional light sources. A schematic diagram of a laser is shown in Fig. 1.7 (13).

The Active Medium

Central to a laser is the light amplifier (or active medium) that provides amplification by the process of stimulated emission of radiation. This process, first described by Einstein (14) in 1917, is one of the ways in which energy can be first stored and then given up by atoms. Energy can be transferred to atoms from a pumping source (see Fig. 1.7) in several ways: (1) by thermal heating; (2) via the absorption of light; or (3) in collisions with electrons in an electrical current. In processes (1) and (3), part of the energy increases the random motion of the atoms and part is absorbed, causing electrons to move to the higher energy levels of the atoms. The former part is not useful in producing amplification, but the latter part (electronic excitation) is extremely useful.

Excited atoms radiate their excess energy in the form of light when the electrons fall back to their lowest energy state as shown in Fig. 1.8 (*middle*). The light that is emitted has a frequency that exactly corresponds to the energy the electrons gave up according to Einstein's formula $E = hf$. In stationary single atoms, the energy states of the electron, and thus the frequency of the emitted light, are precisely defined. For nonstationary atoms, a small amount of broaden-

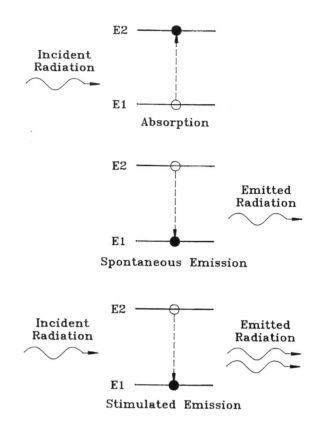

Fig. 1.8 Energy level diagrams for absorption (*top*), spontaneous emission (*middle*), and stimulated emission (*bottom*) of light.

ing is caused by the random motion of the radiators (i.e., a Doppler shift). Nonetheless, single atoms or molecules (such as those in a gas) emit relatively pure frequencies. In liquids and solids the atoms are so closely packed that the interaction with neighbors causes their energy levels to be smeared out. Consequently, molecules in liquids and solids generally emit a broad spectrum of frequencies. In either case (narrow or broad-band), stimulated emission can occur when light interacts with an atom that has energy stored in an excited state as shown in Fig. 1.8 (*bottom*). The incident light must have the exact energy that the radiator can give up when its electron falls to a lower state. If this requirement is satisfied, the atom will emit its light in the same direction as the incident light, and the emitted light will be in step (in phase) with the incident light. In other words, light can be amplified by stimulating atoms to emit radiation. A reverse and competing process, known as absorption, can remove light from the beam by raising electrons from the lower energy state to higher ones as shown in Fig. 1.8 (*top*). Thus, to have net amplification (instead of absorption) when the light passes through the active medium, there must be more atoms with electrons at the higher energy state than at the lower energy state, as shown in Fig. 1.9. This condition is called a *population inversion*.

In most lasers the amplification region is relatively long compared to its transverse dimension. If the intensity of

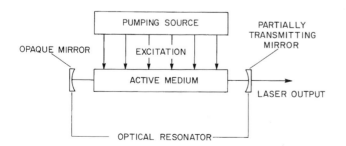

Fig. 1.7 Schematic diagram of a laser illustrating the terminology. (From Patel and Wood [13]; reproduced by permission from Appleton-Century-Crofts.)

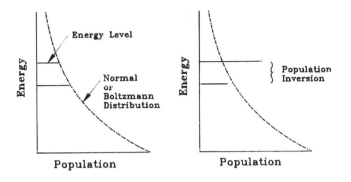

Fig. 1.9 Distribution of populations among energy levels of an atom in thermal equilibrium (*left*) and during a population inversion (*right*).

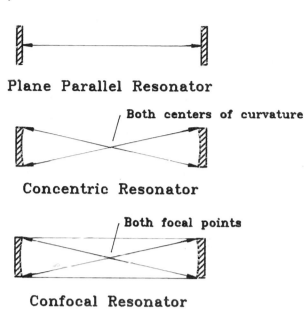

Fig. 1.10 Schematic diagram shows three common optical resonator geometries.

light passing through the length of the amplifier is increased by say 5% (typical of many lasers), the active medium is said to have a gain of 5%. If light from an ordinary light source such as a flashlight were shown through such an amplifier, it would not look much different from the original flashlight beam except in the very narrow region of amplified wavelengths. If mirrors are placed at opposite ends of the amplifier in such a way that nearly 100% of the light leaving the amplifier is reflected back into it (see Fig. 1.7), this light would grow by about 5% every time it passed through the amplifier. After 100 passes, the initial light intensity would be increased approximately 130 times and after 200 passes would be increased over 17,000 times. In any case, only a portion of the beam (that which was reflected by one mirror in such a way that it would arrive at the other mirror after having passed through the amplifier) is preserved in the multiple reflection process. Thus, a few hundred passes would provide a very precise direction to the beam of light. Some of this light could be made available (coupled out) by making one of the resonator mirrors partially transmitting (1% or 2% is typical). The number of times the beam can pass through the active medium before it ceases to grow is limited by the amount of energy stored in the amplifier. When this limit is reached, the amplifier is said to be saturated, and the laser is said to have reached a steady state.

Optical Resonators

The active medium is central to a laser, but without an optical resonator there would be no laser beam and the light emitted would not be nearly so monochromatic, directional, or bright. The 1958 publication by Schawlow and Townes (1) suggested the use of an optical resonator with a relatively long cylindrical geometry bounded at the two ends of the cylinder by flat mirrors and with the remaining walls of the cylinder left open (Fig. 1.10). At that time, it was not entirely clear what modes would be supported in such a resonator or if in fact such a resonator would support modes with sufficiently low loss. By *modes* we refer to

a particular set of electromagnetic field configurations, propagating back and forth along the laser axis, whose pattern over the surface of the mirrors is maintained on completion of each round trip. The computer calculations of Fox and Li (15) and analytical calculations of Boyd and Gordon (16) showed very clearly that the losses for the fundamental modes of a plane parallel mirror (or a spherical mirror) resonator would be much lower than what would be expected from simple considerations and that, in fact, such a resonator would provide a small number of very low loss modes, which could be used to obtain laser action. Because of the relatively long cylindrical geometry of a laser resonator, these electromagnetic field configurations can be separated into transverse and longitudinal modes, which are nearly independent of one another. Laser oscillation is only possible in those modes for which the amplification of the active medium makes up for the total round trip diffraction and transmission losses.

A complete understanding of the modes inside resonators with curved mirrors was obtained by Kogelnik and Boyd (17) in 1962 and later generalized by Kogelnik (18). Boyd and Gordon (16) found that the fundamental transverse mode of a spherical mirror resonator, usually designated with the notation TEM_{00} (transverse electromagnetic wave), has a gaussian distribution with an intensity that is maximum along the laser axis gradually diminishing in the radial direction (Fig. 1.11). Higher order transverse modes have a more complex intensity distribution described mathematically by a product of Hermite and gaussian functions (exhibiting a number of maxima and minima in the radial direction) and occupy a larger area than the fundamental transverse mode (Fig. 1.12 [19]). For the confocal resonator illustrated

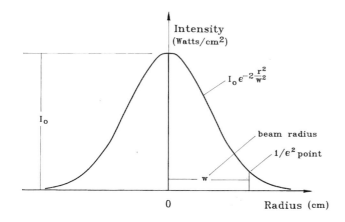

Fig. 1.11 Plot of intensity versus radius for a laser beam with a gaussian cross section.

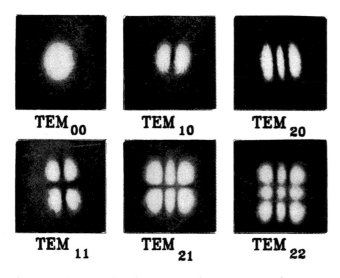

Fig. 1.12 Photographs of some typical transverse mode patterns from a laser. The light regions represent areas where radiation is present. (From Yariv and Gordon [19]; reproduced by permission from the IEEE.)

in Fig. 1.10 (two spherical mirrors separated by a distance, d, equal to their radii of curvature, R), the beam radii of the fundamental gaussian mode, w_0 in the center of the resonator and w_1 on the surface of the curved mirrors, are given by (20)

$$w_0 = (\lambda\, d/2\pi)^{1/2} \qquad (Eq.\ 2)$$

and

$$w_1 = (\lambda\, d/\pi)^{1/2} \qquad (Eq.\ 3)$$

In addition to limiting oscillation to a small number of transverse modes, the optical resonator also determines the exact frequencies at which the laser operates. Laser oscillation is only possible at those frequencies for which the total phase shift after a complete round trip is an integral multiple of 2π. This condition, to a good approximation, leads to oscillating frequencies at $f = nc/2d$

where n is a positive integer and c is the velocity of light in the medium. The different integers n correspond to the longitudinal modes of the resonator. In general, each transverse mode has associated with it a number of longitudinal modes separated in frequency by c/2d.

Focusing Gaussian Beams

As the laser beam propagates through space, the intensity distribution of the fundamental mode remains gaussian in cross section, but its width changes along the direction of propagation. A gaussian beam is a minimum at its waist where the phase front is plane (Fig. 1.13). If one measures distance, z, from such a waist, the law governing the expansion of the beam assumes the simple form (20)

$$w^2 = w_0^2\,[1 + (\lambda z/\pi w_0^2)^2] \qquad (Eq.\ 4)$$

where w_0 is the size of the beam waist and λ is the wavelength. The parameter w is often called the beam radius or "spot size" and 2w is called the beam diameter. As z increases, the beam expands linearly, with a far-field diffraction angle (for small θ) given by

$$\theta = \lambda/\pi w_0 \qquad (Eq.\ 5)$$

When a gaussian beam passes through an ideal lens, a new beam waist is formed. If before passing through the lens, a beam waist of radius w_1 is located at distance d_1 to the left of a lens whose focal length is f, the lens will produce another waist with radius w_2 to the right of the lens at a distance d_2 (Fig. 1.14). The position d_2 and radius w_2 of this new waist are given by (20)

$$\frac{1}{w_2^2} = \frac{1}{w_1^2}\,(1 - d_1/f)^2 + \frac{1}{f^2}\,(\pi w_1/\lambda)^2 \qquad (Eq.\ 6)$$

$$d_2 - f = (d_1 - f)f^2/[(d_1 - f)^2 + (\pi w_1^2/\lambda)^2] \qquad (Eq.\ 7)$$

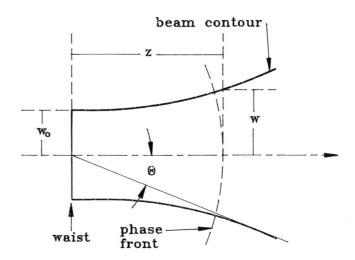

Fig. 1.13 Gaussian beam propagation starting from the waist of a confocal resonator.

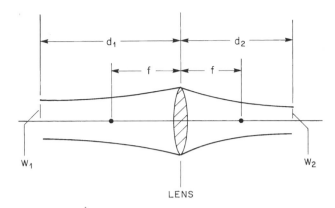

Fig. 1.14 Effect of converging lens on a gaussian beam.

In general, the minimum spot radius w_2 does not occur at the lens focal plane f. However, in cases where the divergence angle is small and the beam radius on entering the lens can be assumed equal to the untransformed waist w_1 and where the second term in Eq. 6 is large, the new waist will occur close to the lens focal plane, f, and its radius will be given by

$$w_2 = f\lambda/\pi w_1 \qquad \text{(Eq. 8)}$$

In practice, one may have little control over the initial beam waist w_1 (e.g., if it is formed by the geometry of the laser resonator). In this case, before entering the focusing lens, a beam expander could be used to increase w_1 before focusing, thus decreasing the size of the focal spot. As an example, for a CO_2 laser ($\lambda = 10.6$ μm) with a 1 m confocal resonator (R − d = 1 meter) providing 1 W of continuous wave (CW) power in the fundamental (gaussian) TEM_{00} mode, we find that the minimum spot radius within the resonator (w_0) is 1.3 mm (from Eq. 2), that the spot radius on either mirror (w_1) is 1.8 mm (from Eq. 3) and that the far-field divergence angle (θ) is 3×10^{-3} radians (from Eq. 5). If this output were brought to a focus with a 25-mm diameter, 25-mm focal length lens located 50 cm from one resonator mirror and a 10× beam expander ($w_1/w_0 = 10$) were used to expand the untransformed waist (1.3 mm) so that it fills the lens, then the radius of the focal spot (w_2) will be 6.5 μm (from Eq. 6). The *peak power density*, or *peak intensity* I_0, obtained within the focused spot can be found from the total power P_0 using the expression

$$I_0 = 2P_0/\pi w_2^2 \qquad \text{(Eq. 9)}$$

Thus, for the 1 W CW CO_2 laser of our example, the peak intensity (I_0) within the focused spot is 1.5×10^6 W/cm^2 (from Eq. 9). It should be pointed out that this value of intensity is more than enough to explosively vaporize water in the focused spot and is sufficient to substantially modify any biologic tissue.

In many applications, the confocal parameter, b, is also important. The *confocal parameter* is the axial distance over which the laser intensity has fallen to half the value that it had at the beam waist and is generally used to indicate the useful working distance. The confocal parameter is given by (20)

$$b = 2\pi w^2/\lambda \qquad \text{(Eq. 10)}$$

For the 1-W CW CO_2 laser example cited above, the confocal parameter is only 25 μm. A longer working distance could, of course, be obtained by avoiding such a tightly focused beam.

Common Surgical Lasers

Laser action or amplified spontaneous emission has now been observed at wavelengths that range from the extreme ultraviolet at around 4 nm to beyond 1000 μm in the submillimeter region of the spectrum. Stimulated emission has been reported on thousands of electronic transitions in the atomic species of over 40 elements and on numerous vibrational-rotational transitions in a wide variety of molecular compounds as well as in a number of liquids and solids. Peak power outputs have now been increased to terawatt (10^{12} W) power levels in several systems. Some of the more prominent members of each type of laser together with their operating wavelengths are illustrated in Fig. 1.15.

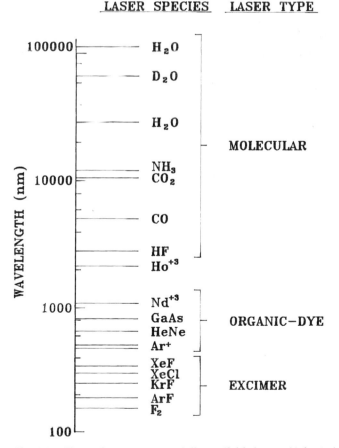

Fig. 1.15 Chart of some commercially available lasers. (Adapted from Patel and Wood [13]; reproduced by permission from Appleton-Century-Crofts.)

Lasers are generally operated in one of the following modes: (1) continuous wave (CW), (2) pulsed, (3) Q-switched, or (4) mode-locked. In the CW mode, illustrated in Fig. 1.16 (*top*), a continuous beam of constant power is emitted by the laser. In pulsed operation, illustrated in Fig. 1.16 (*middle*), pulsed pumping of the active medium results in relatively high-energy output pulses at repetition rates from one to hundreds of pulses per second. The technique of Q-switching (21) and mode-locking (22) are often used when output pulses of extremely short duration are required. The peak power output attainable in these short-pulse modes, illustrated in Fig. 1.16 (*bottom*), greatly exceeds that which can be achieved during CW or pulsed operation. Typical pulse durations range from hundreds of femtoseconds (10^{-15} sec) to hundreds of nanoseconds (10^{-9} sec) depending on the particular laser system and mode of operation.

The technique of Q-switching is illustrated in Fig. 1.17. To Q-switch a laser, the resonator losses must initially be large enough to prevent the buildup of laser oscillation. Then, at some later time, the resonator losses are suddenly

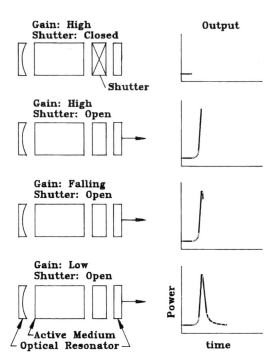

Fig. 1.17 Schematic diagram of a Q-switched laser. (Adapted from Hecht [10]; reproduced by permission from the IEEE.)

reduced (preferably to zero). Because the pumping process continues to create a large population inversion even when the cavity losses are high, the gain greatly exceeds the resonator losses (after they have been reduced) and all of the energy accumulated in the active medium is discharged in a giant pulse.

The most useful technique for generating ultrashort pulses with a laser is called *mode-locking*. In an ordinary laser, if no special precautions are taken, a number of longitudinal modes will usually oscillate simultaneously. The process of mode-locking involves the establishment of a definite phase and amplitude relationship between these modes by active or passive means. Under the right conditions, constructive and destructive interference between these discrete frequencies can lead to a train of very narrow pulses. The uncertainty principle between frequency and time variables limits the width of such pulses to $\Delta t \sim 1/\Delta f$ where Δt is pulse length and Δf is band width representing frequencies over which laser oscillation occurs. The broad-band emission of an organic dye laser, for example, permits the locking of thousands of longitudinal modes and the generation of pulses as short as 10 femtoseconds (10^{-14} sec). Mode-locking also leads to an n-fold increase in the peak power of the pulses where n is the number of coupled modes.

The lasers discussed in this section have been grouped according to whether their active medium is a gas, a liquid, or a solid.

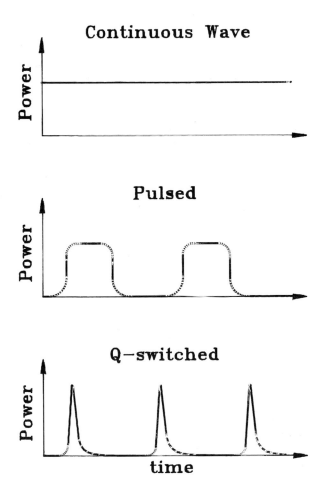

Fig. 1.16 Temporal behavior of laser output during several modes of operation.

Gas Lasers

The active medium of a gas laser, a low or moderate pressure gas, is usually excited with an electrical discharge (either RF or DC).

The Helium-Neon Laser

The helium-neon (HeNe) laser (the first gas laser) is the most common visible-wavelength laser. It was discovered by Javan and colleagues (23) in 1961, shortly after the ruby laser was discovered. The first device was operated in the infrared and produced a power output of the order of 15 mW on several wavelengths near 1 μm. White and Rigden (24) soon found that the same gas mixture could operate on a red transition at a wavelength of 632.8 nm. Virtually all commercial HeNe lasers are now designed to emit only in the red, although HeNe lasers that emit in the green, yellow, and orange are currently in limited production.

The active medium in a HeNe laser is a mixture of helium and neon gases at total pressures between a fraction of a torr and several torr. The gas mixture (5:1 helium to neon) is excited with a few milliamps of DC current at a voltage of a few kilovolts. Electrons passing through the gas collide with both helium and neon atoms, raising them to excited levels. Most of the energy is collected by the helium atoms, which can transfer that energy to neon atoms readily because the two have excited states at about the same energy. Emission is possible on several transitions, as shown in Fig. 1.18.

The internal design for a modern hard-sealed HeNe laser is shown in Fig. 1.19 (25). An electric discharge passing between electrodes at the opposite ends of a gas-filled glass tube excites the gas mixture. Mirrors on each end of the discharge tube form an optical resonator; one is totally reflecting, the other transmits about 1% of the incident light, which emerges as the output beam.

Helium-neon lasers are produced in large quantities and are available in several forms; bare laser tubes, laser head only, or complete laser systems. Standard mass-produced tubes, such as that shown in Fig. 1.20, have operating lifetimes of 20,000 to 25,000 hours. Typical commercially available HeNe lasers are characterized by output powers of 0.5 to 10 mW at 632.8 nm. The overall efficiency of a HeNe laser (defined as the ratio of optical power divided by the electrical power input) is low, typically in the range of 0.01% to 0.1%. Even though a diode laser can generate a 1-mW beam more cheaply and more efficiently, from a much smaller package and without the need for high voltage, HeNe lasers continue to be used because of their better coherence, beam quality,

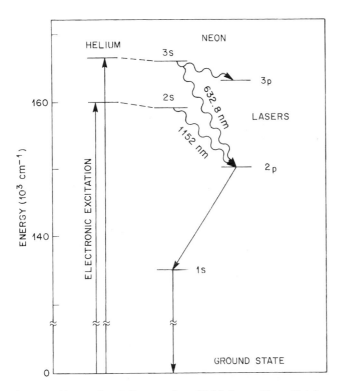

Fig. 1.18 Energy level diagram for a HeNe laser. (From Patel and Wood [13]; reproduced by permission from Appleton-Century-Crofts.)

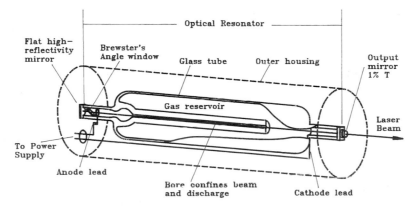

Fig. 1.19 Schematic diagram of the internal structure of a typical HeNe laser. (Adapted from Hecht [25]; reproduced with permission from Tab Books.)

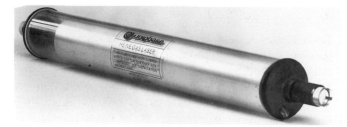

Fig. 1.20 Photograph of an unpackaged HeNe laser tube. (Courtesy of Uniphase, Manteca, CA.)

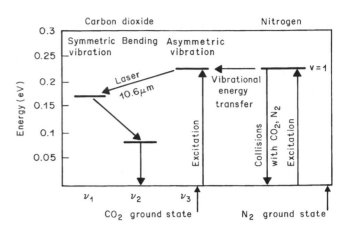

Fig. 1.21 Energy level diagram for a CO_2 laser. (From Patel and Wood [13]; reproduced by permission from Appleton-Century-Crofts.)

and more useful (i.e., shorter) wavelength. HeNe lasers are used for a broad range of applications, the most common being for bar code scanning, holography, alignment and positioning in the construction industry, and for educational demonstrations. HeNe lasers are used in medicine primarily as pointers for infrared or UV surgical lasers.

The Carbon Dioxide Laser

Continuous wave laser operation at 10.6 μm in CO_2 was first announced by Patel in 1964 (26). Since that time, CO_2 lasers have remained of great interest because they give a higher CW output with higher efficiency than any other laser. Commercially available CO_2 lasers can be made to emit radiation at a number of discrete wavelengths between 9 and 11 μm in the infrared, can produce CW powers ranging from under 1 W for scientific applications to many tens of kilowatts for material working, and can also produce short, intense pulses. Custom-made CO_2 lasers can emit CW powers of hundreds of kilowatts for military applications or single nanosecond pulses with more than 40 kJ of energy for fusion research applications.

The active medium of a conventional CO_2 laser is an electrically excited mixture of carbon dioxide, nitrogen, and helium gases. An energy level diagram illustrating the population inversion mechanism in a CO_2 laser is shown in Fig. 1.21. Laser action occurs on a vibrational-rotational transition of the ground electronic state of CO_2. The v = 1 level of N_2 is in close coincidence with the upper laser level ν_3 of CO_2, and rapid energy exchange between the two occurs. The N_2 level, which is readily excited by electron collisions, is metastable and thus provides a reservoir of stored energy for selective and efficient excitation of the ν_3 level of CO_2. The lower laser level decays to the ground state by means of ν_2, and the rate of depopulation of this level can be the rate-limiting process in the laser. Because the ν_2 level lies close to the ground state, the gas temperature must be kept low to prevent this level from becoming thermally populated. The presence of helium in the gas mixture helps to cool the gas and, in addition, increases the relaxation rate of the lower laser level.

Several different internal structures for CO_2 lasers are in practical use (some of which are illustrated in Fig. 1.22):

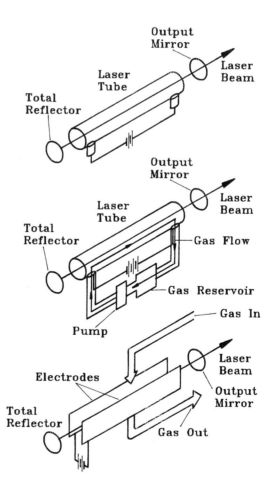

Fig. 1.22 Schematic diagram of the internal structure of CO_2 lasers with various types of excitation: sealed-tube laser with longitudinal DC discharge (*top*), fast axial-flow laser with longitudinal discharge (*middle*), and transverse-flow laser with transverse discharge (*bottom*). (Adapted from Hecht [25]; reproduced by permission from Tab Books.)

sealed-tube lasers, waveguide lasers, flowing-gas lasers of various types, and pulsed transversely-excited atmospheric-pressure lasers. Maximum output depends on the type of CO_2 laser. Commercial waveguide lasers now can produce up to about 40 W CW. Conventional sealed-tube CO_2 lasers can deliver up to a few hundred watts, although powers of 100 W or less are more typical. Slow-flow axial lasers typically generate 50 to 500 W and commercial fast-flow axial lasers generate 500 W to 5 kW. Transverse-flow lasers are available with 3- to 45-kW output powers.

The CO_2 laser is the most versatile and most powerful of commercial lasers. The most common applications of CO_2 lasers are in material processing, cutting, welding, drilling, and heat treating various metals. Medical applications of CO_2 lasers primarily are surgical. A typical multipurpose surgical CO_2 laser system is shown in Fig. 1.23. Surgery can be performed with CW powers of tens of watts at 10 μm, a wavelength at which the water in tissue is highly absorbent. The laser cauterizes tissue as it cuts.

Argon and Other Ion Lasers

Laser action has been obtained in the ions of the noble gases (27), argon, krypton, xenon, and neon. The prime attraction of these so-called ion lasers is their ability to produce tens of watts of CW power in the visible region of the spectrum. The most useful ion laser is the argon laser, first operated by Bridges and his colleagues in 1964 (28).

The active medium of an ion laser is a high current density electrical discharge in a noble gas at a fraction of a torr pressure. In such a discharge, it is possible to ionize (remove one or more electrons from) many of the gas atoms. The pertinent energy level scheme in argon is shown in Fig. 1.24. A high-current DC or RF discharge produces electrons with an average energy of 4 to 5 eV. Because the upper laser levels of the argon-ion laser are about 20 eV above the ground state of the ion, more than one electron collision is required to excite an argon ion to one of these

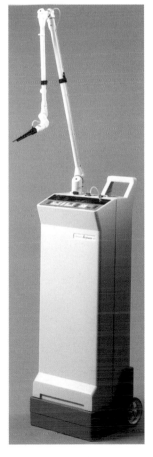

Fig. 1.23 Photograph of the Surgicenter 40 CO_2 laser system. (Courtesy of Sharplan Lasers, Inc., Allendale, NJ.)

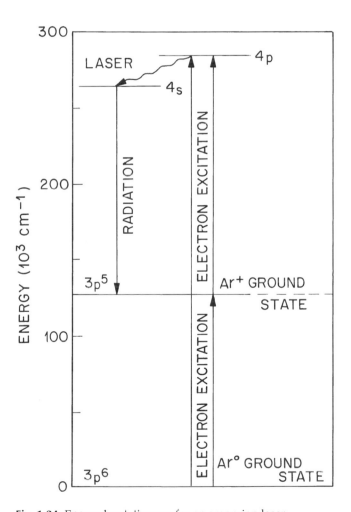

Fig. 1.24 Energy level diagram for an argon-ion laser. (From Patel and Wood [13]; reproduced by permission from Appleton-Century-Crofts.)

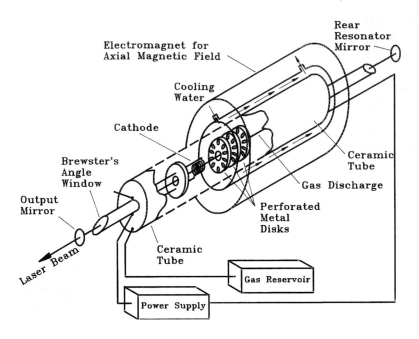

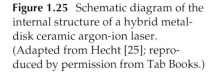

Figure 1.25 Schematic diagram of the internal structure of a hybrid metal-disk ceramic argon-ion laser. (Adapted from Hecht [25]; reproduced by permission from Tab Books.)

levels. Large population inversions can be produced because the lower laser levels, which lie approximately 17 eV above the ion ground state, have negligible population. Furthermore, a population inversion can be produced either on a transient or CW basis because the lower laser levels have very short lifetimes, quickly decaying to the ion ground state.

Noble gas-ion lasers require high electrical input powers, necessitating expensive discharge tubes. The internal structure of a typical high-power ion laser tube, in which the discharge passes through a "bore" defined by holes in the center of a row of metal disks, is shown in Fig. 1.25. Waste heat, a consequence of the low wall-plug efficiencies (0.01% to 0.001%) of these devices, is conducted from these disks through copper cups to a ceramic outer tube and thus to cooling water flowing over the ceramic. A solenoid, which creates a magnetic field parallel to the center of the bore, is used to help confine the discharge current to the center of the bore and increase the ion density without seriously affecting the average electron energy. Most ion lasers have Brewster's angle windows on the ends of the discharge tube, with external mirrors defining the laser resonator. If no dispersive element is inserted into the laser resonator, ion lasers will oscillate in a number of lines simultaneously, some of the most important of which are listed in Table 1.1.

Argon is by far the most important ion laser, commercially accounting for most of the units sold, with krypton in second place, accounting for about 10% of the market (25). Ion lasers carry price tags of a few thousand to as much as $100,000, have tubes with operating lifetimes limited to 1000 to 10,000 hours, and tend to be delicate. Nevertheless, because of their unrivaled CW power in the visible, ion lasers have found uses in ophthalmology, high-speed printing, entertainment (laser light shows),

and data storage applications. Ion lasers tend to be packaged either for laboratory applications or for incorporation into laser systems for specific applications such as high-speed printing or medical treatment. A photograph of a laser photocoagulator incorporating a 4-W water-cooled argon-ion laser designed for applications in ophthalmology is shown in Fig. 1.26.

Table 1.1 Major Wavelengths of Ion Lasers

Argon	Krypton
334.0 nm	337.4 nm
351.1 nm	350.7 nm
363.8 nm	356.4 nm
457.9 nm	406.7 nm
476.5 nm	413.1 nm
488.0 nm (strong)	415.4 nm
496.5 nm	468.0 nm
501.7 nm	476.2 nm
514.5 nm (strong)	482.5 nm
528.7 nm	520.8 nm
1090.0 nm	530.9 nm
	568.2 nm
	647.1 nm (strong)
	676.4 nm
	752.5 nm
	799.3 nm

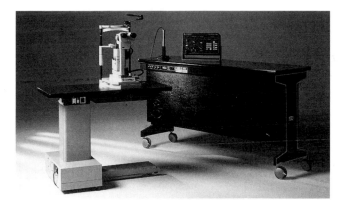

Fig. 1.26 Photograph of the Coherent 920 Argon laser photo-coagulator. (Courtesy of Coherent, Inc., Palo Alto, CA.)

Excimer Lasers

First demonstrated in the mid-1970s, excimers are a family of lasers that emit powerful pulses lasting tens of nanoseconds at average powers in excess of 100 W at wavelengths in or near the UV region of the spectrum. The term *excimer* originated as a contraction of "excited dimer," a description of a molecule consisting of two identical atoms that exist only in an excited state. It is now used in a broader sense for any diatomic molecule in which the component atoms are bound in the excited state, but not in the ground state. The active media of the most important excimer lasers are rare-gas halide (29) compounds such as argon fluoride, krypton fluoride, xenon fluoride, and xenon chloride, which do not occur in nature.

The ground and excited states of a typical rare-gas halide molecule as a function of interatomic spacing are shown in Fig. 1.27. When the molecule is excited, its potential energy is at a minimum when the two atoms are a certain distance apart, that is, trapped in a potential well.

In the lowest energy state there is no binding energy to hold the two atoms together and the molecule falls apart as shown in the lower curve in Fig. 1.27. Excimer lasers are excited by passing a short, intense electrical pulse through a mixture of gases containing the desired rare gas and halogen. Electrons in the discharge transfer energy to the gas mixture, breaking up halogen molecules and forming electronically excited rare-gas halogen molecules. The molecules remain excited for about 10 nsec, then drop to the ground state and disassociate. The molecular kinetics (and to a lesser extent the excitation pulse) limit the laser pulse duration to tens or hundreds of nanoseconds. The emitted photon energies are large, and the output is at UV wavelengths, as shown in Table 1.2.

The internal structure of an excimer laser (Fig. 1.28) is similar to that of other transversely excited lasers except that the excimer laser tube must resist attack by the highly corrosive halogens in the laser gas. The laser tube contains a mixture of gases, the bulk of which is a buffer gas that mediates energy transfer, at total pressures well below 5 atmospheres. Energy is typically deposited in the mixture by a short, high-voltage electrical pulse applied perpendicularly to the laser beam axis. To avoid arcing, the gas is usually "preionized" before the excitation pulse is applied. In commercial excimer lasers, preionization is normally produced by a pulse of UV light, but an electrical discharge pulse, a pulse of x-rays, or a pulse from an electron beam can also be used. Excimer lasers have such high gain that their resonator consists of a fully reflecting rear mirror and an uncoated output window that reflects a few percent of the beam back into the cavity and transmits the rest.

Typical average power output from excimer lasers range from 50 to 100 W although a kilowatt of power has recently been demonstrated in an x-ray preionized XeCl at 308 nm. The bandwidth of an excimer laser is about 0.3 nm, with an output wavelength tunable across 3 nm. Conventional excimer lasers with stable resonator optics typically have rectangular-shaped beams roughly 10 by 20 mm across at the output window. Typical wall-plug efficiency for a discharge-driven commercial KrF excimer laser is 1.5% to 2%. No other commercial laser can generate such high average powers at such short wavelengths.

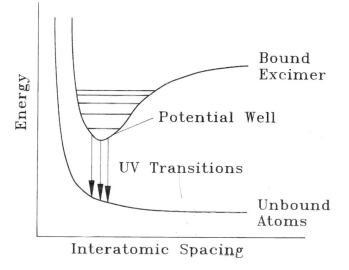

Fig. 1.27 Energy level diagram for an excimer laser.

Table 1.2 Major Excimer Lasers

Type	Wavelength
ArF	193 nm
KrCl	222 nm
KrF	248 nm
XeCl	308 nm
XeF	350 nm

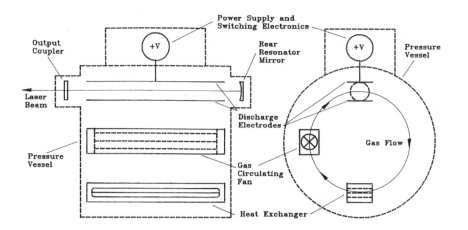

Fig. 1.28 Schematic diagram of the internal structure of an excimer laser.

Scientific applications have long accounted for 90% of the excimer-laser market (25). Major scientific uses include pumping of tunable dye lasers, photochemistry, and materials research. Industrial applications include semiconductor fabrication systems; marking of ceramic, glass, plastic, and metal; precision micromachining and drilling; thin-film deposition; and surface treatment of materials. Medical applications include corneal sculpting, laser angioplasty, and microsurgery. A photograph of a laser system for refractive surgery, incorporating an ArF excimer laser and a holmium laser, is shown in Fig. 1.29.

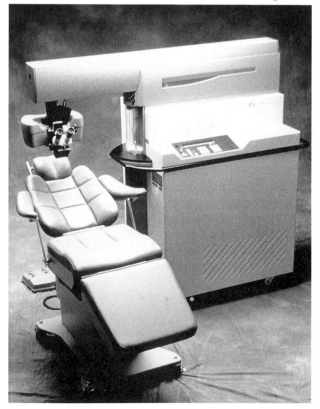

Fig. 1.29 Photograph of the OnmiMed Excimer Laser Refractive Workstation. (Courtesy of Summit Technology, Inc., Waltham, MA.)

Liquid Lasers—The Organic Dye Laser

The active medium of the most important class of liquid lasers, an organic dye dissolved in a liquid solvent, is usually excited by optical pumping with the light from flashlamps or the output from other fixed-frequency lasers. Organic dye lasers, invented by Sorokin and Lankard (30) in 1966, are important today for two reasons. First, their output is tunable in wavelength (tunable dye lasers are available which, when several dyes are used, cover the spectrum from the near UV to the near infrared). Second, their emission bandwidth is broad, facilitating the generation of ultrashort optical pulses.

An energy level diagram for an organic dye laser is shown in Fig. 1.30. The upper laser level is populated by optically pumping dye molecules from their singlet ground state, S_0, to their first excited singlet, S_1. Both of these electronic states are composed of a continuum of vibrational and rotational levels that thermalize separately, resulting in a Boltzmann distribution of occupied levels within each state. Because the Franck-Condon effect shifts the emission band to longer wavelengths than the absorption band, a population inversion can be established between levels at the bottom of the excited singlet state and any of the continuum of unoccupied vibrational and rotational levels in the ground state. After emission of a photon, rapid thermalization of the singlet ground state occurs, emptying the lower laser level.

Dye laser systems are available with a wide variety of optical pumping sources and resonator geometries, two of which are illustrated in Fig. 1.31. The internal structure of a wavelength-tunable dye laser is shown in Fig. 1.31 (*top*). Because most dye lasers operate at visible wavelengths and the pump wavelength must be shorter than the emission wavelength (as mentioned above), visible dye lasers in most cases are pumped with the output from a pulsed laser operating in the ultraviolet or short-wavelength end of the visible spectrum. Typical pump lasers for pulsed dye lasers include frequency

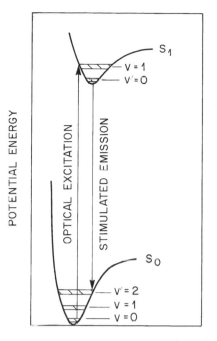

Fig. 1.30 Energy level diagram for an organic dye laser. (From Patel and Wood [13]; reproduced by permission from Appleton-Century-Crofts.)

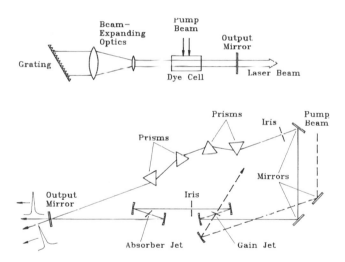

Fig. 1.31 Schematic diagrams of the internal structures of grating-tuned (*top*) and colliding-pulse mode-locked (*bottom*) dye lasers. (Adapted from Hecht [25]; reproduced by permission from Tab Books.)

doubled or tripled neodymium lasers, copper vapor lasers, nitrogen lasers, and excimer lasers. A pulsed dye laser with a broad-band optical resonator usually oscillates with a bandwidth of 5 to 10 nm. Soffer and McFarland (31) were the first to discover that, with the insertion of a frequency-selective element such as a diffraction grating or a prism into the resonator, the broad-band emission could be reduced to a much smaller range (several thousandths of a nanometer) without

appreciable loss in power. If the diffraction grating and the other resonator mirror are arranged so that only one wavelength can oscillate in the laser cavity (other wavelengths are deflected from the axis of the cavity), then simple rotation of the grating results in tuning of the dye lasers emission wavelength. To cover the entire visible spectrum, however, it is necessary to switch among several dyes because each has a limited tuning range.

The internal structure of a colliding-pulse mode-locked dye laser for ultrashort pulse generation is also shown in Fig. 1.31 (*bottom*). In such a continuously-pumped laser, instead of exciting the dye in a sealed cell, the continuous pump beam is focused on the narrowest part of a free-flowing jet of dye solution, avoiding optical damage to the solid windows of a cell. One quarter of the way around the ring from the dye jet, the resonator includes a second jet containing a saturable absorber, which has lowest loss when two opposite-direction pulses (the ring resonator results in pulses going in opposite directions around the ring) pass through it at the same time. The presence of the saturable absorber leads to passive mode-locking of the dye laser (discussed earlier in this section) and the generation of a train of ultrashort pulses. Pulse durations can be under 100 femtoseconds in commercial versions of this laser and tens of femtoseconds in laboratory systems (32).

A variety of dye laser systems are available, each of which offers one of the following features: extremely narrow linewidth, high average power, or ultrashort pulses. The precise range of operating wavelengths depends on choice of dye and pump source. Emission wavelengths from about 310 to about 1200 nm are available. The output power depends on choice of pump laser, design of the dye laser, and choice of dye. Manufacturers usually specify maximum output power with Rhodamine 6G, a particularly efficient dye that can be used with all types of dye lasers and one that has a peak emission wavelength near 600 nm. The efficiency of a laser-pumped dye laser (the fraction of input energy converted to output energy) can exceed 50%. The wall-plug efficiency of a flashlamp pumped dye laser can reach 1%. The prime consumable in a dye laser is the dye solution itself; stated lifetimes range from around an hour to well over 1000 hours depending on the choice of dye and operating conditions. Flashlamps also have a limited lifetime, decreasing rapidly as pulse energy increases. Linear flashlamps can be operated for millions of shots. Even though dye laser systems are expensive, they have found use in high-resolution spectroscopy and in the study of ultrafast phenomena in biologic as well as other systems. In medicine, dye lasers are used to treat skin disorders and to shatter stones in the urinary tract and gallbladder. A photograph of a laser lithotripter based on a flashlamp-pumped dye laser is shown in Fig. 1.32.

tum efficiency into the $^4F_{3/2}$ level, which serves as the upper laser level for a 1.06 μm laser transition between the $^4F_{3/2}$ and the $^4I_{11/2}$ levels. Because the lower laser level, $^4I_{11/2}$, lies well above the ground level, its population is negligible. This leads to the creation of a population inversion with only modest pumping powers.

The internal structure of all Nd lasers, until the mid-1980s, looked very much like that of a ruby laser (the first working laser). Before that date all Nd lasers were pumped by broad-spectrum light sources, continuous tungsten arc lamps, or pulsed flashlamps. For lamp pumping, hollow reflector cavities such as shown in Fig. 1.34 (*top*) were used to couple pump light from one or more lamps to the laser rod. A much more efficient approach has since been developed and involves exciting a 0.8-μm wide spectral band with the output from a gallium-aluminum-arsenide (GaAlAs) semiconductor laser (34) as shown in Fig. 1.34 (*bottom*). The optical resonator for a Nd:YAG laser is designed to extract energy from as much of the laser medium as possible, typically a rod 6 to 9 mm in diameter and several centimeters long. It should maximize both output power and beam quality

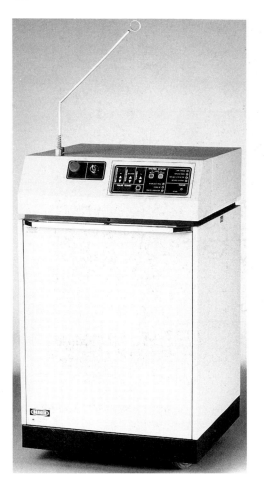

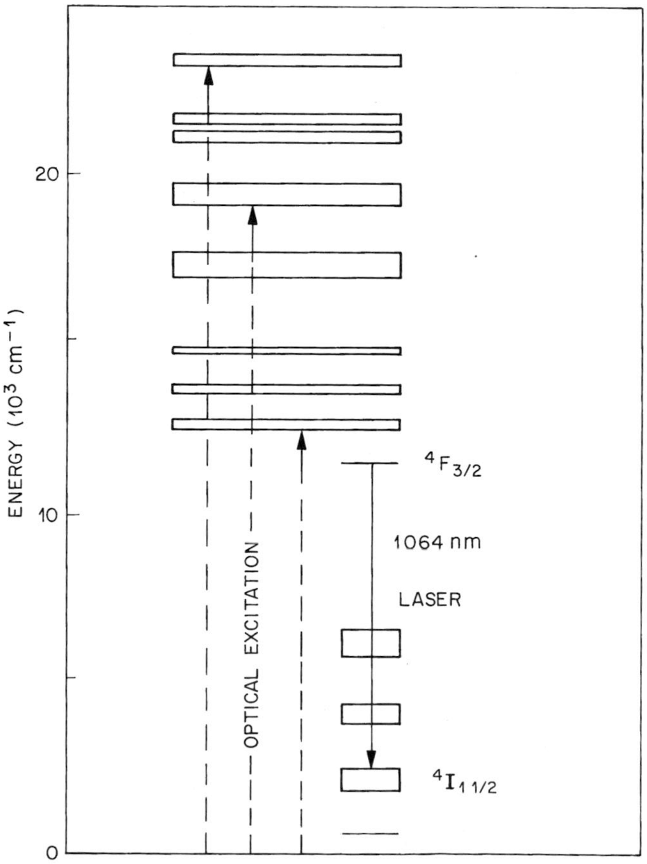

Fig. 1.32 Photograph of the Candela MDL 2000 LaserTripter organic dye laser system. (Courtesy of Candela Laser Corporation, Wayland, MA.)

Solid-State Lasers

The active media of solid-state lasers, ions doped into crystal or glass hosts, are usually excited with light from a flashlamp.

The Neodymium YAG Laser

The 1.06 μm neodymium (Nd) laser, developed by Geusic and his colleagues (33) in 1964, is the most common solid-state laser. Nd lasers can generate continuous beams from a few milliwatts to over a kilowatt, short pulses with peak powers in the gigawatt range, or pulsed beams with average powers in the kilowatt range (25).

The active medium of this laser is the trivalent rare-earth ion Nd^{3+} in a host material of yttrium-aluminum-garnet (YAG). An energy level diagram for Nd ions in a crystalline host is shown in Fig. 1.33. Nd^{3+} ions are optically pumped using a broad-band incoherent source, such as a flashlamp or tungsten lamp, or a semiconductor laser, from the $^4I_{9/2}$ ground level to high-lying levels. These excited ions decay nonradiatively with nearly unity quan-

Fig. 1.33 Energy level diagram for the neodymium-YAG laser. (From Patel and Wood [13]; reproduced by permission from Appleton-Century-Crofts.)

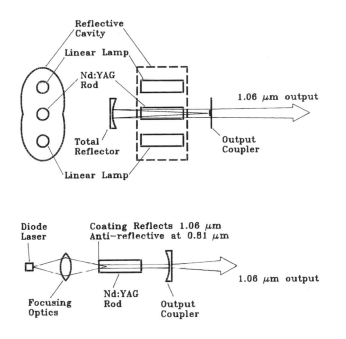

Fig. 1.34 Schematic diagrams of internal structure of flashlamp pumped (*top*) and diode laser pumped (*bottom*) Nd:YAG lasers. (Adapted from Hecht [25]; reproduced by permission from Tab Books.)

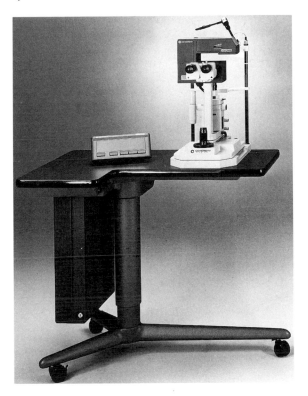

Fig. 1.35 Photograph of Coherent 7970 Nd:YAG Laser system. (Courtesy of Coherent, Inc., Palo Alto, CA.)

and compensate for any thermal lensing caused by uneven heating of the laser rod. Nd lasers can be arranged in series in an oscillator-amplifier configuration to produce pulses whose power is higher than that possible with a laser oscillator alone. Multiple amplifiers can and have been used where extremely high laser powers are required, such as in laser fusion experiments.

A wide range of output powers is available from Nd:YAG, neodymium:yttrium-lithium-fluoride (Nd:YLF), and Nd:glass lasers, depending on configuration, pumping source, and operating wavelength. Average powers in the kilowatt range can be obtained from pulsed or CW lasers. Peak powers available from Nd lasers are much higher and depend on both pulse energy and duration. In general, the shorter the pulse duration the higher the peak power for a given laser rod and pump source. The overall efficiency (wall plug) of a commercial lamp-pumped Nd laser is typically 0.1% to 1%, whereas that of a diode-pumped Nd laser can exceed 10%. Nd lasers can operate in several pulsed modes or deliver a continuous beam. A typical pulse duration from a Q-switched flashlamp-pumped Nd:YAG laser is 3 to 30 nsec. The shortest pulse duration from a mode-locked flashlamp-pumped Nd:glass laser is in the 5 to 20 psec range, although, using a technique called chirped pulse, amplification pulses as short as 1 to 3 psec and terawatt (10^{12} W) levels have recently been achieved (35).

The largest single use of Nd:YAG lasers is in military range finders and target designators (25). Nd:YAG lasers are also used in materials processing applications and as pumping sources for dye lasers. Harmonic generation can shift the wavelength into the green and UV, and Q-switching and mode-locking can generate short pulses and high powers. In medicine, Nd lasers have become the standard tool for performing a posterior capsulotomy. Because the 1-μm wavelength can be transported by standard optical fibers, Nd lasers can be used with endoscopes for gallbladder surgery and for the treatment of gastrointestinal bleeding. A photograph of a Q-switched Nd:YAG laser system designed specifically for posterior capsulotomy is shown in Fig. 1.35.

The Holmium YAG Laser

Laser action from a solid-state holmium (Ho) laser at 2.1 μm was first observed in 1962 by Johnson and colleagues (36) at cryogenic temperatures (about 80° above absolute zero). A major breakthrough in the technology of Ho lasers occurred in 1985, when Antipenko and coworkers (37) reported that co-doping the crystalline host with chromium (Cr^{3+}) and thulium (Tm^{3+}) ions permitted efficient pulsed operation at room temperature. Since that time, the development of Ho lasers has proceeded at a furious pace, motivated to a large extent by its eye-safe emission wavelength. As a result, room-temperature pulsed Ho:YAG lasers with average powers in excess of 40 W at 2.1 μm wavelength are now commercially available.

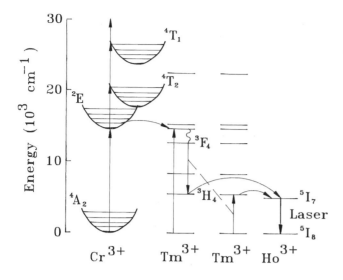

Fig. 1.36 Energy level diagram for a Ho:YAG laser. (Adapted from Quarles et al. [38]; reproduced by permission from the American Institute of Physics.)

The active medium of the 2.1 μm Ho:YAG laser is a trivalent holmium ion (Ho^{3+}) in a YAG crystal that has been sensitized with Cr^{3+} and Tm^{3+} co-dopants. An energy level diagram illustrating both flashlamp and diode laser pumping of a Ho:YAG laser is shown in Fig. 1.36 (38). With flashlamp pumping, light is absorbed by the broad absorption bands of the Cr^{3+} ion. After a nonradiative decay, excitation is transferred from the Cr^{3+} ion to the $^3F_3$ and $^3H_4$ states of the Tm^{3+} ion. Each excited Tm^{3+} then interacts with a ground state Tm^{3+} ion in a cross-relaxation process that gives rise to two Tm^{3+} ions in the $^3H_4$ state. Finally, these Tm^{3+} ions transfer their energy to the $^5I_7$ level of Ho^{3+}, which serves as the upper laser level for the 2.098 μm $^5I_7$ to $^5I_8$ Ho laser transition. With diode laser pumping, the $^3F_4$ states of the Tm^{3+} ion are directly pumped by an AlGaAs diode laser operating near 780 nm. This process is followed by fast spatial energy migration among the Tm^{3+} ions, subsequent transfer to the $^5I_7$ states of Ho^{3+} and finally laser action on the Ho $^5I_7$ to $^5I_8$ transi-

tion. In diode laser pumping, the Cr^{3+} ion plays no active role. The lower laser level of Ho lies within 500 cm^{-1} of the ground level, and, hence, is heavily populated at room temperature. Such a heavily populated lower laser level necessitates a high pumping power and makes a Ho:YAG laser less efficient than a Nd:YAG laser.

The internal structure of a Ho:YAG laser is similar to the internal structure of a Nd:YAG laser. With flashlamp pumping (see Fig. 1.34), a hollow reflective cavity is used to couple broad-band radiation from a lamp to a YAG rod doped with Ho, Cromium, Tm. With diode laser pumping (Fig. 1.37 [39]), the 781.5 nm output from an AlGaAs diode laser is focused into a cavity containing a thin crystal of YAG doped with Ho and Tm. With flashlamp pumping, such a Cr,Tm,Ho:YAG laser rod can provide average output powers up to 42.5 W at 15 Hz repetition rate in 250 μsec duration pulses (the actual output pulse consists of an envelope of microsecond duration spikes). As with Nd:YAG lasers, Ho lasers can be Q-switched to provide shorter duration (200 nsec), higher peak power pulses.

The 2.1-μm Ho wavelength is highly absorbed by water, making it eye safe and potentially important for applications that require atmospheric propagation such as coherent radar and range finding (39). The strong water absorption also makes it an efficient cutting and ablating tool for medical applications. Moreover, 2.1-μm laser radiation can be readily transmitted through practical lengths of flexible, commercially available low-OH fused silica fibers with negligible power attenuation. A photograph of a Ho laser system with a fiberoptic probe delivery system for the treatment of glaucoma is shown in Fig. 1.38. In general surgery, Ho lasers have been used in arthroscopy, percutaneous diskectomy, joint revision surgery, sinus surgery, and temporomandibular joint surgery. In gallbladder surgery, Ho lasers have been used for tissue welding. In ophthalmology, Ho lasers have been used in external filtering surgery for glaucoma and in photothermal keratoplasty for the treatment of hyperopia (40). In the latter case, the 2.1-μm output from a Ho laser

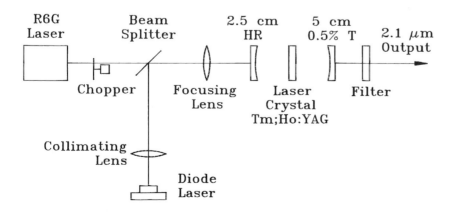

Fig. 1.37 Experimental arrangement for optically pumping a Tm, Ho:YAG crystal with radiation from a GaAs diode laser or a R6G organic dye laser. (Adapted from Fan et al [39].)

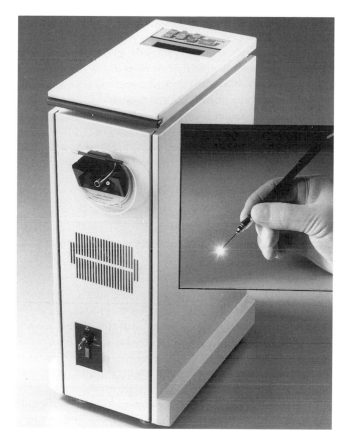

Fig. 1.38 Photograph of gLASE 210 Holmium Laser System for glaucoma. (Courtesy of Sunrise Technologies, Fremont, CA.)

Table 1.3 Major Semiconductor Diode Lasers

Material Type	Wavelength Range
InGaAlP	630–608 nm
GaInP	670 nm
GaAlAs	720–895 nm
GaAs	905 nm
InGaAs	980 nm
InGaAsP	1100–1650 nm
InGaAsSb	1700–4400 nm
PbCdS	2700–4200 nm
PbSnTe	6300–29,000 nm
PbSnSe	8000–29,000 nm

is used to adjust the refractive power of the cornea by shrinking corneal collagen fibers. Although the number of patients treated to date is small, the procedure has been shown to be reasonably predictable and the refractive outcome fairly stable.

Semiconductor Diode Lasers

The first semiconductor diode lasers (41–43) were developed in 1962, only 2 years after the first ruby laser. Today, semiconductor diode lasers are the lowest cost lasers on the market (25). Some of the more important semiconductor laser compounds and their normal wavelength ranges are listed in Table 1.3. The most important semiconductor diode lasers are GaAlAs devices emitting in the 720- to 890-nm wavelength region. These lasers are packaged in arrays that can deliver CW powers of 10 W or more. In 1988 unit sales of semiconductor diode lasers worldwide passed 20 million a year (25). This is compared to less than half a million units for all other lasers combined.

The active medium of a semiconductor diode laser is the boundary zone between two parts of a semiconductor crystal with different impurities (a p-n junction) through which a suitably high current is flowing as shown in Fig. 1.39. Impurities that have fewer electrons than the atoms they replace produce p-type (positive carrier) material, because the doping results in a hole where an electron would otherwise reside. Impurities with extra electrons produce n-type (negative carrier) material. Applying a negative voltage to the n material and a positive voltage to the p material (forward bias) makes the carriers flow toward the junction, resulting in a process called *injection.* At the junction, the free electrons from the n material are trapped by holes from the p material, releasing energy in a process called *electron-hole recombination.* In silicon diodes, most energy is released as heat, and no light is produced. In a GaAs diode, with a direct bandgap of 1.35 eV at room temperature, much of the energy is released as light at 905 nm with a photon energy roughly equivalent to the bandgap. The emission can be moved to shorter wavelengths by adding aluminum. For aluminum concentrations, x, of 0 to 0.45, $Ga_{1-x}Al_xAs$ material can provide emission at wavelengths from 905 nm to as short as 620 nm (25).

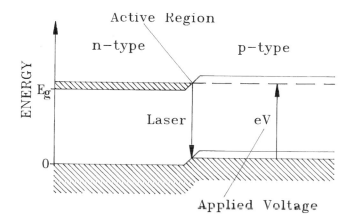

Fig. 1.39 Energy level diagram for the forward-biased p-n junction of a semiconductor diode laser.

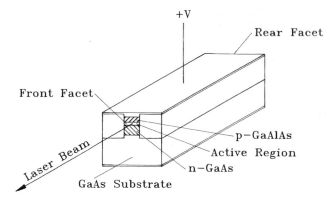

Fig. 1.40 Schematic diagram of the internal structure of a buried heterostructure GaAs diode laser.

In its simplest form, a diode laser consists of a block of semiconductor, less than a millimeter on a side, in which part is n-doped and part is p-doped. In practice, the active layer is usually sandwiched between two layers with larger bandgaps (for electrical confinement) and lower refractive indexes (for optical confinement) in a configuration called a double heterostructure (Fig. 1.40). Smooth facets cut, cleaved, or polished on the edges of the block function as an optical resonator and provide the feedback needed to sustain laser oscillation. As in other lasers, a threshold must be reached before stimulated emission overcomes internal losses and produces laser output. Today, most diode lasers are stripe-geometry types in which the active region is a stripe about 1 μm high and 2 to 10 μm wide (25). GaAlAs lasers with stripes only a few microns wide can generate CW powers to about 100 mW, a 50-μm stripe laser can generate 0.5 W and a 500 μm wide stripe can generate 4 W. The output of single-diode lasers is limited by the volume of the devices, the need to remove excess heat, and optical damage to the laser facets.

The way to reach much higher powers is to fabricate many diode laser stripes on a monolithic substrate. In practice, as many as 200 laser stripes can be fabricated on a 1-cm wide bar. Such an array can generate up to 20 W CW or produce peak powers up to about 100 W in quasi-CW operation (25). Stacking array bars together can generate powers up to a few kilowatts. A good array is about 25% efficient, so it must dissipate three times more power than it emits. This limits CW powers of commercial monolithic arrays to the 10-W range. Diode arrays emit from the entire width of the active area, which means that they have long thin emitting areas and rather asymmetric beams. A single 100-μm wide laser has an emitting area of 100 μm wide by 1μm high. A 1-cm long bar has an emitting area of the same height but 1 cm wide. Stacking bars together increases the height of the emitting area, but the divergence angle remains roughly the same—30° to 40° by about 10°—typical of most diode lasers. While some arrays generate incoherent beams, others have enough optical coupling among stripes to emit a partly coherent beam.

Low cost, high power, and versatility have ensured that GaAlAs lasers are used in a wide range of applications including compact-disc players, short-distance fiberoptic communications, optical data storage, and laser printing. The newly available visible diode lasers, InGaAlP and InGaP types, emitting in the red, are currently used as laser pointers and if their cost can be driven down, they may play a role in photocoagulation systems for ophthalmology. The semiconductor diode lasers, made of indium, gallium, arsenic, and phosphorous, which emit in the 1.1 to 1.65-μm region, are used primarily in fiberoptic communications. The longer wavelength tunable radiation from semiconductor diode lasers fabricated from lead-containing compounds have primarily found use in high-resolution infrared spectroscopy. A photograph of a diode laser photocoagulator incorporating a GaAs diode laser emitting at 805 nm is shown in Fig. 1.41.

KTP Lasers

Second harmonic generation (production of light at twice the laser frequency) was first demonstrated by Franken and colleagues (44) in 1961. Since that time, harmonic gen-

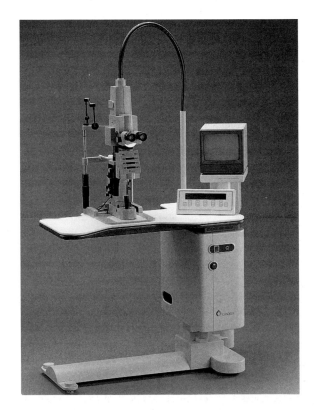

Fig. 1.41 Photograph of the Candela SL 3000 Photocoagulator GaAs diode laser system. (Courtesy of Candela Laser Corporation, Wayland, MA.)

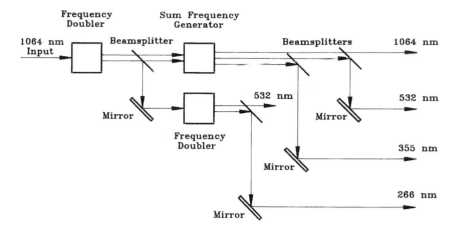

Fig. 1.42 Schematic diagram shows an arrangement of nonlinear crystals to produce second, third, and fourth harmonics from a Nd:YAG laser. (Adapted from Hecht [46]; reproduced by permission from Laser Focus World.)

eration has been used to greatly expand the range of wavelengths at which high laser powers are available, particularly in the visible and ultraviolet ranges. For instance, a nonlinear crystal of potassium titanyl phosphate (KTP) can transform the 1064-nm radiation from a Nd:YAG laser into 532-nm green laser light. Today, harmonic generation from Nd:YAG lasers has become so common that one sometimes refers to "green" Nd:YAG lasers even though the Ndy atom does not emit green light and "KTP" lasers even though KTP crystals do not exhibit laser action.

The production of optical harmonics is possible because all materials are nonlinear at high enough electric fields. When exposed to the oscillating electric field of a monochromatic light wave (a light intensity of 2.5×10^6 W/cm^2 corresponds to an electric field of 3×10^4 V/cm), the bound charges of a crystalline material will tend to vibrate with the same frequency as the electric field. If the electric field is a significant fraction of the field that binds the electrons and ions of the crystal together (about 3×10^8 V/cm), as will be the case with many lasers, the charges no longer respond linearly and instead can give rise to a variety of nonlinear optical effects such as optical rectification, the Pockels effect, second harmonic generation, sum- and difference-frequency generation, optical parametric amplification, etc.

A variety of nonlinear crystals are available for harmonic generation, including potassium dihydrogen phosphate (KDP), lithium niobate (LiNbO$_3$), beta barium borate (BBO) and KTP. The choice of material for a given application depends on the operating wavelength and available power level. For example, KTP is one of the most widely used nonlinear materials for second harmonic generation, frequency mixing, and optical parametric amplification with the 1064- and 1325-nm lines of Nd:YAG. Some of the attractive features that have contributed to its popularity are a high optical damage threshold, a low absorption, a wide spectral transmission range (0.35 to 4.5 μm) and a high second harmonic generation conversion efficiency (45).

The high laser intensities needed to generate optical harmonics with reasonable efficiency can be produced by focusing the laser beam in the crystal or using the high intensities available at the peak of Q-switched or modelocked laser pulses. In the simplest case, illustrated in Fig. 1.42 (46), the laser beam makes a single pass through a nonlinear material located outside the laser cavity. As described above, if the laser intensity is sufficiently high, as the laser beam passes through the crystal, nonlinear interactions between the beam and the material produce the second harmonic. The generation of higher harmonics using nonlinear crystals is usually a multistep process. For example, frequency tripling (also shown in Fig. 1.42) is produced by first generating the second harmonic, then mixing it with the fundamental wavelength in another nonlinear crystal, so that the frequencies add together to produce the third harmonic. To produce the fourth harmonic, the output of a second harmonic generator is passed through a second frequency doubler. The experimental arrangement shown in Fig. 1.42 is most commonly used with the 1064 Nd:YAG laser, producing the 532 nm second harmonic, the 355-nm third harmonic, and the 266-nm fourth harmonic. The generation of still higher harmonics of the Nd:YAG laser in nonlinear crystals is impractical due to poor conversion efficiency and low ultraviolet transmission.

Alternatively, the frequency-doubling crystal can be located either inside the laser cavity itself or inside another resonant cavity using the experimental arrangement shown in Fig. 1.43 (47). In this case, the circulating power within the cavity of a laser, which can be up to 10 times the extracavity power, can efficiently generate the second harmonic of even a low-power laser. Using a slightly more complicated experimental arrangement, the 532-nm second harmonic from a diode-pumped Nd:YAG laser has been produced with nearly 71% optical efficiency (48) The second harmonic power available from such a device probably will not exceed 0.5 W of CW 532-nm output with available 810-nm diode lasers. Nevertheless, for some

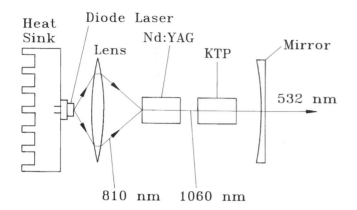

Fig. 1.43 Experimental arrangement for doubling the output of a diode-pumped Nd:YAG laser with a KTP crystal. (Adapted from Messenger [47]; reproduced by permission from Laser Focus World.)

applications, a frequency-doubled diode-pumped solid state provides an attractive alternative to the costly and in-efficient argon laser.

High-power green lasers can now produce more than 28 W of average power at 532 nm. Recently developed applications in the semiconductor industry for such a laser include wafer drilling, cutting of diamond films, removal of gold, and scribing of photovoltaic panels. Frequency-doubled Nd:YAG lasers, when run at CW and quasi-CW modes, can be a reliable alternative to the argon laser in ophthalmology, simultaneously supplying an infrared wavelength for ciliary body coagulation (49). A photograph of a KTP/YAG surgical laser system developed for laser nucleotomy in the treatment of herniated disks and laparoscopic surgery is shown in Fig. 1.44. The 266-nm output from a frequency-quadrupled Nd:YAG laser may someday provide an attractive alternative to the excimer laser in some photoablative applications (49).

Selected Medical Applications of Lasers

Lasers have now been used in ophthalmology, gynecology, gastroenterology, dermatology, oncology, cardiology, orthopedics, otolaryngology, burn therapy, plastic and reconstructive surgery, thoracic surgery, neurosurgery, and urology. A list of all reported circumstances in which lasers have been applied in medicine and surgery would require a bibliography the size of this chapter. Instead, this section briefly describes three specific ophthalmic applications, chosen because they illustrate the unique capabilities of lasers in medicine: photocoagulation of the retina, photodisruption of the posterior lens capsule, and photoablation of the cornea (corneal sculpting).

Retinal Photocoagulation

In the early 1950s, Meyer-Schwickerath (50) collaborated on the design of the first xenon-arc photocoagulator and

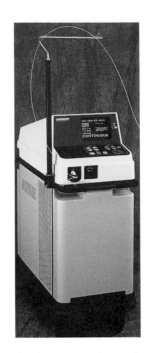

Fig. 1.44 Photograph of Laserscope's KTP/Nd:YAG XP Surgical Laser System. (Courtesy of Laserscope Surgical Systems, San Jose, CA.)

successfully used it in the treatment of retinal tears. In the early 1960s, Koester and coworkers (51) introduced the ruby laser photocoagulator, transforming retinal photocoagulation from an operating room procedure to one that could be performed on an outpatient basis. In the late 1960s, L'Esperance (4) introduced the argon-ion laser photocoagulator, which has now become the preferred instrument for retinal photocoagulation although krypton, organic dye, frequency-doubled Nd:YAG and, recently, diode lasers have been used to explore the clinical possibilities of different wavelengths for retinal photocoagulation (49).

The eye is one of the most accessible human organs, and its media (cornea, aqueous humor, lens, and vitreous) are all transparent to light in the visible spectrum. Curves showing the transmission of the transparent structures of the eye as a function of wavelength (40) are presented in Fig. 1.45 (*top*). On the other hand, many intraocular tissues (the iris, retina, choroid, etc.) are pigmented and, thus, will absorb laser light. Absorption spectra of some of the more absorbing pigments in the retina are also shown in Fig. 1.45 (*bottom*) along with the wavelengths of three commonly used ophthalmic lasers: argon, GaAs diode, and Nd:YAG (40). Because laser light is selectively absorbed in pigmented tissues, such tissues can be selectively heated. The precise effect on the tissue depends on both the magnitude and the rate of the temperature rise. For example, a 0.1- to 1-sec exposure of the retina to 488 and 514.5 nm radiation from an argon-ion laser at an irradiance of approximately

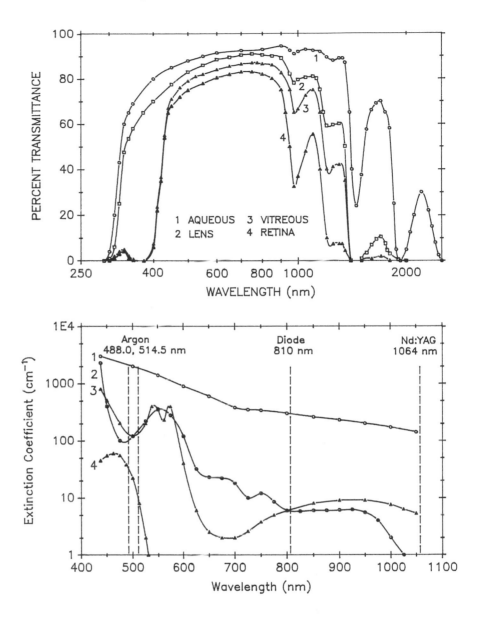

Fig. 1.45 Total transmittance of the entire eye (*top*) and transmission spectra of the major ocular chromophores (*bottom*): melanin (1), reduced hemoglobin (2), oxygenated hemoglobin (3), and macular xanthophyll (4). Also shown are the wavelengths of three commonly used ophthalmic lasers: argon, diode and Nd:YAG. (Adapted from Thompson et al [40]; reproduced by permission from the IEEE.)

100 W/cm² results in a 20° to 30° temperature rise and leads to coagulation of retinal tissue (40).

Photocoagulation has proven most useful in the treatment of proliferative diabetic retinopathy. In this disorder, the retina becomes starved for oxygen and releases chemical agents that cause the proliferation of new blood vessels. By destroying a portion of the peripheral retina with a laser, in a process termed *panretinal photocoagulation* (Fig. 1.46), the stimulus for new vessel formation can be reduced significantly. The side effects of this treatment, the loss of some night vision and constriction of visual field, are far outweighed by the preservation of central vision. The widespread use of argon and krypton lasers by ophthalmologists to treat proliferative diabetic retinopathy has been responsible for preserving the vision of thousands of diabetic patients (40).

The optical arrangement for the slit-lamp laser delivery system used in laser photocoagulation is shown in Fig. 1.47. Energy from a CW argon, krypton, organic dye, Nd:YAG, or diode laser is conducted to the slit lamp by a 500-μm diameter silica fiber and directed toward the eye by means of a coaxial beam splitter. Alternative delivery systems include the indirect ophthalmoscope, which allows treatment of the peripheral retina, fiber delivery used for the endoscopic probe (argon) in vitreoretinal surgery, and fiber delivery used for transscleral ciliary body coagulation (Nd:YAG), and filtering sclerostomy (Ho; 49). The laser, with its ability to preferentially coagulate a target tissue while minimizing thermal damage to surrounding ocular tissue during laser treatment, is ideally suited to retinal photocoagulation. It is no wonder, then, that it has become the instrument of choice for this procedure.

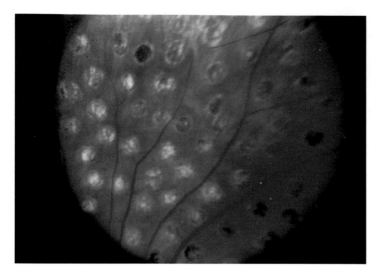

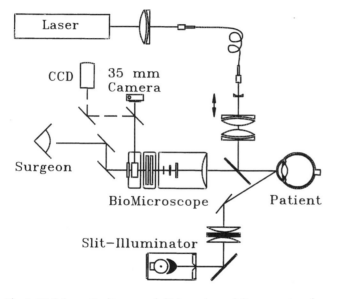

Fig. 1.46 Fundus photograph showing panretinal photocoagulation. (Courtesy of Dr. David B. Karlin.)

Fig. 1.47 Schematic diagram of slit lamp laser delivery system for retinal photocoagulation. (Adapted from Thompson et al. [40]; reproduced by permission from the IEEE.)

Posterior Capsulotomy

The short pulse output from a 1.06-μm Nd:YAG laser (30 psec for mode-locked and 10 nsec for Q-switched) is now being used, in a procedure called *posterior capsulotomy*, to break up the opacified membrane that often forms in the eye following cataract surgery and intraocular lens (IOL) implantation. This procedure, simultaneously introduced by glaucoma specialist Franz Fankhauser (6) in Switzerland and cataract specialist Danielle Aron-Rosa (5) in France in 1980, in most cases eliminates the need for reoperations, is noninvasive, eliminates the risk of IOL dislocation, and in some cases allows cutting of other intraocular tissues (iris, trabecula, vitreous strands, etc.) as well (40).

The implantation of an IOL at the time of cataract surgery is an increasingly common procedure. Typically, a patient receives a plastic IOL immediately following ex-

tracapsular cataract extraction and a careful polishing of the posterior lens capsule, a procedure that leaves the vitreous cavity undisturbed. In an uncomfortably high percentage of cases, however, the posterior capsule begins to opacify soon after the surgery because retained lens epithelial cells proliferate. The patient, who experiences improvement of vision following surgery, suffers slowly declining vision as the capsule opacifies.

Secondary opacification of the posterior capsule can be treated, without any anesthesia, by focusing the output from a mode-locked or Q-switched Nd:YAG laser with a high numerical aperture beam expander focusing lens system (20° to 40° cone angle) through the IOL to a sharp focus (10 to 50 μm diameter focal spot) on the posterior capsule as shown in Fig. 1.48. Using an incident pulse energy at the surface of the cornea of only 3 to 4.5 mJ, a power density as high as 10^{11} W/cm² can be produced at the beam waist. The plasma (a collection of ions and electrons) produced by this high-power density serves two functions: (1) it blocks further energy transmission (a dense plasma can reflect as well as absorb laser light) and thus reduces the

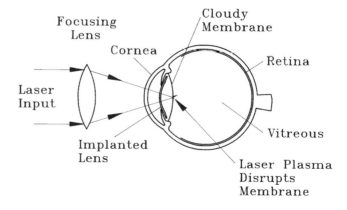

Fig 1.48 Schematic diagram illustrating posterior capsulotomy with the focused output of a Q-switched Nd:YAG laser.

risk of injury to underlying tissue; (2) its rapid expansion results in the formation of a hydrodynamic shock wave in the focal region. This shock wave, with shock-front pressures of 10^7 mm Hg at a distance of 0.1 mm and 10 mm Hg at a distance of 10 mm, is used to mechanically rupture the opacified membrane and clear the visual axis, restoring vision. The use of a highly converging incident beam (20° or more cone angle) reduces the risk of damage to the plastic implant or the cornea. Both the shielding effect of the plasma and the large cone angle beyond the focus reduce the risk of damage to the retina.

Because plasma formation is a threshold phenomenon that depends on the strength of the applied electric field, photodisruption is not dependent on absorption of the laser wavelength by the target tissue. Hence, photodisruption can be used in tissues that are transparent to the incident laser wavelength. Today, most photodisruptors are Q-switched Nd:YAG lasers with a pulse duration of about 10 nsec (40). By far, the most common photodisruptor applications are in posterior capsulotomy. However, they have also been used for cutting vitreous strands in the vitreous cavity and anterior chamber, creating peripheral iridotomies, severing trapped IOL haptic loops and cutting sutures. These lasers allow outpatient surgical treatment and have reduced postoperative complications, such as inflammation and infections, associated with intraocular surgical procedures.

Photorefractive Keratectomy

The short-pulse output from an ArF excimer laser at 193 nm is currently being investigated for its safety and efficacy in refractive surgery of the cornea. This relatively new surgical procedure grew out of work by Trokel and colleagues (52), who demonstrated that precise cuts without subsequent thermal damage could be obtained in biologic material using an ArF excimer laser. Initially, it was suggested that an excimer laser be used to produce precise radial incisions in the periphery of the cornea to correct for refractive errors in the eye in a procedure called radial keratotomy. In 1986, a more promising technique, called *photorefractive keratectomy* (PRK), which makes use of the precise photoablation capabilities of an ArF excimer laser to reshape the cornea as though with a lathe, was described by Marshall and coworkers (7). Refractive correction using this procedure is possible because most of the refractive power of the eye comes from the cornea (80% cornea, 20% lens) and most myopia can be corrected by removing less than 30 μm of the 500 μm thick cornea (40).

Excimer laser photoablation occurs because the cornea has an extremely high absorption coefficient at 193 nm, and the 193-nm photons are energetic enough to break intermolecular bonds interlinking the protein molecules of the cornea. Although the precise ablative process is not yet completely understood, there appears to be both a photo-

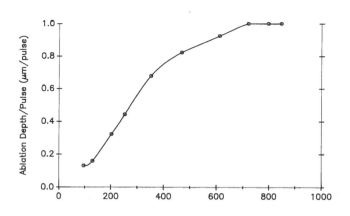

Fig. 1.49 Depth of corneal ablation versus 193-nm excimer laser exposure dose for the human cornea. (From Thompson et al. [40]; reproduced by permission from the IEEE.)

chemical and a thermal component in the ablative process. In any case, a discrete volume of corneal tissue is removed with each pulse of the laser (40), as shown in Fig. 1.49. The depth of ablation depends on the exposure and typically varies from 0.1 to 0.5 μm per pulse at fluences of 50 to 250 mJ/cm².

Several beam delivery systems to homogenize, shape, transmit, and focus the ArF excimer beam for corneal ablation have been developed for PRK. In PRK, the cornea is first scanned, its topography mapped, and the amount of cornea to be removed (generally 20 to 40 μm) calculated. Then, the corneal epithelium is removed by the surgeon. Next, the stromal surface of the cornea is contoured using excimer laser ablation in a procedure that takes less than 60 sec as shown in Fig. 1.50. Following reepithelialization, the anterior corneal curvature is flattened, and the myopia is reduced. Preliminary evidence indicates that the technique is safe and effective for reducing myopia up to 6 diopters. The present delivery systems available are limited to creating simple spherical or spherocylindrical optical corrections. Corneal sculpting has already been tested in over 10,000 eyes worldwide. If approved for

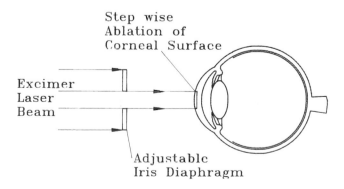

Fig. 1.50 Schematic diagram illustrating photorefractive keratectomy with an excimer laser beam.

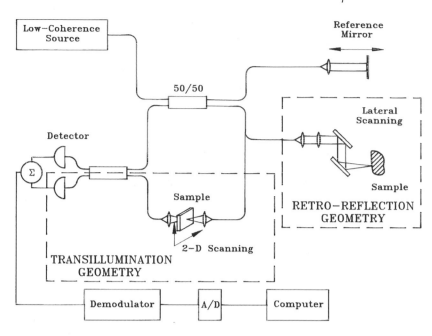

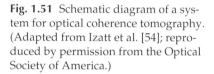

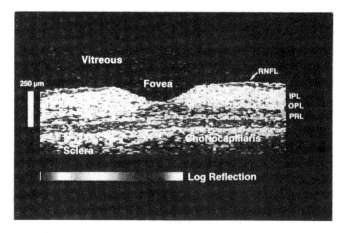

Fig. 1.51 Schematic diagram of a system for optical coherence tomography. (Adapted from Izatt et al. [54]; reproduced by permission from the Optical Society of America.)

Future Directions

More than 30 years have elapsed since the advent of the laser, yet medical laser technology continues to evolve rapidly. The need for more compact, less expensive, and more reliable clinical lasers has accelerated the development of diode-pumped solid-state lasers, semiconductor diode lasers, and mid-IR Ho and Er:YAG lasers and will, without doubt, lead to further improvements in existing lasers. Research into basic laser tissue interactions, in contrast, is pointing the way to two potentially revolutionary developments in the medical laser field. These developments are in (1) optical imaging and diagnostics and (2) laser systems with feedback control.

Optical Imaging and Diagnostics

Recent developments in semiconductor lasers, fiberoptics, and ultrafast laser generation and measurement have led to techniques for noninvasive, high-resolution tissue imaging in the red and near-IR spectral regions (600 nm to 1.3 μm). The fundamental problem with optical tissue imaging is that, in contrast to x-rays, the average optical photon travels less than 100 μm into tissue before scattering. Scattering severely degrades image resolution by randomizing the image information contained in the transmitted or retroreflected light. A number of promising time and frequency domain methods for dealing with scattered light are currently being investigated (53). A tissue imaging technique developed by Izatt and coworkers

(54) called *optical coherence tomography* (OCT) seems particularly promising. In this technique, 500 μW of power at 830 nm from a low-coherence broad-bandwidth superluminescent semiconductor diode is coupled into a single-mode fiberoptic Michelson interferometer illustrated in Fig. 1.51. Light exiting from the sample arm of the interferometer is coupled into a standard slit-lamp biomicroscope and directed onto a patient's retina. Light backscattered from the retina is combined in a fiberoptic beamsplitter with Doppler-shifted light reflected from a scanning reference mirror to give a map of reflectivity versus distance into the retina. A sagittal section through the macular region of a human volunteer recorded by OCT imaging (54) is shown in Fig. 1.52. The fovea is clearly vis-

Fig. 1.52 In vivo retroreflection optical coherence tomographic image of the foveal region of a human subject. (From Izatt et al. [54]; reproduced by permission from the Optical Society of America.)

general use, PRK will offer an alternative to glasses and contact lenses for millions of myopic individuals and could become the most widespread application for lasers in medicine (40).

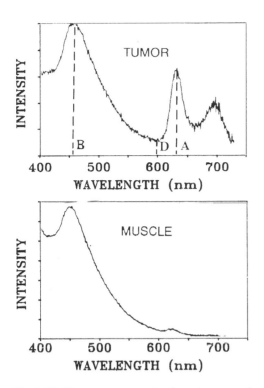

Fig. 1.53 Fluorescence spectra from tumor and adjacent normal muscle tissue of a rat injected with Photofrin. (Adapted from Svanberg [55]; reproduced by permission from the Optical Society of America.)

ible in the center of the image. Lateral to the fovea, layers of alternating high and low scattering reveal the stratified cellular structure of the retina in exquisite detail. OCT is noninvasive and has an axial resolution (13 μm) a factor of 5 to 10 higher than standard ultrasound. This new imaging technique may prove useful in evaluating the condition of the optic nerve in patients with glaucoma.

Recent improvements in the techniques of laser-induced fluorescence (LIF) hold out the possibility of diagnosing disease as well as performing an objective assessment of biologic function. Tissue fluorescence can be due to molecules that are either intrinsic to the tissue or injected from an external source. Intrinsic fluorescence has been shown effective in the differentiation of normal and atherosclerotic arterial tissue and normal and cancerous colon and lung tissue. Extrinsic fluorescence has been used to localize cancerous lesions within the skin, bladder, and lungs. A number of different laser sources have been used to excite the fluorescence; special multifiber catheters have been designed to help image regions of normal and abnormal tissue and optical multichannel analyzers have been used to record the temporal shape of the fluorescent signal. For example, LIF spectra from tumor and adjacent normal muscle tissue of a rat, injected with Photofrin (a hematoporphyrin derivative) is shown in Fig. 1.53 (55). To produce these spectra, radiation from a pulsed nitrogen laser (337 nm) was transmitted

through the biopsy channel of an endoscope. LIF was collected by the same fiber and was brought back to the entrance slit of a small monochromator equipped with an intensified diode array detector, capturing the full fluorescence spectrum in each laser shot. Using Photofrin as a sensitizer, malignant tissue shows up with an increased fluorescence emission in the red spectral region (55; peaks at 630 and 690 nm in Fig. 1.53). In the not too distant future, a combination of optical tissue imaging and LIF could lead to powerful new techniques for the guidance of laser surgery (angioplasty and lithotripsy), the detection of tumors, and the monitoring of drug uptake and clearance (providing information on both kinetics and spatial distributions).

Laser with Feedback Control

The medical laser field is beginning to see the first applications of "smart medical lasers" in which feedback control is capable of guiding the treatment. Pulse-by-pulse monitoring of the fluorescence obtained during excimer laser ablation of arterial tissue has been used to identify the transition from the artheromatous layer to the normal media (56) and could be used for computer control of laser angioplasty. Real-time monitoring of tissue temperature during argon laser welding of vascular tissue has been used to provide the feedback to maintain a quasi-constant tissue temperature during laser-assisted vascular anastomosis (57). Magnetic resonance imaging (MRI) of the brain and ultrasonic imaging of the abdomen during Nd:YAG laser destruction of solid tumor tissue may someday be used to control dynamically the shape of an interstitial laser photocoagulation (ILP) lesion (8). In ILP, first described by Bown (58), the 1.06-μm output from a 2.0 W CW Nd:YAG laser is directed into tissue through

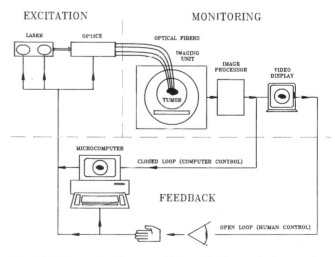

Fig. 1.54 Schematic diagram of interstitial laser photocoagulation monitored using radiologic imaging and controlled by a computer and/or human operator. (Adapted from Wyman et al. [8]; reproduced by permission from the IEEE.)

one or more optical fibers implanted interstitially. Thermal diffusion of the absorbed energy heats cells throughout the target volume to temperatures exceeding protein denaturation thresholds of approximately 60° C, inducing coagulation necrosis. Both abdominal ultrasound imaging and MRI of the brain can produce high-contrast images of ILP lesions in real or near-real time. The investigations conducted to date suggest that accurate feedback control of ILP in the brain might be achievable with MRI (8), as shown in Fig. 1.54. In ophthalmology, real-time measurements of corneal curvature based on the reflected light from a number of light-emitting diodes during refractive surgery may soon be used to control excimer laser ablation in photorefractive keratectomy.

In the last 30 years the contributions of lasers to ophthalmology have been truly revolutionary. In the next 30 years the contributions are unimaginable.

References

1. Schawlow AL, Townes CH. Infrared and optical masers. Phys Rev 1958;112:1940–1949.
2. Maiman TH. Stimulated optical radiation in ruby masers. Nature 1960;187:493–494.
3. Abraham RK, Miller GL. Outpatient argon laser iridectomy for angle closure glaucoma: a two year study. Trans Am Acad Ophthalmol Otolaryngol 1975;79:529–538.
4. L'Esperance Jr FA. Treatment of ophthalmic vascular disease by argon laser photocoagulation. Trans Am Acad Ophthalmol Otolaryngol 1969;73:1077–1096.
5. Aron-Rosa D, Aron JJ, Griesemann M, Thyzel R. Use of the neodymium-YAG laser to open the posterior capsule after lens implant surgery: a preliminary report. Am Intraocular Implant Soc J 1980;6:352–354.
6. Van Der Zypen E, Fankhauser F, Bebie H, Marshall J. Changes in the ultrastructure of the iris after irradiation with intense light. Adv Ophthalmol 1979;39:59–180.
7. Marshall J, Trokel S, Rothery S. Photoablative reprofiling of the cornea using an excimer laser: photorefractive keratotomy. Laser Ophthalmol 1986;1:21–48.
8. Wyman DR, Wilson BC, Malone DE. Medical imaging systems for feedback control of interstitital laser photocoagulation. Proc IEEE 1992;80:890–902.
9. Allen CW. Astrophysical quantities. London: Athlone, 1973.
10. Hecht J. Understanding lasers: an entry level guide. New York: IEEE Press, 1992.
11. Herzberg G. Atmomic spectra and atmomic structure. New York: Dover Publications, 1944.
12. Stone JM. Radiation and optics. New York: McGraw-Hill, 1963.
13. Patel CKN, Wood OR. History of the laser. In: Baggish MS, ed. Basic and advanced laser surgery in gynecology. Norwalk, CT: Appleton-Century-Crofts, 1985.
14. Einstein A. Zur quantentheorie der strahlung. Phys Zeit 1917; 18:121–128.
15. Fox AG, Li T. Resonant modes in a maser interferometer. Bell Sys Tech J 1961;40:453–458.
16. Boyd GD, Gordon JP. Confocal multimode resonator for millimeter through optical wavelength masers. Bell Sys Tech J 1961;40:489–508.
17. Kogelnik H, Boyd GD. Generalized confocal resonator theory. Bell Sys Tech J 1962;41:1347–1371.
18. Koeglnik H. On the propagation of gaussian beams of light through lenslike media including those with a loss or gain variation. Appl Opt 1965;4:1562–1569.
19. Yariv A, Gordon JP. The laser. Proc IEEE 1963;5:4–29.
20. Kogelnik H, Li T. Laser beams and resonators. Appl Opt 1966;5:1550–1567.
21. Hellwarth RW. Advances in quantum electronics. New York: Columbia University Press, 1961.
22. Hargrove LE, Fork RL, Pollack MA. Locking of He-Ne laser modes induced by synchronous intracavity modulation. Appl Phys Lett 1964;5:4–5.
23. Javan A, Bennett WB Jr, Herriott DR. Population inversion and continuous optical maser oscillation in a gas discharge containing a He-Ne mixture. Phys Rev Lett 1961; 6:106–110.
24. White AD, Rigden JD. Continuous gas maser operation in the visible. Proc IRE 1962;50:1695.
25. Hecht J. The laser guidebook. Blue Ridge Summit, PA: Tab Books, 1992.
26. Patel CKNP. Continuous-wave laser action on vibrational-rotational transitions of CO_2. Phys Rev A 1964; 136:A1187–A1193.
27. Bridges WB, Chester AN. Visible and UV laser oscillation at 118 wavelengths in ionized neon, argon, krypton, xenon, oxygen and other gases. Appl Opt 1965;4:573–580.
28. Bridges WB. Laser oscillation in singly ionized argon in the visible spectrum. Appl Phys Lett 1964;4:128–130.
29. Brau CA. Rare gas halogen excimers. In: Rhodes CK, ed. Excimer lasers. Berlin: Springer-Verlag, 1984.
30. Sorokin PP, Lankard JR. Stimulated emission observed from an organic dye, chloro-aluminum phthalocyanine. IBM J Res Dev 1966;10:162–163.
31. Soffer BH, McFarland BB. Continuously tunable narrow-band organic dye lasers. Appl Phys Lett 1967;10:266–267.
32. Fork RL, Brito Cruz CH, Becker PC, Shank CV. Compression of optical pulses to six femtoseconds by using cubic phase compensation. Opt Lett 1987;12:483–485.
33. Geusic JE, Marcos HM, Van Uitert LG. Laser oscillation in Nd-doped yttrium aluminum, yttrium gallium and gadolinium garnets. Appl Phys Lett 1964;4:182–184.
34. Cordova-Plaza A, Fan TY Digonnet MJF. $Nd:MgO:LiNbO_3$ continuous wave laser pumped by a laser diode. Opt Lett 1988;13:209-211.
35. Maine P, Mourou G. Amplification of 1-nsec pulses in Nd: glass followed by compression to 1 psec. Opt Lett 1988;13:467–469.
36. Johnson LF, Boyd GD, Nassau K. Optical maser characteristics of Ho^{3+} in $CaWO_4$. Proc IRE 1962;50:87–88.
37. Antipenko BM, Glebov AS, Kiseleva TI, Pis'menny VA. 2.12-μm Ho:YAG laser. Sov Tech Phys Lett 1985;11: 284–285.
38. Quarles GJ, Rosenbaum A, Marquardt CL, Esterowitz L. High efficiency 2.09 μm flashlamp-pumped laser. Appl Phys Lett 1989;55:1062–1064.
39. Fan TY, Huber G, Byer RL, Mitzscherlich P. Continuous-wave operation at 2.1 μm of a diode-laser-pumped Tm-

sensitized Ho:$Y_3Al_5O_{13}$ laser at 300 K. Opt Lett 1987;12: 678–680.

40. Thompson KP, Ren QS, Parel J-M. Therapeutic and diagnostic application of lasers in ophthalmology. Proc IEEE 1992;80:838–860.

41. Hall RN, Fenner GE, Kingsley JD, Soltys TJ, Carlson RO. Coherent light emission from GaAs junctions. Phys Rev Lett 1962;9:366–368.

42. Nathan MI, Dumke WP, Burns G, Dill FH Jr, Lasher G. Stimulated emission of radiation from GaAs p-n junctions. Appl Phys Lett 1962;1:62–64.

43. Quist TM, Rediker RH, Keyes RJ, et al. Semiconductor maser of GaAs. Appl Phys Lett 1962;1:91–92.

44. Franken PA, Hill AE, Peters CW, Weinreich G. Generation of optical harmonics. Phys Rev Lett 1961;7:118–119.

45. Bierlein J, Vanherzeele H. Potassium titanyl phosphate: properties and new applications. J Opt Soc Am B 1989;6: 622–633.

46. Hecht J. Neodymium lasers prove versatile over three decades. Laser Focus World 1992;28:77–94.

47. Messenger HW. Difficult technology challenges device developers. Laser Focus World 1992;28:95–103.

48. Gerstenberger DC, Tye GE, Wallace RW. Efficient second-harmonic conversion of cw single-frequency Nd:YAG laser light by frequency locking to a monolithic ring frequency doubler. Opt Lett 1991;16:992–994.

49. Trokel SL. Lasers in ophthalmology. Optics & Photonics News 1992;3:11–13.

50. Meyer-Schwickerath G. Light coagulation. St. Louis: CV Mosby, 1960.

51. Koester CJ, Switzer E, Campbell CJ, Ritter MC. Experimental laser retinal coagulator. J Opt Soc Am 1962;52:607.

52. Trokel SL, Srinivasan R, Braren BA. Excimer laser surgery of the cornea. Am J Ophthalmol 1983;96:710–715.

53. Wilson BC, Sevick EM, Patterson MS, Chance B. Time-dependent optical spectroscopy and imaging for biomedical applications. Proc IEEE 1992;80:918–930.

54. Izatt JA, Hee MR, Huang D. Micron-resolution biomedical imaging with optical coherence tomography. Optics & Photonics News 1993;4:14–19.

55. Svanberg S. Optical tissue diagnostics: fluorescence and transillumination imaging. Optics & Photonics News 1992;3:31–34.

56. Papazoglou TG, Papaioannou T, Arakawa K, Fishbein M, Marmarelis VZ, Grundfest WS. Control of excimer laser aided tissue ablation via laser-induced fluorescence monitoring. Appl Opt 1990;29:4950–4955.

57. Springer TA, Welch AJ. Temperature control during laser vessel welding. Appl Opt 1993;32:517–525.

58. Bown SG. Phototherapy of tumors. World J Surg 1983; 7:700–709.

2

Laser Surgery of the Cornea—The Excimer Laser

Francis A. L'Esperance, Jr.
Olivia N. Serdarevic

The use of UV laser irradiation was first suggested by research scientists in the materials processing and integrated circuit industries (1–4). Soon after, UV laser radiation was used by researchers in the life science field, who noted that it could affect the corneal epithelium or delicately damage the superficial layers of the eye (5,6). Lasers in the UV portion of the electromagnetic spectrum were recognized to have the capability, particularly in the area of 193 nm, to interact with human tissues in a new manner. Due to the high photon energy of the laser emissions, the material on which the radiation had an impact could be removed in a highly delicate fashion. The enormous potential of this unique laser–tissue interaction encouraged our research team to design and construct an instrument to investigate the overall capabilities of the far-UV laser spectral emissions for the eventual purpose of creating a photorefractive or phototherapeutic keratectomy.

In 1969, Houtermans (7) first described the concept of a bound-free excimer system as a laser medium. Considerable research was done in various laboratories in the early 1970s and the commercial introduction of excimer lasers eventually occurred in 1976 (1,8). In 1979, Ruderman (2) suggested that excimer lasers were applicable to studying the effects of intense radiation on tissue and additionally emphasized that a single photon from an excimer laser was energetic enough to rupture many chemical bonds within a tissue element.

Although excimer lasers were extremely rudimentary in 1979, the possibility of a new laser–tissue interaction was considered that could have multiple applications in various medical branches. The actual technique of applying this radiation from the ultraviolet portion of the spectrum to various parts of the eye to control a particular disease or remove a precise amount of tissue was devised in the 1980s. It became apparent that the production of a precise corneal incision or a superficial lamellar keratectomy was feasible (9–13). In addition, corneal incisions could be shaped in any manner and to any predetermined width or depth. By producing a superficial lamellar keratectomy, external corneal scars could be removed and various refractive errors of the eye could be decreased or eliminated by applying a variable density of photons to the central or more peripheral portions of the cornea. The reports of Taboada and colleagues (5,6) emphasized that depressions in the corneal epithelium were the result of the laser irradiation even at weak threshold levels and that the high-energy photons involved could interact with corneal tissue in such a manner as to cut or remove tissue in a nondisruptive fashion.

During this time, L'Esperance made three important assumptions and then proceeded to develop the concept of therapeutic controlled-tissue (corneal) erosion or removal.

1. The *first assumption* was that a UV laser, particularly an excimer laser producing an emission at 193 nm, would impact the anterior surface of the cornea and remove a specific volume of anterior corneal tissue.

2. The *second assumption* was that the laser could be manipulated in such a way, by computer control if necessary, to perform a reconstructive superficial keratectomy and possibly to sculpt, reprofile, or recontour the cornea to correct myopic, astigmatic, and hyperopic refractive errors.

3. The *third assumption*, and probably the most tenuous, was that the keratectomy or recontouring procedure, which would remove superficial scarred corneal tissue or sculpt a new curvature on the anterior surface of the cornea involving Bowman's membrane and most probably the anterior stromal area as well (but not necessarily), could be performed without creating minute opacifications and scarring of the remaining anterior stroma or that portion of Bowman's membrane that had not been removed.

Classical teachings at that time (1979–1983) were that any impact, incision, or manipulation of Bowman's membrane and the underlying anterior stroma would, in most cases, result in a moderately dense opacification that would hinder the passage of light rays through the

(Modified from L'Esperance FA Jr.: *Excimer Laser* and Serdarevic: *Corneal Laser Surgery*. In: L'Esperance FA Jr. Ophthalmic Lasers, 3rd ed., St. Louis: 1989, Mosby-Year Book, Inc.)

cornea toward the retina. By the nature of this new technique, the purposeful volumetric removal of a portion of the anterior surface of the cornea in such a way as to remove opacified anterior corneal tissue or create a new curvature for the correction of various refractive errors would necessarily involve the optical zone of the cornea. Therefore, considering the critical corneal area involved, this third assumption—that clarity could be maintained if the removal process was extremely delicate such as provided by the excimer laser—was a considerable departure from the classical teachings of corneal physiology and appeared to be the most monumental obstacle to the success of the project.

During this interval in the early 1980s, the work of Srinivasan and his colleagues (3,4) at the IBM Thomas J. Watson Research Center demonstrated that high-energy UV photons from excimer lasers, primarily the argon-fluoride (ArF) excimer laser at 193 nm, could photoetch plastics such as polyethylene terephthalate, polyimide, and polymethylmethacrylate with great precision without apparent photothermal effects. Soon thereafter, Srinivasan and coworkers (14) and Linsker and colleagues (15) in early 1983 showed that hair, aorta, and cartilage could be etched, incised, or contoured with great accuracy, partially confirming our original concept. In late 1983, ArF excimer laser incisions into enucleated bovine eyes were produced by Trokel and associates (16) and later by Puliafito (17), Seiler (18), and Marshall (19) and their coworkers. The processes of corneal area ablation, excision of the superficial cornea, and reprofiling of the anterior surface of the cornea were later tested in rabbits and monkeys and found to be technically feasible (20). During most investigations concerning this procedure, the ArF excimer laser with an emission at 193 nm was used and produced results in animals that were similar in many ways to those created previously in plastics and described extensively by Srinivasan and his associates (3,21,22).

These basic laser–tissue assumptions and the resulting conceptualization of new surgical techniques, the preliminary studies in the materials and electronics industries, and a knowledge of laser electro-optics led us to consider designing and constructing an excimer laser ophthalmic system that would create accurately delineated corneal incisions, produce a smooth and precise superficial keratectomy, or recontour the anterior surface of the cornea in a delicate and reproducible fashion. L'Esperance gathered together an outstanding team of physicists formerly from the Perkin-Elmer Company in Connecticut to develop and implement this intricate surgical technique (Fig. 2.1). This team of physicists and their associates formed a company named Taunton Technologies, Inc., headquartered in Monroe, Connecticut, and they eventually constructed the ultrasophisticated instrumentation required to successfully remove scarred, calcified, and opacified anterior

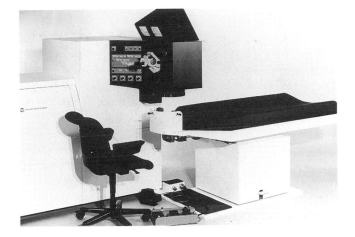

Fig. 2.1 An extremely sophisticated excimer laser instrument designed for the precise volumetric removal of the anterior corneal structures to produce a phototherapeutic keratectomy or a photorefractive keratectomy. (Copyright Taunton Technologies, Inc.)

corneal tissue or recontour the cornea for the accurate correction of corneal refractive errors.

Design, Development, and Use of an Excimer Laser Ophthalmic System for Phototherapeutic or Photorefractive Keratectomy

The ArF Excimer Laser

Although frequency-quadrupled and frequency-quintupled neodymium:yttrium-aluminum-garnet (Nd:YAG) lasers as well as frequency-doubled organic dye lasers and several other families of UV lasers are available to produce laser outputs in the far-UV spectrum (wavelengths shorter than 280 nm), it is the excimer family of lasers that seem to be most easily applicable to corneal incision, excision, or reprofiling. Theoretically, the extremely short *pulse duration* of the excimer laser (12 to 15 nsec) will decrease thermal effects to infinitesimal levels due to the apparent lack of time for thermal diffusion. Secondly, the *pulse-to-pulse energy level* is reproducible within acceptable limits and the repetition rate (Hertz) of the pulses can be varied over a relatively large range, typically 1 to 50 Hz. Thirdly, *sufficient energy* is available (typically up to 450 mJ) so that a large beam can be produced to ablate or reprofile a 4- to 7-mm diameter portion of the central cornea without energy limitations. Despite these apparent advantages, the available excimer lasers are less sophisticated when compared to other existing conventional ophthalmic lasers and extensive modifications are required for clinical application. Special optical delivery systems must also be used (23,24).

Beam Delivery System

Four versions of beam delivery apparatus with progressively improved capability were developed to permit precise amounts or thicknesses of tissue to be ablated at exact locations on the anterior corneal surface without involving normal adjacent or deeper corneal tissue. The fourth version allows the intensity distribution to be delivered to the cornea for the correction of hyperopia or myopia over 7.0-nm diameter areas. In this apparatus, a system of variable apertures is used for myopia and a system of variable peripheral annuli is used for hyperopia correction. All these systems operate under computer control. The apertures are adjusted with great precision so that the required number and density of photons impact the anterior cornea and remove the correct amount of tissue in specific areas (Figs. 2.2 through 2.5). The general configuration of the latest beam delivery apparatus developed by Taunton Technologies, Inc. for a therapeutic or refractive application will be described.

The photoreactive keratectomy (PRK) or phototherapeutic keratectomy (PTK) apparatus consists of a Laser Subsystem, an Optical Subsystem, an Alignment Subsystem, a Measurement Subsystem, and a Control Subsystem (20,25). The Laser Subsystem generates the pulsed coherent UV radiation of suitable energy level. The Optical Subsystem provides a means for conditioning the beam and

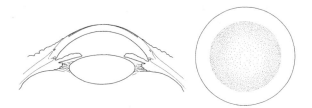

Fig. 2.4 Diagrammatic representation illustrates the excimer laser recontouring (photorefractive keratectomy) of the anterior surface of the central cornea to decrease the radius of curvature and steepen the curvature of the cornea to correct hyperopic refractive errors. (Reproduced by permission from L'Esperance FA Jr [26], p. 892.)

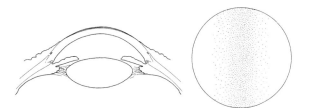

Fig. 2.5 Diagrammatic representation illustrates the excimer laser recontouring (photorefractive keratectomy) of the anterior surface of the central cornea along a particular axis of the cornea for the correction of astigmatism. (Reproduced by permission from L'Esperance FA Jr [26], p. 892.)

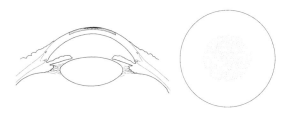

Fig. 2.2 Diagrammatic representation of excimer laser superficial lamellar keratectomy (phototherapeutic keratectomy) to ablate or remove superficial scar tissue from the cornea, thereby permitting optimal clearing of the underlying cornea. (Reproduced by permission from L'Esperance FA Jr [26], p. 891.)

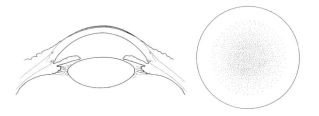

Fig. 2.3 Diagrammatic representation illustrates the excimer laser recontouring or reprofiling (photorefractive keratectomy) of the anterior corneal structures to increase the radius of curvature and flatten the anterior corneal curvature for the correction of myopic refractive errors. (Reproduced by permission from L'Esperance FA Jr [26], p. 891.)

delivering it to the patient's eye as well as a means (Beam Monitor) for characterizing the conditioned laser beam prior to and during its use. The Alignment Subsystem provides a microscope coaxial with the laser beam and having a crosshair reference for sensing lateral alignment of the patient's eye. The Measurement Subsystem provides an integral means for determining the three-dimensional topography of the cornea, in situ, at appropriate times during the procedure. The Control Subsystem provides the computer and electronics circuitry required for monitoring and controlling the apparatus via a user-friendly operator interface. It also automatically monitors safety aspects of the apparatus and maintains a history of the procedure, thus ensuring a safe, predictable, and documented operation.

In the following sections, we summarize the basic functions of these subsystems. For the sake of brevity, the Alignment and Control subsystems will not be described but have been documented elsewhere (26).

Laser Subsystem

The Excimer 2015 system uses a Questék Series 2000 ArF excimer laser as the source of intense pulses of 193 nm radiation. All functions of the laser are software controlled; this simplifies the interfaces to the PRK optical and control subsystems. These lasers have automatic gain compensation, automatic gas replenishing, and other features controlled by an internal microprocessor. Gases and cooling water are obtained from external sources. Sensors constantly monitor temperature, gas pressure, coolant flow, hardware status, and microprocessor function.

Optical Subsystems

Figure 2.6 is a functional optical schematic diagram of the major parts in the Optical Subsystem. The raw laser beam entering at lower left is rectangular with dimensions of approximately 11 × 22 mm as indicated in Fig. 2.7. The intensity profiles in the short and long directions are essentially gaussian and "top hat," respectively, as indicated. Because there are significant "hot spots" at the edges of this beam, we pass it through a 10 × 20 mm aperture mask to "scrape off" these edges. The beam then is expanded anamorphically to form a square 20 × 20 mm beam as shown in Figure 2.8.

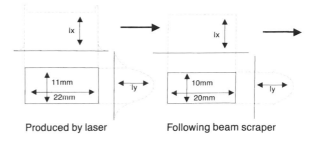

UV Laser Beam Cross-Sections/ Intensity Profiles

Produced by laser   Following beam scraper

Fig. 2.7 Diagrammatic representation of the excimer laser beam as it is manipulated after exiting from a specially designed excimer laser, so as to clip away the "wings" of the partially gaussian beam. (Copyright Taunton Technologies, Inc.)

Commonly used devices for anamorphic beam expansion include cylindrical lens telescopes and refracting prisms. Because of the large amount of spherical aberration introduced by short focal length simple lenses and the desire for ease of alignment without complex designs, we use the prism approach. This works because a refracting prism used at other than minimum deviation has different sized exit and entrance beams and thus introduces magnification in the plane of refraction (27). To eliminate the angular deviation resulting from one such prism, two prisms are used. Aberrations are virtually nonexistent because we are dealing with a monochromatic collimated beam.

Because the expanded laser beam still has different intensity profiles in the principal directions after expansion (see Fig. 2.8), we next pass the beam through a "K-mirror" type beam rotator to time-average the multipulse energy delivered to the cornea.

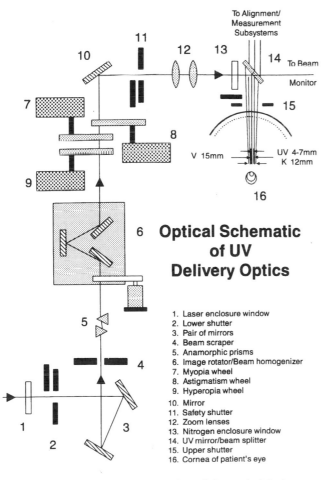

Optical Schematic of UV Delivery Optics

1. Laser enclosure window
2. Lower shutter
3. Pair of mirrors
4. Beam scraper
5. Anamorphic prisms
6. Image rotator/Beam homogenizer
7. Myopia wheel
8. Astigmatism wheel
9. Hyperopia wheel
10. Mirror
11. Safety shutter
12. Zoom lenses
13. Nitrogen enclosure window
14. UV mirror/beam splitter
15. Upper shutter
16. Cornea of patient's eye

Fig. 2.6 Diagrammatic representation of the optical design of the overall excimer laser instrument including anamorphic prisms, a beam homogenizing system, aperture wheels, and a beam-monitoring device. (Copyright Taunton Technologies, Inc.)

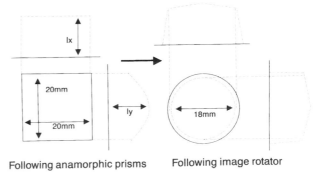

UV Laser Beam Cross-Sections/ Intensity Profiles

Following anamorphic prisms   Following image rotator

Fig. 2.8 Anamorphic prisms convert the rectangular beam to a square beam, which is then homogenized in a beam-image rotator, which converts the beam to a circular configuration. (Copyright Taunton Technologies, Inc.)

The rotating square beam having time-averaged axially symmetric intensity profiles (see Fig. 2.8) is next passed through a set of three aperture wheels spaced along the axis as indicated in Fig. 2.6. One wheel is used for each procedure (myopia, hyperopia, or astigmatism correction) with the two unused wheels being set to a completely open aperture. A stepper motor is used to drive each wheel so as to cycle the different apertures into the beam. The mechanism dwells at each aperture while the laser delivers the appropriate number of pulses as determined by a "recipe" previously entered into the computer to ablate to different depths at various points on the cornea.

The myopia wheel has a series of apertures of decreasing diameter, whereas the hyperopia wheel has a series of annular apertures of decreasing radial width.

Figs. 2.9 and 2.10 illustrate schematically (to exaggerated scale) the ablation profiles achieved with 15 apertures in the myopia and hyperopia cases, respectively. The apparatus used to date is designed to correct at least 10 diopters (D) of either type error over an ablated area as large as 7.0 mm.

The astigmatism wheel has a series of slit-shaped apertures of varying width (Fig. 2.11). Means are provided to adjust the slit orientations about the laser beam axis so as to align the cylindrical ablation axis with the appropriate astigmatism axis of the patient's eye as previously determined with the Measurement Subsystem discussed below. Exposure of the cornea through the series of slits recontours the original toroidal surface into a more nearly spherical one. If the resulting optical power of this ablated surface is then not optimum, the above discussed

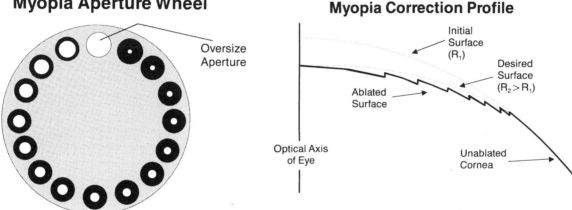

Fig. 2.9 Diagrammatic representation of the myopia aperture wheel (A) that removes more of the central cornea than the peripheral cornea (B) to flatten the corneal curvature by a series of stepwise enlargements of the beam impacting the cornea. The length of time that the aperture opening remains at each of these stations is controlled by a computer whose "recipe" can change for various myopic corrections. (Copyright Taunton Technologies, Inc.)

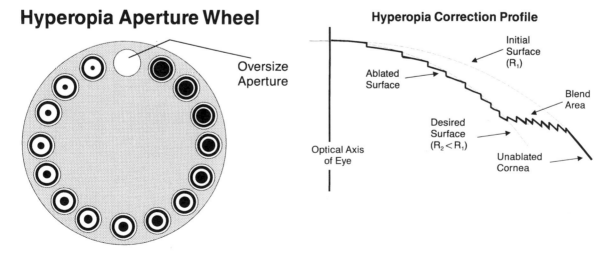

Fig. 2.10 Diagram of the hyperopia aperture wheel constructed so that progressively enlarging annuli (A) remove a greater amount of peripheral corneal tissue than central corneal tissue to steepen the curvature of the cornea (B) to correct the hyperopic refractive condition. (Copyright Taunton Technologies, Inc.)

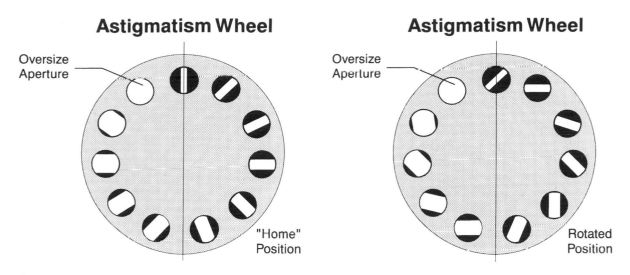

Fig. 2.11 The astigmatism aperture wheel incorporating a series of enlarging rectangles (A) that can be aligned and rotated to coincide with the axis of the astigmatism (B). The astigmatism is reduced in a manner similar to the ablation of the cornea created with the myopic correction profile. (Copyright Taunton Technologies, Inc.)

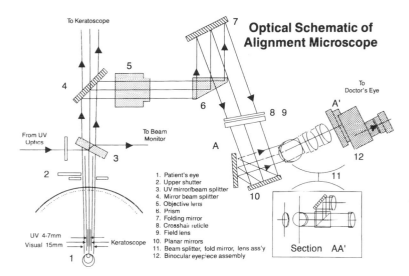

Fig. 2.12 Diagrammatic representation of the alignment microscope that tracks and monitors the corneal photoablation process while part of the beam travels to the keratoscope television monitor. (Copyright Taunton Technologies, Inc.)

myopia- or hyperopia-reducing procedure can be followed to reshape the spherical surface to the desired contour.

The next optical device in the delivery system is a lens (see Fig. 2.6), which focuses the collimated beam as received through the selected aperture in front of the cornea. The diverging beam then falls on the cornea and selectively ablates tissue in accordance with the recipe controlled by the computer located in the Control Subsystem.

The next optical component in the UV optical train of Fig. 2.12 is a beamsplitter plate that reflects most of the UV light onto the eye. The low-intensity sample that leaks through the plate is used by the Beam Monitor. This monitor functions in the manner described in more detail by Telfair and coworkers (28) as a digital beam intensity profilometer. The computer software allows the operator to analyze the intensity profiles of the beam, thereby pro-

viding a check on quality of the homogenized beam before the ablation procedure is started. The quality of the beam is also monitored and recorded during the ablation for documentation purposes.

Measurement Subsystem

A digital keratoscope is incorporated into the PTK (or PRK) apparatus to provide the capability to make quick, accurate measurements of the topography of the cornea prior to and following ablation. The principle of operation of this device (Fig. 2.13) is as follows. A spherical array of light-emitting diodes (LEDs) constitutes a series of "point sources" of visible red light. Beams from these LEDs reflect from the surface to be measured (patient's cornea), which is coaxial to the array. A lens images the reflected

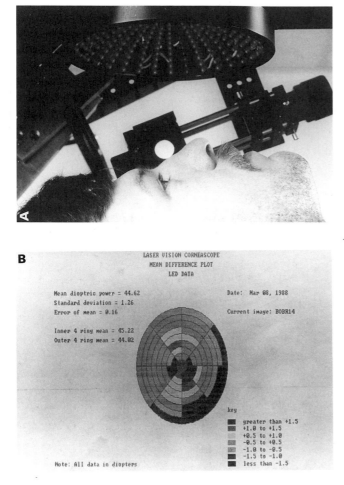

Fig. 2.13 A light-emitting diode keratoscope (A), which is an integral part of the therapeutic excimer laser instrument, captures the corneal image, digitizes it, analyzes it, and provides a printout (B) of the corneal curvature in various colors representing either the radii of curvature or the dioptric powers of the multiple corneal segments. (Copyright Taunton Technologies, Inc.)

beams through a telecentric stop onto a video camera. When the eye is aligned properly, as indicated by the Alignment Subsystem, the operator commands the signal from the camera to be saved. The stored image is analyzed to determine the optical power distribution over the corneal surface. To ensure accuracy of the measurements, the keratoscope incorporates a self-calibration capability. Tests of this instrument indicate repeatability of average power over the sampled area of the order of 0.15 D and accuracy of approximately 0.5 D at each point within a 7-mm diameter area on human eyes.

Phototherapeutic or Photorefractive Keratectomy Procedures

1. At the present time, the various ocular diseases evaluated with excimer laser PTK or PRK are those with corneal opacification and surface irregularities resulting from anterior corneal dystrophies, Salzman's nodular degeneration, spheroidal degeneration, band keratopathy, postinfectious and posttraumatic scars, corneal smoothing following pterygium removal, and the debulking of bacterial and fungal ulcers of the anterior cornea. In most trials in the United States, the patients must be 18 years of age or over and capable of being evaluated by the treating institution. Usually only one eye is treated during the course of the investigative trial. The conditions that would exclude an individual from participating in an excimer laser lamellar keratectomy trial would be pregnancy, an ocular or systemic disease that would influence corneal healing, eyes with extremely thin corneas initially, moderately severe degrees of scars in the posterior stroma, diffuse corneal edema, Fuch's dystrophy, active corneal neovascularization, eyes with uncontrolled glaucoma, blepharitis, uncontrolled iritis or severe keratitis sicca, and those patients who suffer from any degree of immunosuppression.

2. The usual tests during the preoperative period include manifest cycloplegic refraction, pachymetry, slit-lamp examination and photography, specular microscopy, contrast sensitivity, digital keratoscopy, and an otherwise full ophthalmic examination.

3. Prior to the actual excimer laser procedure, patients may be treated with 5 mg Valium orally as a form of preoperative sedation. Electrocardiograph monitoring is usually used, and an anesthesiologist is usually present. A simple chemical antibacterial preparation of the lid is performed, and a topical anesthetic is usually applied to the conjunctiva. A plastic drape over the eye to be treated can be used, and in many cases, the plastic drape extends over the other eye to protect it from any stray radiation.

4. The patient's eye is viewed binocularly through an optical microscope system and positioned so that the central portion of the cornea to be recontoured is aligned to the laser beam axis. The eye is stabilized with a vacuum ring that gently holds the eye in an upright position while the patient is supine. Although fixation of the globe need only be maintained for a few minutes, it is absolutely necessary that the optics of the laser and the eye be perfectly aligned throughout the procedure. Anesthesia of the cornea and anesthesia and akinesia of extraocular muscles are produced by a retrobulbar or peribulbar injection of 2% lidocaine with Wydase added. Care is taken not to inflate the conjunctival area with excessive amounts of lidocaine because the vacuum ring could become less securely attached to the limbal area due to the distorted conjunctiva.

5. The effluent removal apparatus is placed within 2 cm of the eye and turned on. The actual excisional superficial keratectomy or recontouring corneal procedure is performed in a very meticulous manner. Once the eye has been stabilized by the vacuum eye fixation device, the epithelium is then gently removed with a #57 "hockey stick"

Beaver blade to a distance approximately 1 mm outside of the proposed impact site, thereby creating a denuded area 5 to 8 mm in diameter depending on the intended keratectomy zone size. When all fragments of the epithelium have been removed from Bowman's membrane, the eye is aligned to the laser beam axis as represented by a crosshair reticle in the binocular microscope. Once aligned, photoablation starts immediately, at a repetition rate of approximately 10 Hz and with a pulsed energy of 80 to 200 mJ/cm^2 at the cornea. The procedure requires 35 to 45 sec to create an ablation to a depth of 30 to 40 μm in the anterior stroma of the patient's eye.

6. The patient is then examined under the microscope or slit lamp to determine the amount of residual scar. The patient can then be retreated with the appropriate recipe until the satisfactory amount of corneal opacification is removed in the course of a PTK. If the patient's opacification is irregular, it has been shown that the use of 2.5% methylcellulose can be helpful because this viscous liquid ablates at a slower rate than corneal tissue. As the 2.5% methylcellulose spreads over the irregular surface of the scarred cornea, a more suitable surface for corneal ablation is produced. In most cases, the impact site is photographed immediately after exposure and a balanced salt solution is then placed on the ablated area, erythromycin ointment is placed in the conjunctival cul-de-sac, and the upper eyelid is drawn down over the cornea and taped to the lower eyelid. An eye pad is placed over the eye, and the procedure is considered complete at that point.

7. The postoperative regimen as proposed by Sher and Lindstrom (personal communication, 1990) seems appropriate at the present time. They have found that some patients have severe pain, which can be relieved by the use of analgesics such as Percodan or Tylenol #3 orally, when necessary. They have found that a disposable Accuvue soft contact lens can be placed on the eye after the procedure for comfort, and that a combination of fluorometholone (FML), Tobrex, and 5% homatropine should also be used. They continue the FML in decreasing amounts over a period of approximately 4 to 5 months, although the Tobrex and the contact lens can be discontinued when the epithelium has healed, as seen by slit-lamp examination. The preliminary results of Sher and Lindstrom were impressive particularly with the therapeutic patients in which healing proceeded in a relatively normal fashion after the removal of the scarred tissue. They did notice that hyperopic shifts after scar removal were a significant problem, although a "unity recipe" that used a correction for the induced hyperopia seemed to be a solution, although this particular procedure needed refinement. If the patients were myopic, and required removal of scarred tissue, the resulting less myopia and removal of scar tissue seemed most ideal. They also concluded that the excimer laser did not induce significant corneal haze or opacification, perhaps because of the use of cortico-steroids, which may have minimized the corneal haze formation. The removal of irregular astigmatism and some corneal surface irregularities have posed a significant problem, and the solution is still ellusive, although the excimer laser may well solve these particular problems as more intensive research continues.

Clinical Results

Clinical results of the first series of patients treated by lamellar keratectomy showed:

1. There was an increased amount of corneal scattering due to minimal haze at the stromal-epithelial interface and that this haze appeared to heighten at 3 to 6 weeks and then disappeared over a period of 3 to 6 months. The severity of the haze appeared to be related somewhat to the depth of the laser ablation (Fig. 2.14).

2. The epithelium tended to become thicker than normal during the first 1 to 2 months, but this normalized in the range of 4 to 6 months after the initial laser irradiation. The epithelial increase in thickness did not appear to significantly decrease the overall power change.

3. A regression of the dioptric power change occurred during a 4 to 6 month interval after treatment, which appeared to be minimal although variable from eye to eye.

4. No significant effects were noted in the posterior portion of the stroma, Descemet's membrane, or the endothelium.

Histopathologic Results

The corneal tissue that has undergone histopathologic examination has shown variable changes at intervals following the irradiation of the cornea. These tissues were studied by light, scanning, and transmission electron microscopy, and the following histopathologic events have been shown to occur during the healing process.

1. The epithelial layer consists of normal, although elongated, cells with normal hemidesmosomes, and the entire layer was observed to be hyperplastic during the first several months after treatment (Figs. 2.15 through 2.17).

2. There was an attempt within the first 2 to 3 weeks to form a basement membrane beneath the epithelium and this membrane became more defined with the passage of time, with apparent secure attachment of the overlying epithelial cells to it (Figs. 2.18 through 2.20).

3. The stromal zone beneath the stromal-epithelial interface contained vacuoles and was noted to have an increase in keratocytes as well as an increase in keratocytic activity. The active keratocytes were concentrated in an area just beneath the stromal-epithelial interface, and this particular keratocyte activity could not be seen in the deeper layers of the stroma (Figs. 2.21 through 2.25).

4. There is some evidence in the later histopathologic studies at 4 months following irradiation that the stroma had regrown into the area of irradiation, and this was

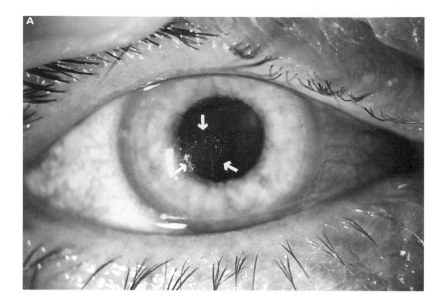

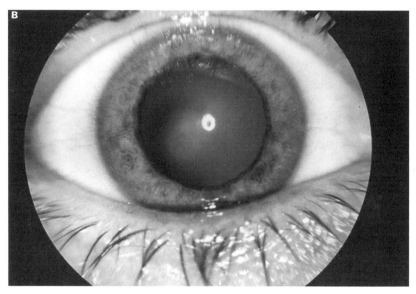

Fig. 2.14 Excimer laser keratectomy performed to a depth of approximately 40 μm from the surface of Bowman's membrane in a 4-mm excision area (*delimiting arrows*) as noted one day postsurgery (A), and 7 days following the laser treatment (B). (Reproduced by permission from L'Esperance FA Jr, et al. [11].)

thought to be consistent with the regression of the initial dioptric power change of the cornea in some eyes.

5. There is no evidence of any inflammation or other untoward event in any other areas of the cornea.

6. The deep stroma, Descemet's membrane, and endothelium underlying the zone of excimer laser irradiation were entirely normal histopathologically.

The use of ArF excimer laser irradiation to produce a superficial lamellar keratectomy has been successful in relatively long-term studies showing considerable corneal stability and clarity, although some discrepancies in corneal regression patterns still exist. The results of human studies (11–13) and animal studies (16,17,19,29,30) during the past several years have corroborated the original concept of removing a precise volume of tissue by UV radiation from the anterior cornea to be used to excise ab-

normal or opacified corneal tissue, or to correct various refractive errors by establishing a new radius of curvature of the anterior portion of the cornea. Phototherapeutic lamellar keratectomy involving the precise volumetric removal of anterior scarred corneal tissue by laser irradiation followed by photorefractive techniques to maximize the resulting visual acuity while minimizing the refractive error have been used in a two-step procedure. PRK involving the precise volumetric removal of anterior corneal tissue by laser irradiation to create a new anterior corneal curvature to correct refractive errors has also been successful with a relatively high degree of corrective precision and minimal regression.

The laser's interaction with the cornea seems to stimulate several tissue processes. One obvious response to excimer laser irradiation of the stroma is the ability of the

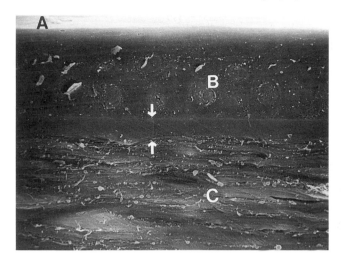

Fig. 2.15 Scanning electron microscopy of eye enucleated within 14 days of excimer laser treatment shows normal corneal architecture in a nonablated area. Note surface of epithelium (A), epithelial cells (B), delimitation of thickness of Bowman's membrane (*arrows*), and stromal lamellae (C). X600. (Copyright Taunton Technologies, Inc.)

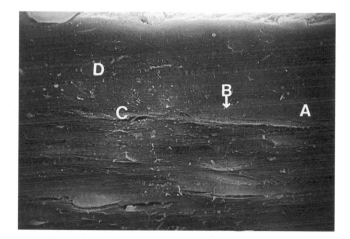

Fig. 2.16 Scanning electron microscopy, taken 12 days after laser keratectomy, shows presence (A), partial sloping ablation (B), and absence (C) of Bowman's membrane. In the ablation zone (C), the epithelium (D) is in direct contact with the irradiated (ablated) anterior stroma. X600. (Copyright Taunton Technologies, Inc.)

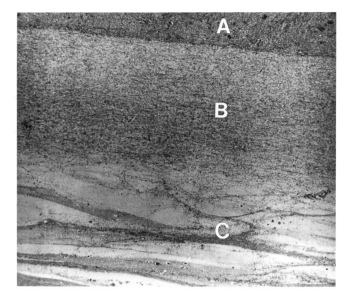

Fig. 2.17 Normal transmission electron microscopy of the non-irradiated portion of the cornea shows epithelium (A) above normal Bowman's membrane (B) and the normal stromal lamellae (C) below. X4000. (Copyright Taunton Technologies, Inc.)

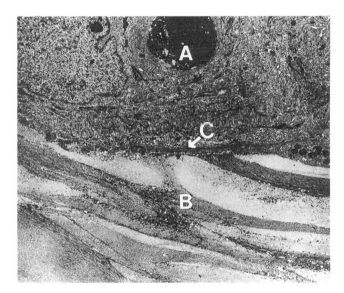

Fig. 2.18 Transmission electron microscopy, taken 3 days after laser keratectomy, shows a large epithelial cell (A) in direct apposition to the corneal lamellae (B) in the ablation area, with a suggestion of a slightly electron-dense epithelial-stromal interface layer (C). X4000. (Copyright Taunton Technologies, Inc.)

keratocytes, after a 3- to 5-week latent inactive stage, to synthesize proteinaceous material, presumably collagen, into a tissue that remodels the laser-shaped corneal curvature, possibly into a new curvature. The mechanism of the remodeling, the degree of remodeling, the consistency and predictability of the remodeling from cornea to cornea, and the degree of regrowth of the surface tissue at various points within the ablated area must be accurately determined but are, as yet, poorly understood or unknown. The tissue regrowth, if not done uniformly across the ablated zone, may affect the dioptric power of the newly contoured cornea in such a way that a portion of the dioptric power, as originally profiled on the cornea by the excimer laser radiation, could be lost.

During the phase of apparent increased keratocyte activity (3 to 6 weeks following laser irradiation), a faint fibrillar haze developed at the epithelial-stromal interface. The haze usually increased in severity until 6 to 10 weeks

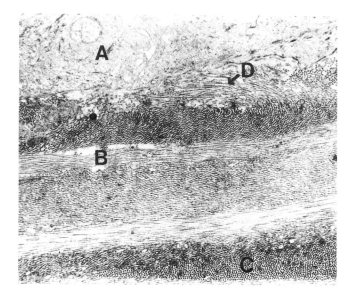

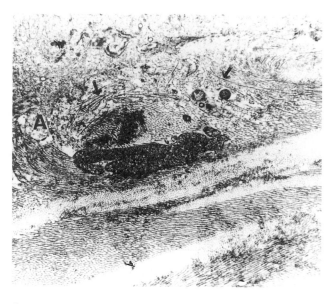

Fig. 2.19 Transmission electron microscopy of the epithelial-stromal interface (*arrows*) 7 days after laser keratectomy shows direct adhesion of the overlying epithelium (A) to the underlying ablated stroma (B). Note well-organized packets of collagen fibrils below (C) with disorganization and splaying of fibrils in the region of excimer laser impact (D), which is now covered by epithelium. X10,000. (Copyright Taunton Technologies, Inc.)

Fig. 2.20 Transmission electron microscopy of the epithelial-stromal interface 7 days after laser keratectomy shows more pronounced disorganization of the irradiated stromal surface, with wide splaying of the collagen fibrils (*arrows*) intertwined with the epithelium (A). X10,000. (Copyright Taunton Technologies, Inc.)

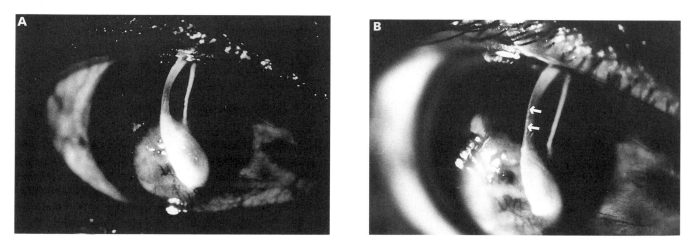

Fig. 2.21 Preoperative appearance of the right cornea (A) of a 46-year-old woman who had sustained a perforating injury in childhood. The appearance of the cornea 4 weeks after excimer laser ablation to the normal corneal area above the scar, with flattening of the cornea apparent in the treated area (B). Trace epithelial-stromal interface haze (*arrows*) can be observed by slit-lamp photography. The eye subsequently underwent corneal transplantation 4 months after the laser treatment, and the excised corneal button was evaluated histopathalogically. (Copyright Taunton Technologies, Inc.; courtesy of Daniel M. Taylor, MD, New Britain, CT.)

after irradiation, when it stabilized or became less apparent. This increase in clarity and decrease in fibrillar haze may coincide with a decrease in keratocytic activity that was seen on some of the 4-month human sections. The interface-speckled haze may be due to the random collagen alignment, to irregular separation of the collagen fibrils, or to a combination of vacuolization and protein deposition that could produce various degrees of light scatter-ing. It is unknown whether the keratocytes and their initial activity during the first few months after the laser treatment are the key cells that must be controlled. Pharmacologic agents may be capable of interacting early in the course of the keratocyte activity to ameliorate or control the activity. For both the phototherapeutic lamellar keratectomy and the photorefractive lamellar keratectomy, it is essential that the speckled haze be minimized

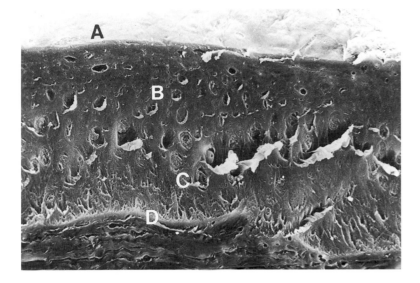

Fig. 2.22 After corneal transplantation, 4 months after laser keratectomy, the excised corneal button shows the surface of the epithelium (A), more numerous than normal structurally intact superficial epithelial cells (B), elongated basal epithelial cells (C) that contribute to the increased thickness of the epithelium is lying in apposition (D) to the stromal layers, without evidence of Bowman's membrane. X750. (Copyright Taunton Technologies, Inc.)

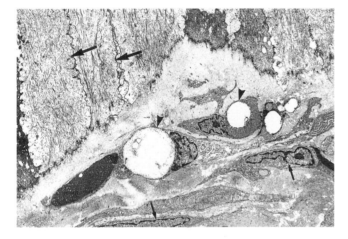

Fig. 2.23 Transmission electron microscopy from the corneal button taken from same patient as in Fig. 2.21 shows the periphery (*right edge*) of the portion that underwent excimer laser keratectomy, resulting in considerable cellular debris and fibroblastic activity. Bowman's layer is absent. Arrows indicate numerous extremely elongated basal epithelial cells, an increased number of spindle-shaped fibroblasts (*arrows*) in the subepithelial tissue, and numerous vacuoles within cells and outside cells (*arrowheads*). X2500. (Copyright Taunton Technologies, Inc.)

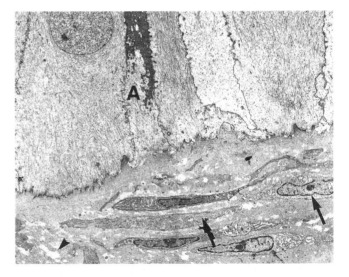

Fig. 2.24 Transmission electron microscopy of central ablated cornea in same patient as in Fig. 2.21, taken 4 months after laser keratectomy. There are numerous elongated basal epithelial cells (A). Arrows indicate an increased number of fibroblasts beneath the epithelium and an increased amount of extracellular electron-lucent materials (*arrowhead*). X10,000. (Copyright Taunton Technologies, Inc.)

or eradicated and the remodeling of the cornea be eliminated or at least maintained at a consistent and predictable level.

The basic properties of tissue photoablative decomposition that are fundamental to this type of investigational surgery were demonstrated in eye bank eyes, in animals, histopathologically and, later, in human beings. The limited penetration of the cornea by UV radiation at 193 nm (1.0 to 3.0 μm) can restrict the photoablative effect of each laser pulse to a superficial layer (0.2 to 0.5 μm), with only a narrow zone of conduction damage (0.2 to 0.3 μm) re-

sulting in the adjacent tissues (16). In this regard, the amount of tissue removed per laser pulse is energy dependent once the ablation threshold has been reached (31). Therefore, it is possible to remove predictable increments of tissue from the target surface. This delicate removal of the tissue surface by controlled photoablation creates an exceptionally smooth surface, leaving a suitable substrate for optimal regrowth of the overlying epithelium.

Ultraviolet radiation is capable of ablating biologic tissue with minimal damage to surrounding tissue because of its high absorption by organic molecules and limited

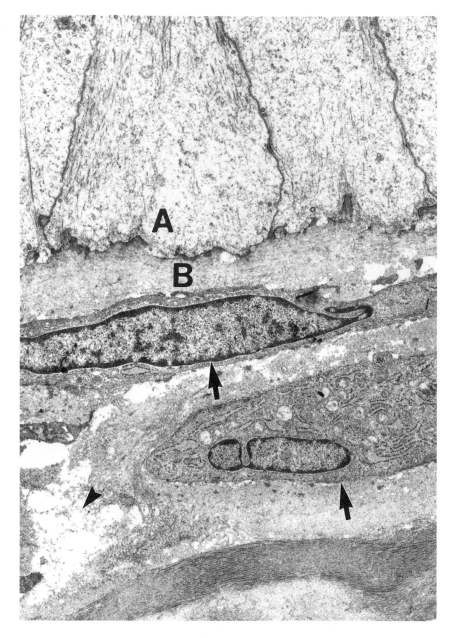

Fig. 2.25 Transmission electron microscopy of the central portion of the laser keratectomy region in same patient as in Fig. 2.21 (taken 4 months after laser keratectomy) shows the corneal epithelium (A) adhering to the underlying stroma (B). High magnification of two active fibroblasts with prominent endoplasmic reticulum and dense staining is noted by the arrows. Arrowheads indicate much electron-lucent material in the extracellular spaces. X10,000. (Copyright Taunton Technologies, Inc.)

penetration. The ablation process is believed to be a photodecomposition of peptide molecular bonds (29,32). Each photon of emitted UV irradiation, at 193 nm, is highly energized, at 6.4 eV, and is easily capable of cleaving the peptide and carbon-to-carbon intramolecular bonds that are held together by a binding energy of approximately 3.4 eV (32). Most investigators (17,29) have documented that the optimal UV wavelength for laser ablation is 193 nm. Longer wavelengths (248 nm, 308 nm) within the UV range have higher penetration, resulting in unwanted destruction of surrounding tissue, in part due to thermal effects. In addition, these longer wavelengths are similar to some solar UV wavelengths known to be mutagenic or carcinogenic.

During photoablative corneal surgery, the ArF excimer laser creates an ablation area that is uniquely smooth with little or no effect, thermal or otherwise, on adjacent tissues (17,19,21,29,33,34). The initial application of the excimer laser to create superficial lamellar keratectomies in human corneas has been shown to be effective, but the long-term corneal stability and clarity and the basic corneal pathophysiologic reactions to excimer laser irradiation are still being evaluated.

Phototherapeutic Keratectomy

Lamellar Keratectomy and Keratoplasty

Lamellar keratectomy and keratoplasty are performed for optical, therapeutic, or tectonic purposes. Optical indications for lamellar surgical techniques include central opacification and surface irregularities resulting from anterior corneal dystrophies, Salzmann's nodular degeneration, spheroid degeneration, posttraumatic scars, and postinfectious leukomas (35–38). Therapeutic lamellar keratectomy with or without a lamellar graft is useful in the management of pterygium, squamous cell carcinoma, epithelioma, and Mooren's ulcer (35–37). In fungal keratitis unresponsive to medical therapy, lamellar keratectomy can be helpful as a debulking procedure to remove fungal plaques or infiltrates, allowing for deeper penetration of topical antimycotic medications (39). Lamellar keratoplasty usually is contraindicated in corneal infections because the extent of corneal involvement is difficult to ascertain and a lamellar graft could prevent adequate penetration of topical antimicrobial therapy for eradication of underlying residual organisms (39). Tectonic lamellar grafts are used to repair areas of corneal thinning or peripheral corneal perforations (35–37).

Lamellar keratoplasty has been used with decreasing frequency over the past few decades because meticulous stromal dissection is required to prevent irregularities and scarring (35–38). Even when corneal disease does not involve the endothelium, penetrating keratoplasty often is performed instead of lamellar keratoplasty because many surgeons attain better visual results with the former procedure (36–38,40). Lamellar keratectomy and keratoplasty generally are performed using traditional techniques consisting of partial-thickness mechanical trephination and stromal lamellar dissection with a blade or spatula. Control of dissection can be challenging in heavily scarred, necrotic, or vascularized corneas. In skilled hands, an electromechanical microkeratome allows for a smoother, more regular keratectomy surface (38,41). However, loss of suction or imperfect positioning of the microkeratome or perilimbal suction ring results in an irregular keratectomy and possible corneal perforation. Moreover, the mi-

crokeratome follows the irregularity of an astigmatic corneal contour and, in such cases, causes the keratectomy surface to be astigmatic (38).

Historical Aspects

In 1984, Serdarevic and associates were the first to apply the ArF excimer laser for therapeutic lamellar keratectomy. They chose an experimental fungal keratitis model to evaluate the potential of the excimer laser for creating a precise, controlled lamellar keratectomy in an inflamed, necrotic cornea. Rabbit corneas with *Candida albicans* fungal lesions 2 to 5 mm in diameter were irradiated with the excimer laser at energy densities varying from 300 to 330 mJ/cm^2. Both ArF and KrF laser outputs were evaluated at pulse rates of 10 and 20 Hz, respectively. The laser beam was focused through circular slits and masks, and the exposure time ranged from 30 to 90 sec, depending on the depth (between one half to nearly full thickness of the cornea) required to remove all clinically visible infiltration (Fig. 2.26). The ArF excimer laser was effective, probably because infected tissue was removed totally by photochemical ablation. The precise lamellar keratectomy obtained with the ArF excimer laser was shown to heal with minimal scarring that became less visible with time, so that the cornea was almost completely clear after 4 months (Fig. 2.27).

The fact that the cornea healed without surface irregularities and with almost no scarring after ArF excimer laser deep lamellar keratectomy for fungal keratitis led to intensive investigation of this unique lamellar procedure for therapeutic and refractive indications. Ultrastructural studies in eye bank eyes confirmed the smoothness of the ArF excimer laser keratectomy beds that had irregularities of less than 1 μm as compared with the rough undu-

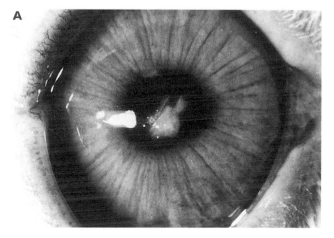
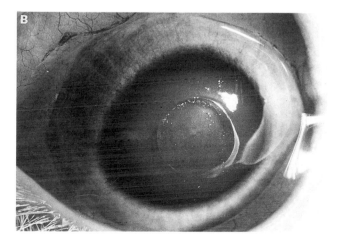

Fig. 2.26 A, *Candida albicans* keratitis 2 days after inoculation. B, Cornea immediately after treatment with ArF excimer laser. (Reproduced by permission from Serdarevic ON et al. [97]. Published with permission from The American Journal of Ophthalmology. Copyright by the American Ophthalmic Publishing Company.)

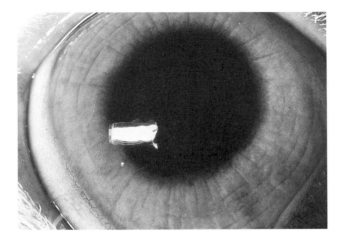

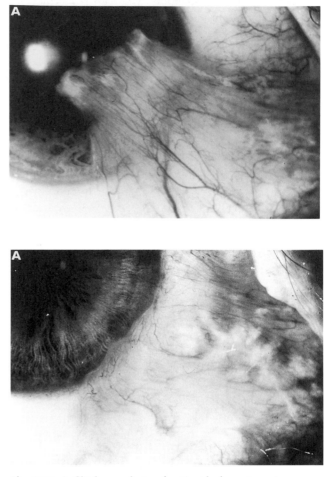

Fig. 2.27 Rabbit cornea that is almost transparent 4 months after treatment with an ArF excimer laser for fungal keratitis. (Reproduced by permission from Serdarevic ON et al. Am J Ophthalmol 1985;99:534–538. Published with permission from The American Journal of Ophthalmology. Copyright by The Ophthalmic Publishing Company.)

Fig. 2.28 A, Slit-lamp photo of patient before pterygium removal. B, Slit-lamp photo of same patient following excimer laser corneal smoothing. (Courtesy of Theo Seiler, MD.)

lations greater than 10 μm observed in the uneven and distorted keratectomy beds obtained by freehand dissection (42). No significant endothelial damage occurred when corneal ablations were performed more than 40 μm away from Descemet's membrane (29). Wound-healing studies in nonhuman primates demonstrated that, despite the ablation of Bowman's membrane, smooth epithelial resurfacing of the keratectomy bed occurred with the production of normal-appearing epithelial attachment complexes (29). There was minimal alteration of the anterior corneal stroma at low fluences; superficial stromal vacuoles containing remnants of degenerating collagen fibers were observed within and between lamellae extending 10 to 15 μm beneath the basal membrane of epithelial cells in the keratectomy beds. Stromal reorganization and eventual disappearance of the vacuoles were noted during the healing process. Recent experimental studies have shown the excimer laser to be effective in killing bacteria in culture (43) and suggest that the excimer laser may have a role in the treatment of the most challenging organisms in bacterial microbial keratitis. However, Stark and associates (44) demonstrated the possibility of inadequate elimination of organisms despite a clear postlaser clinical appearance and the risk of laser-associated perforation in infected corneas.

Seiler in Germany performed the first ArF excimer laser therapeutic keratectomy in patient in 1986 (Fig. 2.28). He smoothed the corneal surface after pterygium excision by irradiating through an appropriate size slit in a polymethylmethacrylate mask that was held in place over the eye by a suction ring. A thin layer of viscous fluid was applied to fill the corneal "valleys" and allow the laser beam to progressively ablate the corneal "peaks" to the level of the liquid until a smooth surface was obtained.

Indications

Clinical studies of PTK commenced in the United States in 1989 and are being monitored by the Food and Drug Administration. On the basis of studies to date, it seems feasible to use the excimer laser for lamellar keratectomy at least for all indications for which conventional surgical keratectomy is performed presently. Nevertheless, this laser's exact clinical role remains to be determined. Better and more predictable visual results would expand the application of lamellar keratectomy in cases of anterior corneal disease where penetrating keratoplasty is performed currently, so that the higher rejection rate of penetrating keratoplasty and the complications of intraocular surgery could be avoided. Stark and coworkers have predicted that PTK may delay or prevent the need for conventional penetrating keratoplasty in 10% of cases (44).

Phototherapeutic keratectomy has been performed in patients with anterior corneal degenerations and dystrophies, recurrent erosions, superficial corneal scarring, corneal neoplasia, and corneal infection. Excimer laser removal of as much as 300 μm in depth of stromal tissue has been accomplished without grafting, but most therapeutic keratectomies have been performed with excision of less than one third of the corneal depth.

Operative Technique

The fluence and repetition rates depend on the type of ArF excimer laser used and vary from 100 to 500 mJ/cm² and 5 to 20 Hz, respectively. Determination of ablation zone diameter is based on the area of corneal pathology and the type of laser used. Fluence and beam homogeneity are monitored before each laser treatment. The computer is programmed for the desired ablation diameter and depth; the laser then is calibrated for these settings. Before laser treatment, 1% pilocarpine may be applied to constrict the pupil. The iris shields the lens from possible UV-B exposure from secondary radiation. Topical anesthetic drops with or without retrobulbar or peribulbar injections and sedation are administered; a speculum is inserted between the lids. Fixation is maintained by the patient or with a limbal suction device.

Smoothing of the Anterior Corneal Surface

Mechanical debulking of large surface irregularities, such as elevated scars in Salzmann's nodular degeneration and pterygia, is beneficial prior to laser therapeutic keratectomy. Cautery of potential bleeding sites must be performed because any blood on the surface could preclude adequate corneal absorption of laser radiation. The epithelium can be abraded with a knife or spatula prior to laser treatment, but some investigators believe that laser ablation of the epithelium enhances surface smoothing effects (45). Stark and colleagues have reported that in patients with Reis-Buckler's dystrophy, for example, laser ablation of the epithelium results in a very smooth surface, whereas mechanical abrasion of the epithelium prior to laser keratectomy results in "golf ball-like" surfaces (45). When the anterior surface is irregular, a viscous fluid, such as 1% methylcellulose diluted with saline solution, is placed on the cornea to mask underlying tissue while protruding irregularities are ablated. Experimental studies have demonstrated that corneas treated with 0.3% hydroxypropylmethylcellulose 2910 and 0.1% dextran 70 have fewer surface irregularities on scanning electron microscopic examination than corneas treated with 1% carboxymethylcellulose and 0.9% saline. The viscous fluid is applied drop by drop on moistened Weck-cel sponges and reapplied after every few laser pulses until the surface is smooth.

Removal of Corneal Opacities

Determination of the depth of corneal opacification is accomplished with an optical pachymeter prior to laser treatment (46; Fig. 2.29). The corneal thickness of the area to be ablated is measured with an ultrasonic pachymeter to prevent perforation during laser treatment. If the depth of opacification is less than one third of the corneal thickness, the computer is set for a depth slightly greater than that measured. If the depth of opacification is greater than one third of the corneal depth, the degree of opacification of the posterior two thirds of the cornea is assessed; laser ablation of the anterior one third is indicated if the opacification is substantially less dense in the posterior two thirds than the anterior one third so as to allow an improvement in visual function and prevent or delay more invasive surgery. The laser ablation rate is set at 0.2 to 0.3 μm per pulse depending on the stromal ablation rate for the laser used. However, because of the unequal density of scar tissue, ablation rates of opacified tissue will be variable and calculations will be less precise than those for normal stromal tissue.

Treatment of Recurrent Erosions

Recurrent erosions that are unresponsive to lubrication and hypertonic salt solutions and involve reduplications of basement membrane may be treated by laser ablation of the epithelium and basement membrane. Because the total thickness of the basement membrane is about 4 μm, only about 15 pulses are necessary to complete ablation.

Treatment of Corneal Infections

Laser treatment of corneal infections may be indicated in cases unresponsive to medical treatment. The depth of the corneal ulcer is ascertained with the slit lamp and, if possible, with an optical pachymeter. The laser also may be used to debulk fungal plaques and allow penetration of medications into deeper tissue. Very deep infections in necrotic tissue should not be photoablated because of the increased risk of perforation.

Postoperative Management

The cornea is irrigated immediately after lasing to remove any debris. Topical or subconjunctival antibiotics and steroids are applied. The optimal postoperative medication regimen to facilitate reepithelialization and to minimize haze formation has not yet been determined. The eye may be pressure patched for a few days until reepithelialization. Alternatively, a bandage contact lens or collagen shield soaked in antibiotics may be placed on the cornea. Topical steroids may be administered for up to several months postoperatively to decrease corneal remodeling.

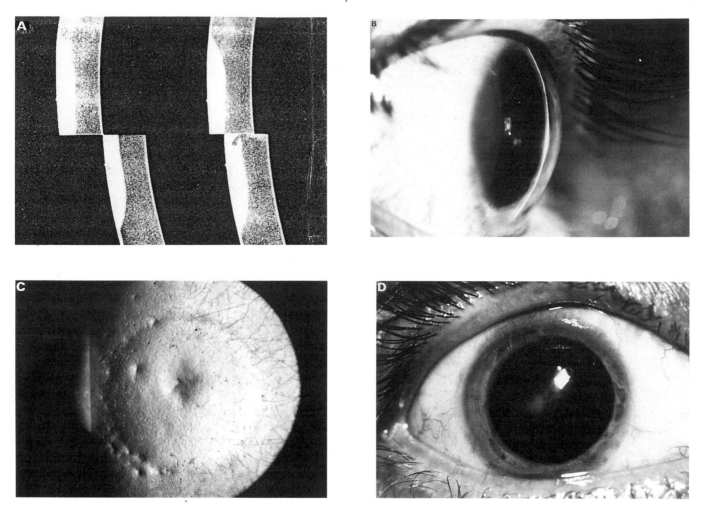

Fig. 2.29 A, (*Left*) Pachymetry of corneal thickness by alignment of upper field endothelium with epithelium of the lower field. (*Right*) Pachymetry of anterior corneal scar aligning the posterior extent of the lesion with the epithelium of the lower field. B and C, Preoperative appearance of the cornea with lattice dystrophy. Preoperative best corrected visual acuity was 20/300. Measured depth of more opaque corneal opacity was 120 μm including the epithelium. D, Postoperative appearance of same eye after excimer laser photoablation to a depth of 125 μm. Diameter of ablated area is 5.5 mm. The majority of opacity has been removed. Posttreatment best corrected visual acuity improved to 20/30. (Reproduced by permission from Stark WJ et al. [46].)

Complications

Possible complications include infectious keratitis, endophthalmitis, intraoperative or postoperative corneal perforations, and cataract formation, but none of these have been reported to date. Corneal ectasia is another possible complication, but probably will not occur when less than one third of the corneal thickness is removed. Corneal scarring with fine reticular haze formation has been noted (Fig. 2.30) by all investigators but does not interfere significantly with the improvement in visual function observed in many patients (44,45,47–49). Recurrence and progression of corneal dystrophies have been reported, particularly in cases where the area of corneal involvement extends beyond the depth of laser treatment (45). Most patients heal with no epithelial abnormalities. Zabel, though, has reported some cases of slow epithelial healing after deep PTKs (47). Complications following treatment of recurrent erosions have not been reported. However, it is not yet known whether excimer laser treatment of recurrent erosions offers substantial improvement over mechanical keratectomies for erosions associated with basement membrane dystrophies or multiple puncture techniques for traumatic and idiopathic erosions. Not enough patients have been followed for extended time periods to determine whether laser smoothing of the surface after pterygium removal prevents pterygium recurrence. Sher and coworkers have reported that irregular astigmatism persists in some patients with corneal scars even after PTK (48). Devices to accurately measure irregular astigmatism have not yet been developed; postlaser irregular astigmatism may be predicated on preexisting irregularities but probably is different and related to variable ablation rates of scar tissue and to ablation techniques with various surfacing agents. The most frequent complication following

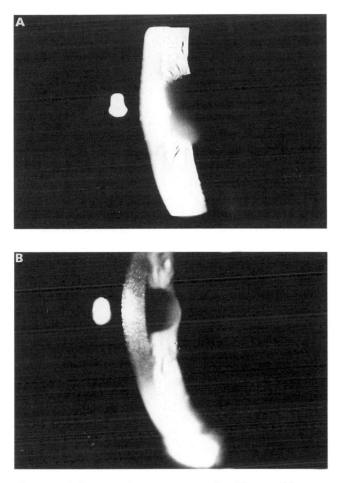

Fig. 2.30 A, Preoperative appearance of an 85-year-old man with a central corneal scar from infectious keratitis. B, Six weeks postoperatively. Note decreased haze. Vision did not improve due to preexisting optic atrophy. (Courtesy of Neal Sher, MD, Arch Ophthalmol, 1991;109(4):491–498.)

PTK keratectomy is hyperopia in nonmyopic patients (44, 45,47–49). However, it is hoped that, with changes in ablation algorithms and techniques, the tremendous advantage of using the laser to perform simultaneous therapeutic and refractive lamellar keratectomies with predictability and stability will be realized.

Penetrating Keratoplasty

Astigmatism is a significant problem after penetrating keratoplasty. Although corneal surgeons are becoming increasingly successful in maintaining clear grafts, high and irregular astigmatism precludes satisfactory visual acuity in up to 10% of postkeratoplasty patients (50). Despite advances in mechanical trephine design and suturing techniques, mean postoperative astigmatism is reported to be between 3 and 5 D in large keratoplasty series after suture removal (50–56). Imprecise trephination is considered a major factor in postkeratoplasty astigmatism (50,52,53,57–59). Currently available mechanical

trephines cause varying amounts of disparity between donor button and recipient wound configuration (60,61). This disparity results from irregular cutting, corneal topographic distortion, and poor centration.

Historical Aspects

In 1987 Serdarevic and collaborators first evaluated the potential of the excimer laser for improving corneal trephination (62,63). Using a delivery system with rotating curvilinear slits that projected a hollow circular beam onto the cornea (Fig. 2.31), they achieved noncontact corneal trephination that was distinctly more precise than that obtainable by mechanical devices. Depending on the thickness of the cornea and the stability of the eye, the exposure time until perforation in one area (with the rest of the cornea trephined down to Descemet's membrane) varied from 30 sec to a few minutes when the fluence was 110 mJ/cm^2. Pulse energies at the cornea were between 4 and 6.6 mJ, and repetition rates were 15 and 20 Hz. The trephination diameter could be varied from 4 to 8 mm, depending on the distance of the cornea from the spherical lens. Complete visualization during trephination allowed for perfect centration with the helium-neon (HeNe) aiming beam. On microscopic examination (Fig. 2.32), the excimer laser created a much more sharply defined, regularly cut edge in eye bank eyes and in animal eyes in vivo than even the Hanna suction trephine, which is reported to create the most regular mechanical trephination (53,64). Thinner trephination sections were possible with less disruption of tissue when the corneas were trephined with the laser rather than manually. Irradiated incisions as thin as 10 μm were possible, but eye movements sometimes led to wider sections. There was minimal alteration of surrounding tissue; deposition of electron-dense material was sometimes

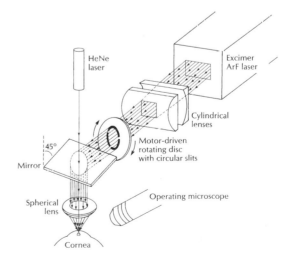

Fig. 2.31 Schematic diagram of the rotating-slit delivery system for ArF excimer laser corneal trephination. (Reproduced by permission from Serdarevic ON et al. [62].)

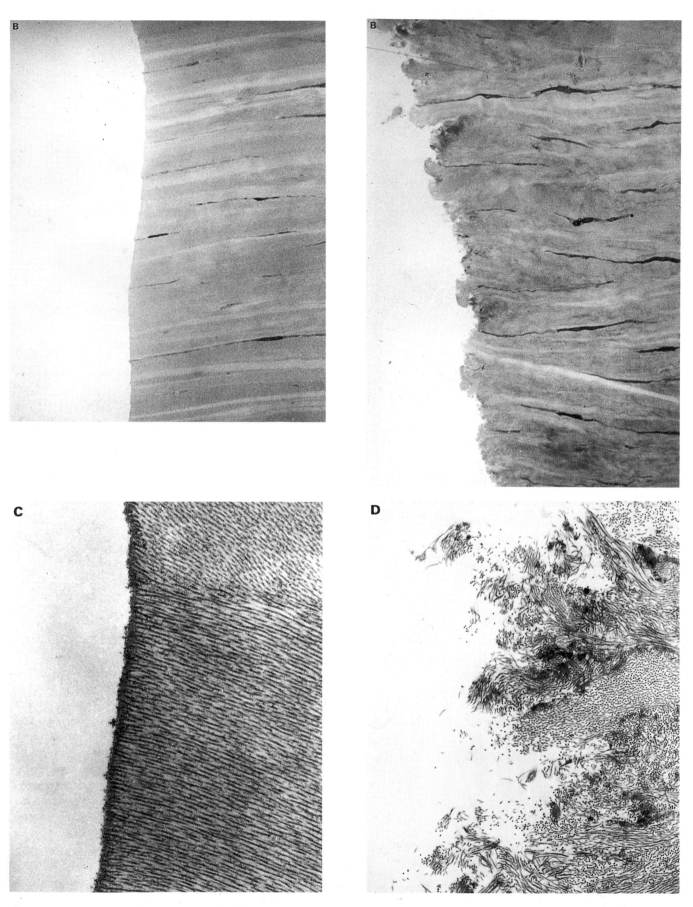

Fig. 2.32 Light micrographs of the corneal stromal edge in human eye bank eyes after trephination with an ArF excimer laser (A) and a Hanna suction trephine (B). Note the more regularly cut edge obtained with the laser. Toluidine blue; X40. C, Transmission electron micrograph of human corneal stroma after ArF excimer laser trephination. The normal structure of stromal collagen is preserved. X18,800. D, Transmission electron micrograph of human corneal stroma after manual trephination. There is significant disruption of stromal lamellae. X12,000. (Reproduced by permission from Serdarevic ON et al. [62].)

evident at the wound edges in an area of only 0.02 to 0.08 μm wide. Scanning electron microscopic examination demonstrated less endothelial cell loss and damage at the edge of Descemet's membrane after excimer laser trephination than after manual trephination. On morphologic examination at 6 hours to 3 months after penetrating keratoplasty in an animal autograft model, there was no evidence of any latency or adverse alteration of wound healing processes, including cellular migration, proliferation, and production of new tissue. In 1989, Lang and associates developed an open mask system for circular and elliptical corneal trephination (65). A metal mask with a large central opening was attached with suction to the globe and a large laser spot was rotated around the edge of the opening. In that same year, Lang and associates performed the first excimer laser corneal trephination in patients using a modified delivery system without suction (65; Fig. 2.33).

Operative Technique

Before trephination of the recipient cornea, 1% pilocarpine may be applied to constrict the pupil and shield the lens from secondary radiation. A thin, elliptical metal mask is centered on the cornea of the donor globe. The excimer laser spot beam is positioned on the outer edge of the mask, half on the mask and half on the cornea. The beam then is directed manually 360° along the edge of the mask until perforation occurs. The recipient mask designed to create an opening of the same size or a 0.1-mm smaller opening (7.0/8.0 mm recipient bed for a 7.1/8.1 mm donor button) is centered on the patient's cornea. The excimer beam then is positioned on the inner edge of the mask, half on the mask and half on the cornea. The beam is directed around the edge of the mask until aqueous appears. Both the donor and recipient corneas must be dried with Weck-cel sponges before lasing because fluid on the

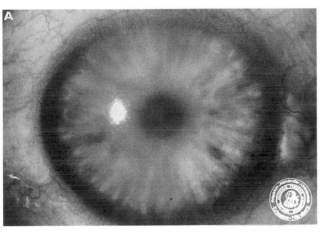
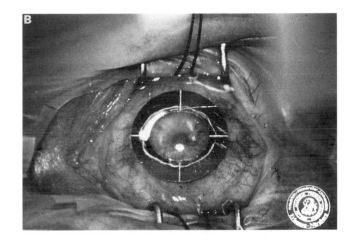

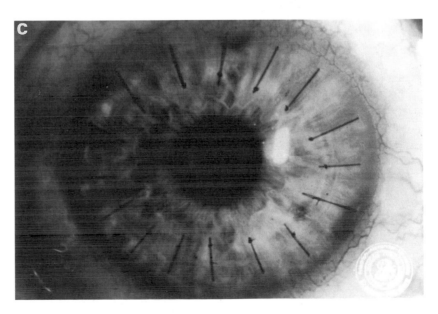

Fig. 2.33 Elliptical corneal transplantation with an excimer laser in a 63-year-old white man. A, Preoperative status: posttraumatic bullous keratopathy with diffuse corneal scarring. Best corrected visual acuity was 20/200 and keratometry readings were 41.00 × 42.00 at the 0° axis. B, The open mask for the recipient trephination is well centered to the pupil. The excimer laser beam (*arrow*) is positioned half on the mask and half on the cornea and is directed by hand along the mask until perforation occurs. C, Six months after elliptical excimer laser keratoplasty (7.0/8.0 mm for the corneal graft). Sixteen interrupted 10-0 nylon sutures were put in place with knots buried in the crystal-clear graft. Best corrected visual acuity was 20/30 and keratometry readings were 42.25 × 44.00 at the 160° axis. (Reproduced by permission from Lang GK et al. Arch Ophthalmol 1990; 108:914–915.)

cornea will absorb laser radiation and prevent adequate laser penetration by the cornea.

Complications

No complications have been reported to date, but only about 10 patients have undergone excimer laser corneal trephination and there has been only a year of follow-up of the first patients. Damage to intraocular structures during trephination is less likely than with manual techniques, because after corneal perforation, the aqueous absorbs the laser radiation. Secondary radiation may cause some UV-B radiation to be absorbed by the lens if it is not shielded by the iris. It is not yet known whether the theoretical advantage of improving trephination precision actually translates into clinically significant reductions in astigmatism. According to Lang and associates, elliptical trephination should decrease postoperative astigmatism because the donor button should fit snugly into the recipient bed and less torsion should occur than with the circular buttons (65). Although evaluation of existing mechanical trephination systems has confirmed that the donor and recipient corneas should be cut at the same angle from the epithelial surface to the endothelial surface to obtain the best approximation of donor button and recipient bed shape and size (60), the ideal cutting direction for laser trephination has not yet been determined. A tighter closure might be achieved by making the cut divergent. This may be desirable to prevent wound leak because the edges are much smoother than those obtained with mechanical devices. The use of an axicon lens, a diverging prismatic lens that has been incorporated into carbon dioxide (66) and hydrogen fluoride (67) laser experimental trephination designs, would allow the cut to be convergent, thereby more closely approximating wound edges. However, differences in irradiation properties of the excimer laser compared to the infrared lasers increase the difficulty of successful incorporation of an axicon lens for excimer laser trephination. Simultaneous trephination of 360° of the whole cornea may be preferable to rotating a laser spot around the edge. Exposure time would be shorter and there would be less risk of corneal distortion by trephining one area before another. However, in corneas with areas of severe thinning, the rotation technique that allows "spot" treatment may be advantageous.

Trephination imprecision, although a major factor, is not the only one causing postkeratoplasty astigmatism. Recipient corneal disease affecting curvature, thickness, and elasticity is another factor. Advances in corneal imaging and modeling systems now offer the possibility for real-time analytic evaluation of corneal structure (68,69). Technologic developments using holographic interferometry will enable calculation of stress lines within the cornea (70,71). High-precision analysis of recipient corneal parameters would facilitate intraoperative determination of the ideal donor button shape and size to correct for preexisting astigmatism. A distinct advantage of laser versus mechanical trephination would be in allowing for precise, noncircular trephination of any shape to match these desired parameters.

If the objective of intraoperative correction of astigmatism were to be realized, the problems of suture-induced astigmatism and irregular wound healing would need to be addressed. Pharmacologic agents, such as epidermal growth factor, have been found to accelerate stromal wound healing in experimental models (72–77). These agents currently are being investigated for their ability to enable earlier suture removal and decrease wound healing variability. Ideally, they would be combined with a corneal adhesive (78) that would obviate the need for sutures and eliminate suture placement and tightening errors.

Large spherical errors may occur following penetrating keratoplasty, particularly after grafting for keratoconus or grafting combined with cataract extraction and intraocular lens implantation; excimer laser corneal profiling may prove to benefit these patients postoperatively (79).

Photorefractive Keratectomy

Lamellar Refractive Keratectomy and Keratoplasty

Although lamellar refractive surgery has been performed since the 1960s and has been modified with improved results over the past three decades, its clinical indications and acceptance remain limited because of variable visual results, slow visual rehabilitation, corneal complications, or technical difficulty (80–92). Autoplastic lamellar procedures in which the anterior portion of a patient's cornea is removed, reshaped, and then replaced in a corneal bed include keratomileusis (KM) and planar lamellar refractive keratoplasty (PLRK). Homoplastic lamellar procedures in which a donor cornea is reshaped and either sutured onto the front surface of the patient's deepithelialized or keratectomized cornea or placed intrastromally include KM, PLRK, keratophakia (KF), and epikeratophakia. In alloplastic lamellar KF, a synthetic lenticule is placed into an intrastromal pocket or between the patient's excised anterior cornea and keratectomized bed and modifies the cornea's refractive power either by altering the anterior corneal curvature, as in other lamellar procedures, or by increasing the stromal refractive index. Lamellar refractive surgery generally is indicated only for high myopia, high hyperopia, aphakia, and keratoconus. But, whenever possible, these conditions first are treated nonsurgically with spectacles or contact lenses or, in the case of aphakia, surgically with intraocular lenses (IOL). Lamellar refractive procedures require a high degree of accuracy in corneal carving. However, with current cryolathing technique, the ability to carve lenticules that result in the desired refraction in KM and KF is still not at the level of contact lenses or IOL. The accuracy usually is within ±2 D (86,89). There is about a 1-D change in refraction for every 10-μm change in thickness. In autoplastic procedures, intraoperative cryolathing can lead to lathing errors of the order of microns that cause greater inaccuracy or possible perforation of the lenticule, necessitating donor tissue. The microkeratome often produces too thin, too thick, or irregular sections, thus contributing to inaccuracy in dioptric power and producing irregular astigmatism and interface scarring (85–89,93).

Corneal freezing or lyophilization in KM, KF, and epikeratophakia induces fractures of Bowman's membrane, kills keratocytes, and alters collagen interfibrillar distance and fiber structure (80,81,82,84,90). This damage often results in slow visual recovery and corneal complications due to prolonged or incomplete healing. PLRK eliminates freeze-induced damage and the accuracy of this technique matches that of cryolathing, but with faster visual recovery. However, the retention of cellular viability in donor tissue may contribute to rejection.

Alloplastic lamellar procedures avoid the complications associated with donor tissue but are still investigational. Thin thermoplastic materials are easy to implant into an intrastromal pocket but are water impermeable and cause nutritional problems unless modified (94). Microfenestration of polysulfore lenses may allow for adequate nutrition and optically satisfactory results (95). Thicker hydrogel implants are highly water permeable but require a microkeratome resection for insertion and, because of their compressibility, may result in unpredictable results (94). Many new materials are being investigated for epikeratophakia lenticules. These lenticules are made from collagen, collagen-hydrogel polymers, coated hydrogels, bioactive synthetics, or gelatin. Biocompatibility remains a big problem. Many of these materials are unstable, incite host corneal tissue reaction, or lead to poor epithelial attachment. Suturing in these procedures can lead to twisting and bending of the lenticule. Bioengineered glues to fixate lenticules are under investigation (78).

Direct mechanical reshaping of the corneal surface to avoid problems related to donor and synthetic lenticules and lenticule attachment has been attempted but has not been pursued because of inadequate control of tissue removal with mechanical devices.

Laser Anterior Keratomileusis

Historical Aspects

In the course of their studies of PTKs, Serdarevic and collaborators (96) noted that the corneas healed with very little scarring and no epithelial resurfacing problems, indicating the possibility of performing these procedures not only for therapeutic indications, but also for refractive purposes. During further investigation of excimer laser

keratectomies, Marshall and collaborators (29) noted significant photokeratoscopic changes even after very shallow ablations and suggested correcting refractive errors by varying the energy distribution in the laser beam for precisely controlled removal of a thin layer of corneal tissue on a microtopographic basis.

In 1987, Renard and coworkers (97), Hanna and colleagues (98), and McDonald and collaborators (99), using enucleated human eyes (97,98) or rabbit eyes (99), were the first to report results of lamellar keratectomies for myopia correction using two different prototype excimer lasers. Both systems were designed to decrease central corneal curvature and thus to decrease central corneal refractive power by ablating more tissue centrally and progressively tapering the ablation to zero toward the edge. The amount and shape of tissue ablation required for correction of myopia has been determined on the basis of mathematical analyses (32; Fig. 2.34). Several types of laser delivery systems have been designed using progressively closing diaphragms, apertures on rotating discs, rotating slits, translating slits, scanning slits, ablatable masks, and gas cell filters. Pouliquen (100), Renard and coworkers (97), McDonald and colleagues (99), among others, have demonstrated in experimental models that, with the early prototype systems, epithelial hyperplasia and subepithelial keratocyte activation resulting in substantial subepithelial fibrosis occurred. To obtain more uniform ablation, research was directed toward creating the smoothest surface. As surface irregularities were diminished and as more gradual corneal curvature changes were produced, more corneas appeared clear and had excellent epithelial resurfacing and little fibrosis (100–104). Better understanding of the impact of beam homogeneity, fluence, total energy, energy orientation, and repetition rate on corneal ablation and wound healing led to better laser and delivery system designs (12,99,104,105). The

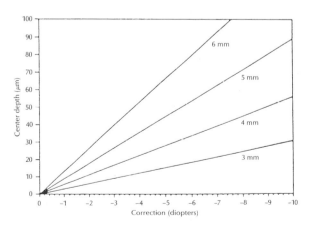

Fig. 2.34 Maximum depth of a cut calculated from an equation for myopic correction. Each line represents the depth of the cut on the optical axis for a given-size treatment zone. (Reproduced by permission from Munnerlyn CR et al. [32].)

excimer laser-corneal interaction did not create a new type of wound healing mechanism; it decreased normal wound healing responses.

L'Esperance and Taylor in 1987 (11,13) were the first to perform refractive corneal sculpting in human beings in blind eyes (Fig. 2.35). The corneas appeared clear on direct illumination, but a slight subepithelial haze that developed at 4 to 6 weeks postoperatively was visible on slit-beam and diffuse illumination. This haze decreased with time, but there were several diopters of refractive regression resulting from new collagen formation and epithelial hyperplasia (Fig. 2.36). With improvements in all the excimer laser systems, better results were obtained (Fig. 2.37). Clinical study of laser anterior KM for myopia in sighted eyes commenced in 1989.

Laser delivery systems to correct hyperopia have been designed (106) to remove more tissue peripherally than centrally. Very few patients have been treated to date and all have demonstrated almost complete loss of re-

fractive effect over time (48,106), resulting from "filling in" of the ablated areas. Different approaches need to be investigated.

Anterior KM laser treatment of astigmatism, consisting of more laser ablation of the steep corneal meridian than the flat meridian, has been performed in only a few patients with postoperative astigmatism. Results are too preliminary for assessment of clinical efficacy.

Operative Technique

The fluence and repetition rates depend on the type of excimer laser used and vary from 100 to 500 mJ/cm^2 and 5 to 20 Hz, respectively. Determination of optical and ablation zones is based on the amount of correction required, the pupil size, the age of the patient, and the type of laser used. Fluence and beam homogeneity are monitored before each laser treatment. The computer is programmed for desired ablation diameter, depth, and rate. The pa-

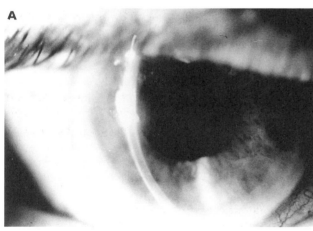

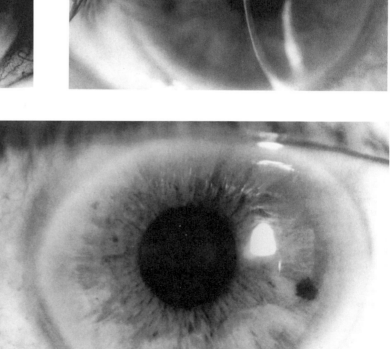

Fig. 2.35 A, Slit-lamp photograph of the *seventh* human eye to be treated with the ArF excimer laser before nonuniform lamellar keratectomy for myopic correction. B, Slit-lamp photograph 4 months postoperatively demonstrates central corneal flattening. C, Four months postoperatively, the cornea appears clear with direct illumination. Slight subepithelial fibrillar haze is visible only on slit-beam examination. (Copyright Taunton Technologies, Inc.; courtesy of Daniel M. Taylor, MD, New Britain, CT.)

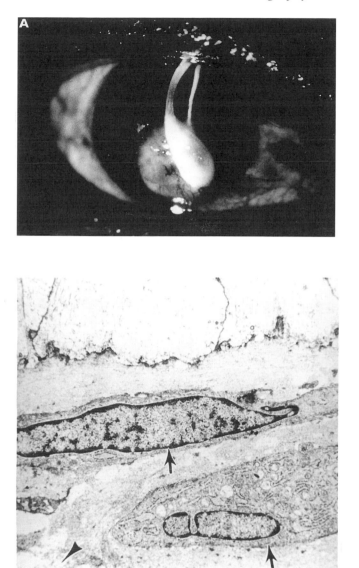

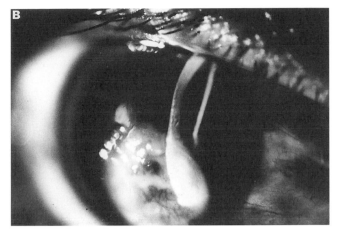

Fig. 2.36 A, Preoperative slit-lamp photograph of a human eye with corneal leukoma. B, Slit-lamp photograph shows corneal flattening 4 weeks after ArF excimer laser nonuniform lamellar keratectomy performed superior to the leukoma. There is a trace fibrillar haze at the epithelial-stromal interface. C, Transmission electron micrograph of the cornea with slight haze 4 months postoperatively. Note the active subepithelial keratocytes (*arrows*) and disorganized collagen (*arrowhead*). (Copyright Taunton Technologies, Inc.; (A) and (B) also courtesy of Daniel M. Taylor, MD, New Britain, CT.)

tient's spherical equivalent refraction and keratometry measurements are entered for correction of spherical errors. The laser then is calibrated for these settings. Before laser exposure 1% pilocarpine may be instilled to constrict the pupil. Topical anesthetic drops with or without retrobulbar or peribulbar injections and sedation are administered. A speculum is inserted between the lids. Fixation is maintained by the patient or with a limbal suction device. The cornea is irrigated after lasing.

Postoperative Management

Topical or subconjunctival antibiotics and steroids are applied. The optimal postoperative medication regimen to facilitate reepithelialization and to minimize haze formation has not yet been determined. The eye may be pressure patched for a few days until reepithelialization. Alternatively, a bandage contact lens or collagen shield soaked in antibiotics may be placed on the cornea. Topical steroids may be tapered for up to several months postoperatively to decrease corneal remodeling or may be titrated according to refractive effect.

Complications

Results to date indicate that laser anterior KM reduces myopia in patients without prior corneal surgery (48,107,108). However, for this procedure to replace glasses or contact lenses, all patients will have to be within 1 D of emmetropia and have excellent visual function. This procedure is not yet predictable. Nevertheless, despite reports of over- and undercorrections, results are encouraging. Most investigators have observed some overcorrections during the first few weeks postoperatively with subsequent myopic shifts starting at about a month after laser treatment and resulting from epithelial hyperplasia and new stromal tissue production. Best corrected visual acuities are achieved in 3 to 12 weeks and are reported to be equal to or better than preoperative visions in almost all cases. Most patients have no increased astigmatism of greater than 1 D (48,107,108).

Many thousand sighted patients have been treated worldwide, but little is known about long-term stability. Preliminary results suggest that this procedure is most predictable for patients with low and moderate myopia (48,107,108). Experimental (109) and clinical (48,108) studies have shown that topical steroids administered

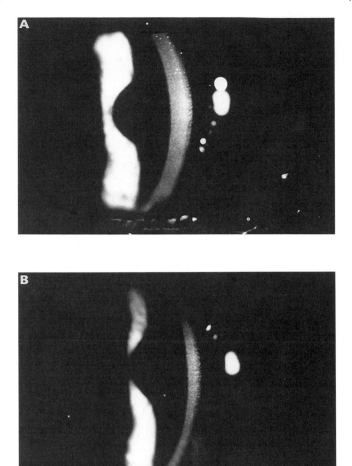

Fig. 2.37 A, Preoperative appearance of 5-D myope. B, Six weeks postoperatively. Note minimal subepithelial haze. (Courtesy of Neal Sher, MD.)

post-operatively increase the procedure's predictability and stability. Sher has reported (48) that, with more than a year follow-up in their series, adjunct steroid treatment has resulted in refractive results within 1 D of emmetropia in patients with preoperative myopia under 8 D and stable refraction following cessation of steroid administration at 3 to 5 months postoperatively. Few high myopes have been treated with the excimer laser. In most cases between 10 and 15 D, regression of more than 1 D has been noted. The deeper laser ablation necessary for correction of higher myopia with the same optical zone diameter results in a more marked difference in curvature between the ablated and nonablated areas and, thus, in a more abrupt curvature change in the transition zone. Better results may be obtained if the transition zone were enlarged and were to have a more gradual ablated profile contour and if pharmacologic agents were to substantially decrease regression. However, Pouliquen (personal communication, September 1990) has suggested that the greater ablation depths necessary for the correction of high my-

opia may lead to corneal steepening and refractive regression possibly because of anterior bowing of the cornea resulting from sliding of lamellae that are not interdigitated in the posterior two thirds of the cornea. Laser anterior KM probably will not be the procedure of choice for very high myopia of over 20 D. Laser posterior KM or epikeratoplasty may be alternative approaches. Recurrent erosions or other clinical manifestations of epithelial resurfacing and adhesion abnormalities have not been reported. Subepithelial reticular haze has been demonstrated in all patients to varying degrees depending on the type of laser and delivery systems used, the ablation depth, corneal wound healing, preexisting corneal pathology, and steroid dose. Pharmacologic acceleration of re-epithelialization that would influence epithelial-stromal interactions may decrease subepithelial haze. Pharmacologic inhibition of inflammatory and stromal cellular elements is important in decreasing wound healing responses, and thereby decreasing subepithelial corneal remodeling to clinically insignificant levels. Current data suggest that the stromal haze usually does not affect vision as measured by Snellen visual acuity charts, but effects on other aspects of visual function, such as contrast sensitivity and glare disability, have not yet been evaluated adequately. The haze decreases over time and has been observed to disappear completely in some cases (110). Study of the correlation between the quality of contrast sensitivity and scarring, optical zone centration, and the range of optical zone surface power is necessary. Preliminary results of Maguire and colleagues have demonstrated that corneal topography after laser sculpting may be compatible with poor to excellent contrast sensitivity (111). Optical zone decentration has occurred with current fixation techniques (Fig. 2.38). More sophisticated laser-eye coupling devices may prove beneficial. Glare disability has occurred following anterior KM using small optical zones in patients with large pupil diameters (108). The correlation between glare and optical zone size, ablation zone size, pupil size, corneal power, peripheral field angle, and anterior chamber depth must be determined (112,113). Presbyopic patients who are treated for myopia with the laser may require glasses for reading. Future excimer laser applications may include sculpting to create multifocal corneas according to the age and visual needs of the patient. Specular microscopy of the corneal endothelium has not revealed any damage from laser anterior KM (49). Intraocular damage secondary to acoustic waves, shock waves, or secondary radiation has not been observed. Complications secondary to steroid use after PRK have not been reported, but need to be avoided. Myopic patients are more vulnerable to developing posterior subcapsular cataracts. Steroid-dependent glaucoma also may occur. Therefore, the role of nonsteroidal anti-inflammatory agents, antimetabolites, and other cell inhibitors must be investigated. More complete under-

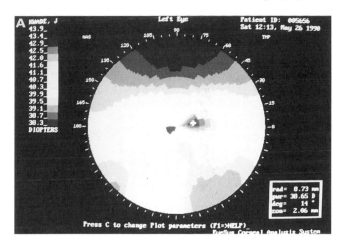

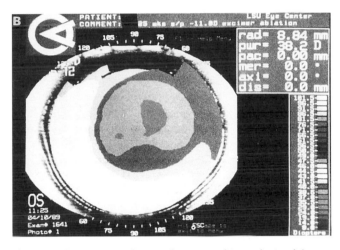

Fig. 2.38 Computerized corneal topographic analysis of the anterior corneal surface following excimer laser sculpting in a 5-mm zone for myopia. Note decentration of laser ablation. (Courtesy of Joe Wakil, MD, EyeSys Laboratories)

standing and control of inflammatory cell, epithelial cell, and stromal cell interactions during wound healing will increase the safety, predictability, and stability of laser anterior KM.

Laser Posterior Keratomileusis

Historical Aspects

In 1987 Hanna and associates first performed excimer laser posterior KM (98,114). They reshaped with the laser instead of with a cryolathe the stromal surface of the anterior portion of a fresh eye bank cornea that had been resected with a microkeratome. The resected disc was placed on a concave suction punch block and the stromal surface was ablated more centrally than peripherally by a rotating slit-shaped laser beam. The energy parameters were the same as those used for anterior KM.

In 1989, Rama and coworkers (115) performed laser sculpting with a progressively closing diaphragm system of the posterior surface of microkeratome-excised plano discs in three patients. Results are too preliminary to compare laser and mechanical techniques. Also in 1989, Pallikaris (116) used the laser combined with a scanning slit delivery system for in situ KM in rabbits. A lamellar, plano flap of cornea was raised with a modified microkeratome and the stromal bed was carved with the laser. The wounds were reported to heal without complications.

Laser Epikeratoplasty

Historical Aspects

In 1987 Lieurance and associates (117) cut epikeratophakia lenticules from human eye bank corneas that had been stored in McCarey-Kaufman medium. The convex epithelial surface of the donor cornea was held by capillary attraction against the concave surface of a sintered glass mold that had been shaped to produce a lenticule of the desired dioptric power. The laser was focused along the horizontal base of the mold, which was rotated on a turntable at 5 rpm to ablate all corneal tissue outside the concave surface of the mold. The energy levels were 15 to 30 J/cm², and the exposure time varied from 2.5 to 4 min. The cut surface of the lenticule was smoother on scanning electron microscopic examination than that obtained by cryolathing (Fig. 2.39). Light and transmission electron microscopic examination demonstrated intact epithelium, Bowman's membrane, keratocytes, and stromal collagen. The lenticules that were grafted onto rabbit eyes were clear in the first week after surgery, and there were no epithelial abnormalities or haze at the graft-host interface.

Laser-Adjusted Synthetic Epikeratoplasty

Historical Aspects

In 1989, Thompson and associates (118) evaluated the effect of lasering the surface of synthetic epikeratoplasty lenticules to smooth the surface to remove debris and irregularities and to adjust both preoperatively and postoperatively refractive power (Fig. 2.40) After removing the epithelium over an 8-mm area, they performed mechanical circular trephination in a 4-mm optical zone to a depth of 0.3 mm in monkey corneas. Following shallow lamellar dissection, they inserted a 7- to 7.5-mm diameter collagen intravenous lenticule that had been lased with the excimer (Fig. 2.41). Although no epithelial attachment problems or host tissue necrosis occurred, enzymatic degradation of the collagen intravenous lenticule resulted in subepithelial erosions and focal thinning. Lenticules made of other types of collagen, as well as other synthetic materials, are being investigated for long-term stability. If

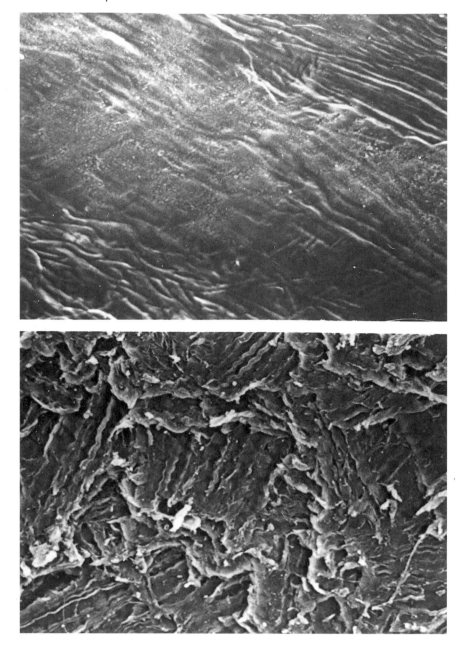

Fig. 2.39 Scanning electron micrographs of human epikeratophakia lenticules obtained by ArF excimer lasing (*top*) and cryolathing (*bottom*). The posterior surface of the laser-cut lenticule is much smoother. X80,000. (Reproduced by permission from Lieurance RC et al. [117]; courtesy of David Schanzlin, MD, St. Louis, MO. Published with permission from The American Journal of Ophthalmology. Copyright by The Ophthalmic Publishing Company.)

the problems associated with lenticular biocompatibility and attachment were to be solved, this procedure would become an important addition to the refractive surgeon's armamentarium.

Noncentral Refractive Keratectomy

Refractive keratotomy and keratectomy procedures that are performed in the midperipheral and peripheral cornea have been designed to correct myopia, hyperopia, or astigmatism by alteration of the central corneal curvature. These techniques consist of various patterns, numbers, lengths, and depths of radial, parallel, transverse, and arcuate incisions and excisions. Sutures sometimes

are used to compensate for or to enhance the effects of corneal relaxing incisions or to approximate wound edges after corneal excision. Radial keratotomy for the correction of mild and moderate myopia is the most frequently performed refractive procedure. Depending on the amount of correction desired, four or more deep radial incisions are made from the edge of the optical zone to the limbus or from the limbus to the optical zone, which is between 3 and 5 mm in diameter. The radial incisions cause the midperipheral and peripheral cornea to weaken and bulge outward, thereby flattening the central optical zone and relatively steepening the midperipheral zone (119–121). Hexagonal keratotomy corrects mild hyperopia. Interrupted circumferential incisions in the midpe-

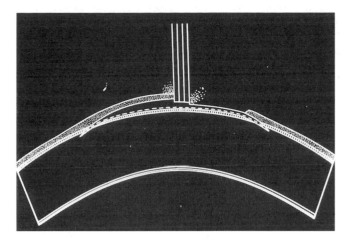

Fig. 2.40 Schematic diagram of laser-adjustable synthetic epi keratoplasty (LASE). The excimer laser is used to correct the refractive power of the synthetic lenticule. (Courtesy of Keith Thompson, MD.)

riphery destabilize the central cornea, causing it to bow forward and steepen (122,123).

In most keratotomy procedures for the correction of astigmatism, the cornea is incised in the steepest meridian. Multiple parallel or grouped radial incisions extending from a central optical zone have been advocated for the correction of mild myopic astigmatism because midperipheral corneal bulging in one meridian leads to a greater central corneal flattening in that meridian than in other meridians (124). Symmetric transverse midperipheral incisions are performed to correct mild and moderate astigmatism. Transverse incisions transect corneal collagen bundles, leading to meridianal corneal flattening (119,124,125). Increased astigmatic correction has been achieved with multiple transverse (124,125) or arcuate incisions (126–128). The amount of spherical equivalent correction after these procedures has been shown to be related to the length of the transverse or arcuate incision because of a coupling effect. Incising the steeper meridian circumferentially not only causes it to flatten, but also causes the flatter meridian 90° away to steepen. Therefore myopic or hyperopic astigmatism can be corrected, depending on the chosen incisions and optical zone (124,125). For moderate and high astigmatism, transverse incisions have been combined with radial incisions to increase astigmatic correction and to reduce the coupling effect (124,125,129–131). Corneal wedge resection is performed for correction of very high degrees of astigmatism. Removal of a peripheral crescentic wedge of tissue that is centered on the flattest meridian and suturing of the wound result in central corneal steepening with peripheral corneal flattening in the area of resection (61,125).

Refractive keratotomy and keratectomy procedures are constantly evolving. Over the past 10 years, widespread interest in these techniques has necessitated and generated numerous experimental and clinical studies that have increased the corneal surgeon's understanding of refractive procedures and have led to many technical refinements. Although many intraoperative and postoperative complications have been reported (132,133), the incidence of severe complications is low, and recent improvements in surgical design and instrumentation have led to decreased complication rates (120,132–135). Significant changes in surgical technique, including the abandonment of intersecting radial and transverse or arcuate incisions, the execution of radial incisions toward the corneal periphery, but not across the limbus, fewer radial incisions, as well as improved pachymeters and high-quality, calibrated gem knives, have rendered these procedures relatively safe.

Nevertheless, these techniques do not allow for retention of best-corrected visual acuity in all cases. In the Prospective Evaluation of Radial Keratotomy (PERK)

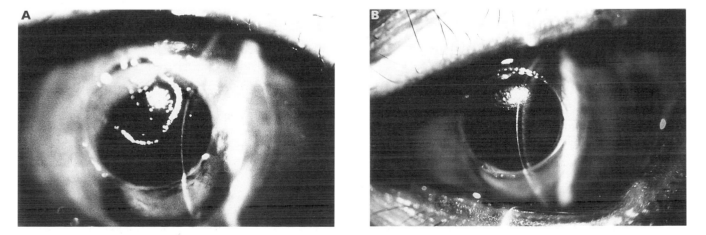

Fig. 2.41 A, Slit-lamp photo of monkey cornea immediately following LASE. B, Slit-lamp photo of monkey cornea at 11 days following LASE. Note corneal reepithelialization. (Reproduced by permission from Thompson K et al. [118].)

Study, a multicenter clinical trial, 2% of eyes had a decrease of two or more lines in best-corrected acuity at 4 years after surgery (136). Although very few patients develop a permanent decrease in best-corrected vision, visual impairment such as glare, distortion, monocular diplopia, or fluctuating vision can occur (132,133, 135–137). Despite the fact that many refractive incisional and excisional procedures have been shown to reduce refractive errors, the unpredictability and instability of these techniques are still of concern (132–134, 136–139). Accurate prediction of outcome in individual eyes is not possible with current techniques (137). Although low myopes (between −2.00 and −3.12 D) have been reported to have 20/40 or better visual acuity in 94% of eyes and refractive error between −1.00 and +1.00 D in 73% of eyes at 4 years postoperatively (136), of all myopes between −2.00 and −8.00 D, only 55% of eyes had a refractive error between −1.00 and +1.00 D in the same series. Another study (135) of radial keratotomy performed in myopes with a mean spherical equivalent refraction of −5.00 ± 2.9, demonstrated that 37% of eyes had 20/20 uncorrected visual acuity and 76% of eyes had at least 20/40 uncorrected visual acuity at 5 years after surgery. There has been no multicenter prospective clinical trial of keratotomy or keratectomy procedures performed mechanically for the correction of hyperopia or astigmatism. Clinical observations of multiple researchers, however, have not yet demonstrated predictable and stable results with any of these techniques (61,124,125,130,140–143).

Several factors relating to surgical technique and response of the operated eye affect the predictability and stability of these procedures. With current instrumentation, the depth of the incision is the most difficult surgical factor to control (138,144). When incisions are performed with metal knives and thickness is measured by optical pachymetry, the depth of cuts has been reported to range from 30% to 100% of corneal thickness (145–147). When incisions are created by diamond knives and thickness is measured by ultrasonic pachymetry, the predictability of incision depth is improved, but variations in incision depth of 61% to 98% of corneal thickness have been found (148). It has been calculated that keratotomy incisions require an accuracy of within 20 μm between desired and attained cutting depth (134). Freehand corneal cutting does not allow for this precision. However, even with high-quality, micrometer-calibrated knives, accurate depths are inconsistently attained. Tilting of the blade to the side or in the forward-backward direction, variation in pressure exerted on the knife or in the speed with which the incisions are executed, and poor eye fixation cause differences in incision depth (120,134,144). Even if gem knives are used, microscopic defects of the cutting edge, micrometer inaccuracy, and faulty foot plate design can lead to significant errors (134).

Radial Keratotomy

Historical Aspects

In 1983, Trokel and associates (16) first suggested applying the excimer laser in radial keratotomy. In 1985 Cotliar and others evaluated the laser in human cadaver eyes for use in radial keratectomy, as the procedure should be termed, because excimer laser photoablation always involves removal of tissue. The laser beam was focused to produce a rectangular beam 70 μm wide on the corneal surface that was shielded with a contact lens to spare the central 3.5-mm optical zone and allow two 3.5-mm excisions of the peripheral cornea. Two additional excisions were performed on the cornea by reexposing the surface after 90° rotation of the laser beam. The laser output was 100 mJ/pulse at a frequency of 10 Hz. Depending on the depth desired, the exposure time was varied from 10 to 45 sec. The edges of the excision sites were extremely smooth. Corneal flattening ranging from 0.12 to 5.35 D was obtained. The depth of the corneal excisions and the degree of central corneal flattening were found to correlate with the energy delivered. Steinert and Puliafito used a slit lamp-delivered excimer beam to perform radial keratectomies one at a time in a rabbit in vivo (149). Photokeratoscopy one day after laser exposure confirmed central flattening and midperipheral steepening at each of the excision sites.

In 1987, Aron-Rosa and others (150, 151), and Tenner and others (152) investigated laser radial keratectomies in blind eyes. In the slit-lamp delivery system used by Aron-Rosa and associates (150,151), the laser beam was directed by prisms through an articulated arm to be coaxial with the slit-lamp illumination and the HeNe aiming beam, and was transmitted through an adjustable slit that could be rotated 360°. The size of the slit could be varied from 50 to 500 μm in width and up to 5 mm in length. The fluence was 370 mJ/cm² with a frequency of 20 Hz. The total number of pulses was computer controlled and was determined by the desired excision depth. The slit was set for a width of 70 μm, and the depth was programmed for either 50% or 90% of corneal thickness. The patient's eye was stabilized by retrobulbar anesthesia. A metal blocking mask with a 70 μm-wide slit was placed on the cornea to further control the size of the excision, but patient movement sometimes led to step-shaped edges. The excision depth was determined histologically and by slit-lamp examination to be 85% or less of the programmed depth. The relatively shallow depths were attributed to poor beam quality, poor eye stability, and the presence of ejected photoablation remnants that might have acted as a shield when pulses were directed repeatedly at the same area. Corneal flattening measured by pachymetry at one day postoperatively was reported to be stable when remeasured 3 weeks later. Wound healing was followed for as long as 3 weeks postoperatively. Light and electron microscopy demonstrated progressive healing of the excisions (Fig. 2.42). Shroder and associates (153) developed a delivery system with special design features to decrease eye motion artifacts and improve cutting precision (Fig. 2.43). The laser was encased underneath a bed, allowing the patient to remain supine during laser beam delivery through an articulated arm. To further minimize errors due to eye movement, a plastic suction mask incorporating a metal plate with 70 μm-wide slits, was held to the eye by a slight vacuum (Fig. 2.44). Constant air flow within the mask cooled the mask and removed molecular remnants to improve laser absorption. Increasing the

depth of field of the image also allowed for more constant absorption over the entire excision site.

Tenner and associates (152) reported on radial keratectomies performed on blind eyes. The number of pulses required to attain a desired depth was calculated based on measured corneal thickness and on assumed ablation depth of 2 μm/pulse. To ensure safety, the depth was preset for only 60% of corneal thickness. Completion of eight radial excisions that were performed one at a time required 5 to 7 min. On slit-lamp examination, the excisions appeared smooth and straight (Fig. 2.45) and were estimated by several observers to extend through 60% of corneal thickness. The degree of corneal flattening attained compared favorably with that achieved by radial

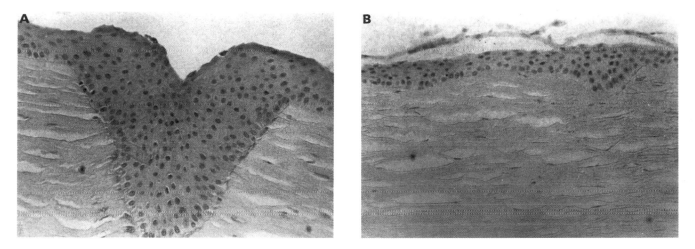

Fig. 2.42 A, Light micrograph of human cornea 14 days after 70-μm-wide ArF excimer laser radial keratectomy. Note the V-shaped epithelial plug. Hematoxylin, eosin, and safran. B, Light micrograph of human cornea 21 days after 70-μm-wide excimer laser radial keratectomy. The epithelial plug is smaller than at 14 days. Hematoxylin, eosin, and safran. (Reproduced by permission from Aron-Rosa DS et al. [151].)

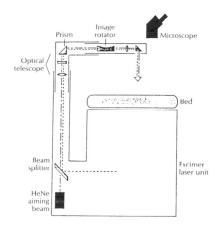

Fig. 2.43 Schematic diagram of the delivery system for ArF excimer laser radial keratectomy. (Reproduced by permission from Schroder E et al. [153]. Published with permission from The American Journal of Ophthalmology. Copyright by The Ophthalmic Publishing Company.)

Fig. 2.44 Schematic diagram of a suction mask with slits for ArF excimer laser radial keratectomy. (Reproduced with permission from Schroder E et al. [153]. Published with permission from The American Journal of Ophthalmology. Copyright by The Ophthalmic Publishing Company.)

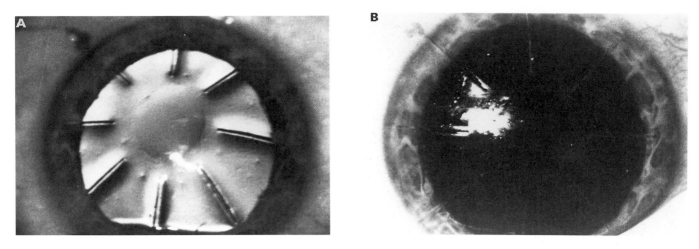

Fig. 2.45 A, Photograph taken through a surgical microscope of a human eye immediately after ArF excimer laser radial keratectomy with a 5-mm optical clear zone. Incision length, 3 mm; incision width, 70 μm; incision depth, 300 μm, corresponding to 60% of the corneal thickness. B, Slit-lamp photograph 30 min postoperatively. (Reproduced by permission from Tenner A et al. [152].)

keratotomy procedures using diamond knives and the same parameters. Six-month follow-up of two patients, though, did not demonstrate regression of initial effect, as has been observed with conventional techniques. The excision sites healed without any notable infiltrate or reaction (Fig. 2.46). With wound healing, excision width decreased and the cut ends of Bowman's membrane were almost reapposed by 18 months, suggesting wound contraction (154). Bansal and others demonstrated that, although excimer radial excision appears to be wider than incisions made with diamond blades, the wound healing responses appear to be similar. In their study, healing was still incomplete after 18 months (154).

Clinical trials were begun in Europe in sighted eyes, but published reports of the results are not available. Theoretically, the laser should offer more control of excisional depth than conventional instruments and should, therefore, increase the predictability of radial keratectomy techniques. However, the wider laser excisions produced with available systems might cause greater instability of the eye and provoke increased glare and fluctuation of visual acuity. Because of the tremendous interest generated by the surface ablation refractive techniques, very little work has been done recently on improving radial keratectomy delivery systems. Randomized clinical trials comparing radial keratotomy and laser anterior KM will need to be done to evaluate whether reliability problems due to wound healing and corneal instability will cause one of these techniques to replace the other in the future.

Transverse and Arcuate Keratectomy

Historical Aspects

Seiler and associates were the first to perform transverse (Fig. 2.47) and arcuate keratectomies with the excimer laser in blind eyes and sighted eyes with astigmatic errors. They used a system incorporating the ArF excimer laser coupled to an operating microscope that provided for coaxial laser delivery at a fluence of 165 mJ/cm² and a repetition rate of 30 Hz. The beam was shaped by two 150-μm wide transverse or arcuate slits in a polymethylmethacrylate contact lens that was coated with a metal foil to reflect UV radiation. The posterior surface of the contact lens contained grooves to minimize capillary forces, thereby allowing for the maintenance of a dry corneal surface and preventing excision site accumulation of tear fluid that has been shown to decrease tissue absorption of laser energy and to decrease excision depth predictability. The procedure was performed with the patient supine. After instillation of topical anesthesia, the contact lens was centered on the cornea and the eye was stabilized with a Thornton ring. Each slit was irradiated separately for less than 1 min. The number of pulses was precalculated and microprocessor controlled. Although excision depth correlated in a linear fashion to the total number of pulses (155), the ablation depth obtained per pulse in the epithelium was approximately twice that obtained in the stroma (18,155). Therefore, the ablation rate and desired ablation depth of both the epithelium and stroma were considered during calculation of pulse number. The ultrasonically measured central corneal thickness was multiplied by 1.18 before determination of desired incision depth to correct for increased peripheral corneal thickness and for nonperpendicular alignment of the laser beam at the irradiated surface.

As compared with conventional techniques, the ArF excimer laser led to less deviation between intended and attained excision depth. Histologic examination of the enucleated eyes demonstrated that the depth was within ±5% of the intended value. Analysis of slit-lamp micrographs revealed attainment of accurate depths within the

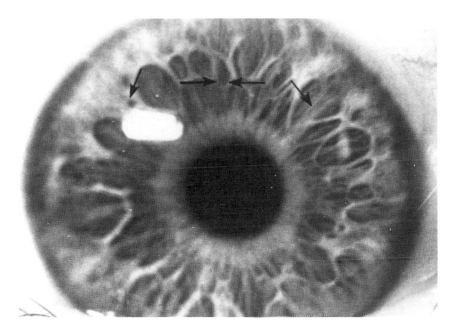

Fig. 2.46 Slit-lamp photograph of the same eye as in Fig. 2.45 several weeks postoperatively. There was 2 D of central corneal flattening. Arrows identify some of the incisions. (Reproduced by permission from Tenner A et al. [152].)

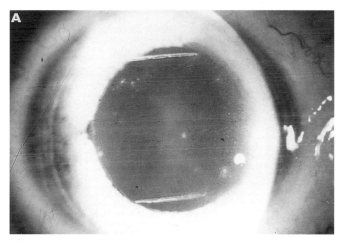

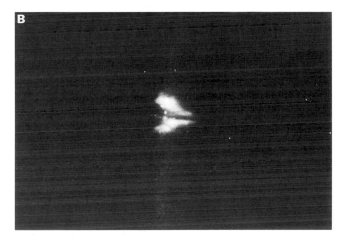

Fig. 2.47 A, Slit-lamp photograph of a human eye after ArF excimer laser transverse keratectomy. B, Slit-lamp photograph 5 weeks postoperatively. The excision depths were estimated to be 90% ± 8% of the corneal thickness. (Reproduced by permission from Seiler T et al. [18]. Published with permission from the American Journal of Ophthalmology. Copyright by The Ophthalmic Publishing Company.)

measurement error of ±8%. According to Seiler and Wollensak's biomechanical model (156), astigmatic changes were predicted to be very dependent on incision depth. The clinical results obtained with ArF excimer laser transverse keratectomy correlated well with the theoretical curve (Fig. 2.48), although actual total astigmatic changes were slightly greater than predicted. Following transverse keratectomy, steepening of the flat meridian was greater than flattening of the steep meridian, thereby inducing a myopic shift. Biconcave arcuate excisions produced astigmatic changes similar to those obtained with transverse excisions, but with no change in the spherical equivalent. Biconvex arcuate excisions have been suggested by Seiler (157) to be the method of choice to correct high hyperopic astigmatism; this procedure caused a myopic shift similar to that produced with transverse excisions but created a one- to sixfold higher astigmatic shift.

Following laser keratectomy, large fluctuations in astigmatism were noted during the first few days and were attributed to stromal edema (18). Stabilization was achieved at approximately 2 weeks, and no regression was noted over the 6-month follow-up period. Patients complained of foreign body sensations and photophobia during the first week postoperatively. These symptoms generally resolved by the following week. Glare persisting for up to 2 months was noted by some patients. Rapid reepithelialization over the first few days was found biomicroscopically and histologically (Fig. 2.49). Epithelial plugs persisted for variable time periods.

In the United States, clinical trials of this procedure were begun by Hunkeler and Fenzl in 1989. After performing ultrasonic pachymetry, they programmed the laser at 70% to 95% depth and delivered the beam through aluminum-coated masks with slits 15 × 4500 μm, with the

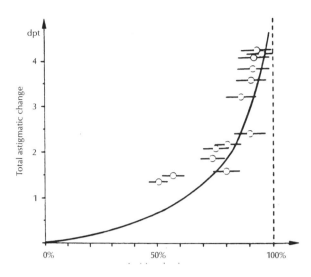

Fig. 2.48 Total astigmatic changes after ArF excimer laser transverse keratectomy as a function of excision depth compared with a theoretical curve. (Reproduced by permission from Seiler T et al. [18]. Published with permission from The American Journal of Ophthalmology. Copyright by The Ophthalmic Company.)

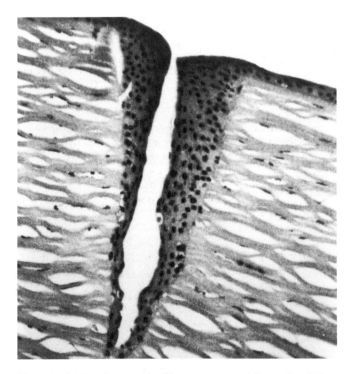

Fig. 2.49 Light micrograph of human cornea 4 days after 150-μm-wide ArF excimer laser transverse keratectomy. Epithelium covers the surface of the excision. (Reproduced by permission from Seiler T et al. [18]. Published with permission from The American Journal of Ophthalmology. Copyright by The Ophthalmic Publishing Company.)

patient under topical or local anesthesia. They treated patients with greater than 3 D of astigmatism. Complications including undercorrection, overcorrection, and perforation have been reported. Imprecise energy calculation, imprecise depth gauging systems, and excess fluid on the cornea have been cited as factors contributing to unreliable results (D Durrie, personal communication, February 1990). Published reports of the predictability and stability of this procedure are not available to properly assess its potential. Preoperative computerized corneal topography analysis and modification of laser techniques to allow variation of excision length according to the circumferential extent of steepening delineated on colorcoded maps may improve this procedure's accuracy. However, recent studies (JM Parel, personal communication, October 6, 1990) have suggested that hydration effects may preclude accurate refractive results and that other laser techniques should be investigated and compared with transverse and arcuate keratectomies.

References

1. Rhodes CK. Excimer lasers. Top Appl Phys, 1979;30:130.
2. Ruderman W. Excimer lasers in photochemistry. Laser Focus 1979;May:68–69.
3. Srinivasan R, Leigh WJ. Ablative photodecomposition: action of far-ultraviolet (193 nm) laser radiation on [poly(ethylene terephthalate)] films. J Am Chem Soc 1982;104:6784–6785.
4. Srinivasan R, Mayne-Banton, V. Self-developing photoetching of poly(ethylene terephthalate) films by far-ultraviolet excimer laser radiation. Appl Phys Lett 1982;41:576–578.
5. Taboada J, Archibald CJ. An extreme sensitivity in the corneal epithelium to far-UV ArF excimer laser pulses. In: Proceedings of the Aero Space Medical Association, 52d Annual Meeting. Washington, DC: Aerospace Medical Association, 1981:8–9.
6. Taboada J, Mikesell GW, Reed RD. Response of the corneal epithelium to KrF excimer laser pulses. Health Phys 1981;40:677.
7. Houtermans FG. Uber Maser-Wirkung im optisschen Spektralgebiet und die moglichkeit absolut negafizer Asorption fur einige Falle zon Molekulspektren (Light-Lawine). Helv Phys Acta 1969;33:933.
8. Rhodes CK. Excimer lasers. Top Appl Phy, 1979;30:180.
9. L'Esperance FA Jr. Method for Performing Ophthalmological Surgery. U.S. Patent 4,669,466; issued June 2, 1987.
10. L'Esperance, FA Jr. Method and Apparatus for Ophthalmological Surgery. U.S. Patent 4,665,913; issued May 19, 1987.
11. L'Esperance FA Jr, Taylor DM, Warner JW. Human excimer laser keratectomy: short term histopathology. Refract Surg 1988;4:118.
12. L'Esperance FA Jr, Warner JW, Telfair WB, et al. Excimer laser instrumentation and technique for human corneal surgery. Arch Ophthalmol 1989;107:131.
13. L'Esperance FA Jr, Taylor DM, Delpero RA, et al. Human excimer laser corneal surgery: preliminary report. Trans Am Ophthalmol Soc 1988;86:208–275.
14. Srinivasan R, Wynne JJ, Blum SE. Far-UV photoetching of organic material. Laser Focus 1983;19:62.

15. Linsker R, Srinivasan R, Wynne JJ, Alonso DR. Far-ultraviolet laser ablation of atherosclerotic lesions. Lasers Surg Med 1984;4:201–206.
16. Trokel SL, Srinivasan R, Braren B. Excimer laser surgery of the cornea. Am J Ophthalmol 1983;96:710–715.
17. Puliafito CA, Steinert RF, Deutsch TF, et al. Excimer laser ablation of the cornea and lens: experimental studies. Ophthalmology 1985;92:741–748.
18. Seiler T, Bende T, Wollensak J, et al. Excimer laser keratectomy for correction of astigmatism. Am J Ophthalmol 1988;105:117–124.
19. Marshall J, Trokel S, Rothery S, Schubert H. An ultrastructural study of corneal incisions induced by an excimer laser at 193 nm. Ophthalmology 1985;92:749–758.
20. Martin CA, DelPero RA, Telfair WB, Warner JW, Yoder PR Jr. Use of the excimer laser in corneal surgery. Presentation to CLEO, 1988.
21. Srinivasan R. Ablation of polymers and biological tissue by ultraviolet lasers. Science 1986;234:559.
22. Srinivasan R, Braren B, Seeger DE, et al. Photochemical cleavage of organic solids: details of the ultraviolet laser ablation of two organic polymers at 193 nm and 248 nm. J Am Chem Soc 1986;19:916.
23. Mandel E, et al. ARVO Proceedings. Abstract 6, 275, 1987.
24. Seiler T, Marshall J, Rothery S, et al. The potential of an infrared Hydrogen Fluoride (HF) laser (3.0 m) for corneal surgery. Lasers Ophthalmol 1986;1:49–60.
25. Yoder PR Jr, Telfair WB, Warner JW, Martin CA, Bennett PS. Beam delivery system for UV laser ablation of the cornea. Proc SPIE 1988;908.
26. Martin CA, Warner JW, DelPero RA, Yoder PR Jr. Corneal sculpting using an excimer laser delivery system. Proc SPIE 1988;908.
27. L'Esperance FA Jr, ed. Ophthalmic lasers. St. Louis: CV Mosby, 1989.
28. Veldkamp W, Van Allen E. Compact, collinear, and variable anamorphic-beam compressor design. Appl Opt 1982;21:7.
29. Telfair WB, et al. Characterization of UV laser beams using fluorescence. Proc SPIE 1987;888.
30. Marshall J, Trokel S, Rothery S, Krueger RR. Photoablative reprofiling of the cornea using an excimer laser: photorefractive keratectomy. Lasers Ophthalmol 1986;1:21–48.
31. Tuft S, Marshall J, Rothery S. Stromal remodeling following photorefractive keratectomy. Lasers Ophthalmol 1987;1:177–183.
32. Krueger RR, Trokel S. Quantitation of corneal ablation by ultraviolet laser light. Arch Ophthalmol 1985;103:1741–1743.
33. Munnerlyn CR, Koons SJ, Marshall J. Photorefractive keratectomy; a technique for laser refractive surgery. J Cataract Refract Surg 1988;14:46.
34. Marshall J, Trokel S, Rothery S, et al. A comparative study of corneal incisions induced by diamond and steel knives and two ultraviolet radiations from an excimer laser. Br J Ophthalmol 1986;70:482.
35. L'Esperance FA Jr, ed. Ophthalmic lasers. St. Louis: CV Mosby, 1989: chaps. 23 and 24.
36. Arentsen JJ. Lamellar grafting. In: Brightbill FS, ed. Corneal surgery: theory, technique, and tissue. St. Louis: CV Mosby, 1986.
37. Casey T. The lamellar graft. In: Casey T, Mayer D, eds. Corneal grafting: principles and practice. Philadelphia: WB Saunders, 1984.
38. Erlich MI, et al. Techniques of lamellar keratoplasty, Int Ophthalmol Clin 1988;28:24.
39. Rich LF, MacRae SM, Fraunfelder FT. An improved method for lamellar keratoplasty. CLAO J 1988;14:42.
40. Mandelbaum S, Udel IJ. Corneal perforations associated with infectious agents. In: Abbott RL, ed. Surgical intervention in corneal and external diseases. New York: Grune & Stratton, 1987.
41. Boruchoff SA. Therapeutic keratoplasty. In: Smolin G, Thoft RA, eds. The cornea: scientific foundations and clinical practice. Boston: Little, Brown, 1983.
42. Rich LF. A technique for preparing corneal lamellar donor tissue using simplified keratomileusis. Ophthalmic Surg 1980;11:606.
43. Kerr-Muir MG, Trokel SL, Marshall J, et al. Ultrastructural comparison of conventional surgical and argon fluoride excimer laser keratectomy. Am J Ophthalmol 1987;103:448–453.
44. Keates RH, Drago PC, Rothchild EJ. Effect of excimer laser on microbiological organisms. Ophthalmic Surg 1988;19:715–718.
45. Stark WJ, Gilbert ML, Goodman GL, et al. Excimer laser phototherapeutic keratectomy. Ophthalmology (in press).
46. Stark WJ, Gilbert ML, Goodman GL, et al. Phototherapeutic keratectomy preliminary report. Invest Ophthalmol Vis Sci 1990;31:245.
47. Stark WJ, Gilbert ML, Gottsch JD, Munnerlyn C. Optical pachometry in the measurement of anterior corneal disease: an evaluative tool for phototherapeutic keratectomy. Arch Ophthalmol 1990;108:12–13.
48. Zabel RW. Oral communication. International Corneal Laser Society, May 1990.
49. Sher NA, Bowers RA, Zabel RW, et al. The clinical use of 193 nm excimer laser in the treatment of corneal scars. Arch Ophthalmol 1991;109(4):491–498.
50. Rowsey JJ. Excimer lasers exciting and expensive. Paper presented at The American Society of Cataract and Refractive Surgery Annual Meeting, Los Angeles, March 4–7, 1990.
51. Perlman EM. An analysis and interpretation of refractive errors after penetrating keratoplasty. Ophthalmology 1981;88:39–45.
52. Binder PS. Selective suture removal can reduce postkeratoplasty astigmatism. Ophthalmology 1985;92:1412–1416.
53. Heidemann DG, Sugar A, Meyer RF, et al. Oversized donor grafts in penetrating keratoplasty: a randomized trial. Arch Ophthalmol 1985;103:1807–1811.
54. Moro-Besson J. Astigmatisme postkeratoplastie transfixiante: interet de l'utilisation due micro-kerato-trepan, these, Paris, 1987, Dactylo-Sorbonne.
55. Troutman RC, Storch RL, Draga A, et al. Postkeratoplasty corneal topography analysis comparing Krumeich suction to manual trephination. Invest Ophthalmol Vis Sci 1990;31:575.
56. Mader TH, Yuan R, Lynn MJ, et al. Changes in keratometric astigmatism following suture removal more than one year after penetrating keratoplasty. Invest Ophthalmol Vis Sci 1990; 31:574.
57. McNeill JI, Wessels IF. Adjustment of single continuous suture to control astigmatism after penetrating keratoplasty. Refract Corneal Surg 1989;5:216–223.
58. Olson RJ. Corneal curvature changes associated with penetrating keratoplasty: a mathematical model. Ophthalmic Surg 1980;11:838–842.
59. Olson RJ. Prevention of astigmatism in corneal transplant surgery. Int Ophthalmol Clin 1988;28:37–45.
60. Mahjoub SB, Au Y. Astigmatism and tissue-shape disparity in penetrating keratoplasty. Ophthalmic Surg 1990;21:187.

61. Denham DB, Barraquer E, Loertscher H, et al. Evaluation of manual motorized and laser trephines by shadow photogrammetric analysis. Invest Ophthalmol Vis Sci 1988; 29(suppl):452.

62. Lindstrom RL, Lavery QW. Correction of postkeratoplasty astigmatism. In: Sanders DR, Hofmann RF, Salz JJ, eds. Refractive corneal surgery. Thorofare, NJ: Slack, Inc. 1986.

63. Serdarevic ON, Hanna K, Gribomont AC, et al. Excimer laser trephination in penetrating keratoplasty: morphologic features and wound healing. Ophthalmology 1988;95:493–505.

64. Serdarevic ON, Hanna K, Gribomont AC, et al. Excimer laser trephination in penetrating keratoplasty. Ophthalmology 1987;94:126.

65. Van Rij G, Waring GO. Configuration of corneal trephines opening using five different trephines in human donor eyes. Arch Ophthalmol 1988;106:1228–1233.

66. Lang GK, Naumann GOH, Koch JW. A new elliptical excision for corneal transplantation using an excimer laser. Arch Ophthalmol 1990;108(1):914–915.

67. Beckman H, Rota A, Barraco R, et al. Limbectomies, keratectomies, and keratostomies performed with a rapid-pulsed carbon dioxide laser. Am J Ophthalmol 1971;71:1277–1283.

68. Loertscher H, Mandelbaum S, Parel JM, et al. Noncontact trephination of the cornea using a pulsed hydrogen fluoride laser. Am J Ophthalmol 1987;104:471–475.

69. Gormley DJ, Gersten M, Koplin RS, et al. Corneal modeling. Cornea 1988; 7:30–35.

70. Klyce SD. Computer-assisted corneal topography, high resolution graphic presentation and analysis of keratoscopy. Invest Ophthalmol Vis Sci 1984;25:426–435.

71. Bille JF, et al. 3-D corneal imaging using the laser tomographic scanner. Invest Ophthalmic Vis Sci 1987;28:223.

72. Smolek MK. Real-time holographic interferometry of bovine eyes. Invest Ophthalmol Vis Sci 1988;29:389.

73. Mathers WD, Jester JV. Full thickness corneal wound strength enhancement by epidermal growth factor. Invest Ophthalmol Vis Sci 1988; 29:312.

74. Petrousos G, Sebag J, Courtois Y. Epidermal growth factor increases tensile strength during wound healing. Ophthalmic Res 1986; 18:299–300.

75. Rich LF, Weimer VL, Squires EL, et al. Stimulation of corneal wound healing with mesodermal growth factor. Arch Ophthalmol 1979;97:1326–1330.

76. Woost PG, Brightwell J, Eiferman RA, et al. Effect of growth factors with dexamethasone on healing of rabbit corneal stromal incisions. Exp Eye Res 1985; 40:47–60.

77. Leibowitz HM, Morello S, Stern M, Kupferman A. Effect of topically administered epidermal growth factor on corneal wound strength. Arch Ophthalmol 1990;108:734.

78. Serdarevic O, Menasche M, Ben-Rayana N, et al. Stimulation of stromal macromolecular biosynthesis after penetrating keratoplasty by human epidermal growth factor. Invest Ophthalmol Vis Sci 1990;31:226.

79. DeToledo AR, Witlock DR, Kaminski LA, et al. Preliminary evaluation of a new collagen-derived bioadhesive. Invest Ophthalmol Vis Sci 1990;31:317.

80. Lewis JS, Foulks GN, Mandel J. Excimer laser corneal contouring and the triple procedure. Lasers and Light in Ophthalmology 1989;2:259.

81. Binder PS, Zavala EY. Why do some epikeratoplasty cases fail? Arch Ophthalmol 1987;105:63–69.

82. Zavala EY, Binder PS, Krumeich J. Laboratory study of freeze and nonfreeze lamellar refractive keratoplasty. Arch Ophthalmol 1987; 105:1125–1128.

83. Binder PS, Zavala EY, Baumgartner SD, et al. Combined morphologic effects of lathing and lyophilization on epikeratoplasty lenticules. Arch Ophthalmol 1986;104:671–679.

84. Krumeich JH, Swinger CA. Nonfreeze epikeratophakia for the correction of myopia. Am J Ophthalmol 1987;103:397–403.

85. Schanzlin DJ, Jester JV, Kay ED. Cryolathe corneal injury. Cornea 1983;2:57.

86. Swinger CA. Keratomileusis for myopia. In: Sanders DR, Hofmann RF, Salz JJ, eds. Refractive corneal surgery. Thorofare, NJ: Slack, Inc., 1986.

87. Swinger CA. Keratophakia and keratomileusis for hyperopia. In: Sanders DR, Hofmann RF, Salz JJ, eds. Refractive corneal surgery. Thorofare, NJ: Slack, Inc., 1986.

88. Swinger CA, Krumeich JH, Cassiday D. Planar lamellar refractive keratoplasty. J Refrac Surg 1986;2:17.

89. Swinger CA, Villasenor RA. Myoptic keratomileusis: evaluation of published results. In: Brightbill FS, ed. Corneal surgery: theory, technique, and tissue. St. Louis: CV Mosby, 1986.

90. Villasenor RA. Homoplastic keratomileusis myopia. In: Sanders DR, Hofmann RF, Salz JJ, eds. Refractive corneal surgery. Thorofare, NJ: Slack, Inc., 1986.

91. Zavala EY, Binder PS, Deg JK, et al. Refractive keratoplasty: lathing and cryopreservation, CLAO J 1985;11:155–162.

92. Maxwell WA, Nordan LT. Optical and wound complications of keratomileusis: incidence and treatment. In: Cavanagh HD, ed. The Cornea-Transactions of the World Congress on the Cornea III. New York: Raven Press, 1988:597.

93. Buratto L, Ferrari M. Retrospective comparison of freeze and non-freeze myopic keratophakia, J Refract Corneal Surg 1989;5:94–99.

94. Schanzlin DJ, Nesburn AB. Refractive keratoplasty. In: Smolin G, Thoft RA, eds. The cornea: scientific foundations and clinical practice. Boston: Little, Brown, 1983.

95. McCarey BE. Synthetic keratophakia: theory and major variables in success or failure. In: Brightbill FS, ed. Corneal surgery: theory, technique, and tissue. St. Louis: CV Mosby, 1986.

96. Lane SS. The current status of polysulfone intracorneal lenses. Paper presented at the XXVI International Congress of Ophthalmology, Singapore, March 18–24, 1990.

97. Serdarevic O, Darrell RW, Krueger R, et al. Excimer laser therapy for experimental *Candida* keratitis. Am J Ophthalmol 1985;90:534–538.

98. Renard G, Hanna K, Saragouss, JJ, et al. Excimer laser experimental keratectomy: an ultrastructural study. Cornea 1987;6:269–272.

99. Hanna K, Chasting JC, Pouliquen Y, et al. A rotating-slit delivery system for excimer laser refractive keratoplasty. Am J Ophthalmol 1987;103:474.

100. McDonald MB, Beverman R, Falzoni W, et al. Refractive surgery with the excimer laser. Am J Ophthalmol 1987;103:469.

101. Pouliquen Y. Wound healing after excimer laser keratomileusis. Paper presented at the International Cornea Laser Society Meeting, Dallas, November 7, 1987.

102. Goodman GL, Trokel SL, Stark WJ, et al. Corneal healing following laser refractive keratectomy. Arch Ophthalmol 1989;107:1799–1803.

103. Hanna KD, Pouliquen Y, Waring GO, et al. Wound healing after excimer laser keratomileusis (photorefractive keratectomy) in monkeys. Arch Ophthalmol 1989;107:895.

104. Fantes F, Hanna KD, Waring GO, et al. Wound healing after excimer laser keratomileusis in monkeys. Arch Ophthalmol 1990;108:665.

105. Waring GO. Development of a system for excimer laser corneal surgery. Trans Am Ophthalmol Soc 1989;LXXXVII:854.

106. Holme RJ, Fouraker BD, Schanzlin OJ. A comparison of en face and tangential wide-area excimer surface ablation in the rabbit. Arch Ophthalmol 1990;108:876–881.

107. Seiler T, Bende T, Matallana M, Wollensak J. Photorefractive keratectomy for hyperopia. Invest Ophthalmol Vis Sci 1990;31:246.

108. McDonald M, Liu J, Andrade H, et al. Clinical results of 193 nm excimer laser central photorefractive keratectomy (PRK) for myopia: the partially sighted and sighted studies. Invest Ophthalmol Vis Sci 1990;31:245.

109. Seiler T, Kahle G, Kriegerowski M. Excimer laser (193 nm) myopic keratomileusis in sighted and blind human eyes. J Refract Corneal Surg 1990;6:165–173.

110. Talamo JH, Gollamudi S, McDonnell PJ, et al. The influence of mitomycin C and corticosteroids on corneal wound healing after excimer laser photoablation. Invest Ophthalmol Vis Sci 1990;31:244.

111. McDonald MB, Kaufman HE, Frantz JM, et al. Excimer laser ablation in a human eye. Arch Ophthalmol 1989;107:1563–1565.

112. Maguire LJ, Zabel RW, Camp J, et al. Raytracing analysis following myopic excimer laser photorefractive keratectomy. Invest Ophthalmol Vis Sci 1990;31:245.

113. Uozato H, Guyton DL: Centering corneal surgical procedures. Am J Ophthalmol 1987;103:264–275.

114. Koester CJ, Roberts CW. Optical zone of the cornea. Invest Ophthalmol Vis Sci 1990;31:481.

115. Hanna KD, Chastang JC, Pouliquen Y, et al. Excimer laser keratectomy for myopia with a rotating-slit delivery system. Arch Ophthalmol 1988;106:245.

116. Rama G, Buratto L, Ferrari M. Keratomileusis by excimer laser. Paper presented at the combined meeting of the International Society for Refractive Keratoplasty and the European Refractive Surgery Society, March 16–17, 1990.

117. Pallikaris I. Laser in situ keratomileusis. Lasers Surg Med 1990;10(5):463–468.

118. Lieurance RC, Patel AC, Wan WL, et al. Excimer laser cut lenticules for epikeratophakia. Am J Ophthalmol 1987;103:475–476.

119. Thompson K, Hanna K, Waring G. Emerging technologies for refractive surgery: laser adjustable synthetic epikeratoplasty. J Refract Corneal Surg 1989;5:46–48.

120. Hays JC, Rowsey JJ. Corneal topography. In: Brightbill FS, ed. Corneal surgery: theory, technique, and tissue. St. Louis: CV Mosby, 1986.

121. Mandelbaum S, Lynn MJ. Theory, case selection, and major variables in success or failure of radial keratotomy. In: Brightbill FS, ed. Corneal surgery: theory, technique, and tissue, St. Louis: CV Mosby, 1986.

122. Rowsey JJ, Balyeat HD, Monlux R, et al. Prospective evaluation of radial keratotomy: photokeratoscope corneal topography. Ophthalmology 1988;95:322–344.

123. Gilbert ML, et al. Hexagonal keratotomy in human cadaver eyes. J Refract Surg 1988;4:12.

124. Geady FJ. Hexagonal keratotomy for corneal steepening, Ophthalmic Surg 1988;19:622–623.

125. Hofmann RF. The surgical correction of idiopathic astigmatism. In: Sanders DR, Hofmann RF, Salz JJ, eds. Refractive corneal surgery. Thorofare, NJ: Slack, Inc., 1986.

126. Lindstrom RL, Lindquist TD. Surgical correction of postoperative astigmatism. Cornea 1988;7:138–148.

127. Duffey RJ, et al. Quantification of paired arcuate keratotomy in human cadaver eye. Invest Ophthalmol Vis Sci 1988;29:392.

128. Forstot SL. Modified relaxing incision technique for postkeratoplasty astigmatism. Cornea 1988;7:133–137.

129. Rubinstein JB, Merck MD, Keys CL. Transverse versus arcuate keratotomy for reduction of astigmatism. Invest Ophthalmol Vis Sci 1988;29:392.

130. Arrowsmith P. Astigmatism correction by paired quantitative T-incisions. In: Brightbill FS, ed. Corneal surgery: theory, technique, and tissue. St. Louis: CV Mosby, 1986.

131. Merck MP, Williams PS, Lindstrom RL. Trapezoidal keratotomy: a vector analysis. Ophthalmology 1986;93:719–726.

132. Terry MA, Rowsey JJ. Dynamic shifts in corneal topography during the modified Ruiz procedure for astigmatism. Arch Ophthalmol 1986; 104:1611–1616.

133. Binder PS. Radial keratotomy in the United States. Arch Ophthalmol 1987;105:37–39.

134. Cross WO, Head WJ III. Complications of radial keratotomy. In: Sanders DR, Hofmann RF, Salz JJ, eds. Refractive corneal surgery. Thorofare, NJ: Slack, Inc., 1986.

135. Hofmann RF, Lindstrom RL. Sources of error in keratotomy knife incision. J Refract Surg 1987;3:215.

136. Arrosmith PN, Marks RG. Visual, refractive, and keratometric results of radial keratotomy. Arch Ophthalmol 1989; 107:506–511.

137. Waring GO, Lynn MJ, Fielding B, et al. Results of the prospective evaluation of radial keratotomy (PERK) study 4 years after surgery for myopia. JAMA 1990;263:1083.

138. Board of Directors of the ISRK Statement on radial keratotomy in 1988. J Refract Surg 1988;4:80.

139. Lynn MJ, Waring GO, Sperduto RD, et al. Factors affecting outcome and predictability of radial keratotomy in the PERK study. Arch Ophthalmol 1987;105:42–51.

140. Lynn M, et al. Prospective evaluation of radial keratotomy (PERK) study: results four years after surgery, Invest Ophthalmol Vis Sci 1988;29:310.

141. Krachmer JH, Fenzl RE. Surgical correction of high postkeratoplasty astigmatism, relaxing incisions vs. wedge resection. Arch Ophthalmol 1980;98:1400.

142. Mandel MR, Shapiro MB, Krachmer JH. Relaxing incisions with augmentation sutures for the correction of post keratoplasty stigmatism. Am J Ophthalmol 1987;103:441–447.

143. Terry MA, Rowsey JJ. Clinical applications of the modified Ruiz procedure for astigmatism. Invest Ophthalmol Vis Sci 1988;29:392.

144. Troutman RC, Swinger C. Relaxing incision for control of postoperative astigmatism following keratoplasty. Ophthalmic Surg 1980; 11:117–120.

145. Villasenor RA, Salz J, Steel D, et al. Changes in corneal thickness during radial keratotomy. Ophthalmic Surg 1981; 12:341–342.

146. Jester JV, Steel D, Salz J, et al. Radial keratotomy in non-human primate eyes. Am J Ophthalmol 1981;92:153.

147. Jester JV, Venet T, Lee J, et al. A statistical analysis of radial keratotomy in human cadaver eyes. Am J Ophthalmol 1981;92:172–177.

148. Salz JJ, et al. Radial keratotomy in fresh human cadaver eyes. Ophthalmology 1981;88:742.

149. Salz JJ, Lee T, Jester JV, et al. Analysis of incision depth following experimental radial keratotomy. Ophthalmology 1983; 90:655–659.

150. Steinert RF, Puliafito CA. Corneal incisions with the excimer laser. In: Sanders DR, Hofmann RF, Salz JJ, eds. Refractive corneal surgery. Thorofare, NJ: Slack, Inc., 1986.

151. Aron-Rosa DS, Boerner CF, Bath D, et al. Corneal wound healing after excimer laser keratotomy in a human eye. Am J Ophthalmol 1987;103:454–464.

152. Aron-Rosa DS, et al. Wound healing following excimer laser radial keratotomy. J Cataract Refract Surg 1988;14:173.

153. Tenner A, et al. Excimer laser radial keratotomy in the living human eye: a preliminary report. J Refract Surg 1988;4:5.

154. Schroder E, Dardenne MV, Neuhann T, et al. An ophthalmic excimer laser for corneal surgery. Am J Ophthalmol 1987;103:472–473.

155. Bansal S, Salz JJ, Tenner A, et al. Clinicopathologic study of healing excimer laser radial excisions. Refract Corneal Surg 1990;6:188.

156. Seiler T, Wollensack J. In vivo experiments with the excimer laser: technical parameters and healing processes. Ophthalmologica 1986;192:65–70.

157. Seiler T, Wollensack J. Zur theorie der T-inzision der kornea. Klin Monatsbl Augenheilkd 1987;191:120–126.

158. Seiler T. Clinical aspects of laser keratectomy, linear and elliptical incisions in the cornea. Paper presented at the Laser Symposium, CLAO-ISRK Annual Meeting, Las Vegas, January 16, 1988.

Acknowledgments

The authors wish to acknowledge the exceptional assistance of Linda Kampley and Elizabeth Mooney.

3

Laser Surgery in Glaucoma

Maurice H. Luntz
Raymond Harrison
Andrea F. Katz

Angle Closure Glaucoma

Laser Peripheral Iridectomy

Peripheral iridectomy by the use of a laser is preferred to invasive surgery because the operation can be performed as an outpatient or office procedure and the globe is not opened surgically. It is indicated in angle closure glaucoma when pupillary block is diagnosed. Apart from acute and chronic angle closure glaucoma, other indications are aphakic and pseudophakic pupillary block; subluxated lens; combined mechanism glaucoma; completion of a previous surgical iridectomy in which the pigment lamina has been retained; nanopthalmos; eyes with anatomically narrow angles when there has been acute angle closure in the fellow eye; and critically narrow angles with iris bombe configuration or plateau iris configuration, especially when a darkroom provocative test is positive. In the latter two groups, prophylactic laser peripheral iridectomy is preferred to long-term miotic therapy, which often fails to prevent chronic angle closure. Only 10% of eyes with narrow angles, however, develop angle closure. Contraindications to laser iridectomy include corneal edema or opacities, hazy anterior chamber, flat anterior chamber, and lack of patient cooperation. It is rarely necessary to resort to opening the eye unless a sector iridectomy is required. An acute attack of angle closure glaucoma should be controlled and terminated by medical therapy and inflammatory reaction eliminated before laser iridectomy is attempted. Two types of laser are currently used for the procedure: the argon and neodymium: yttrium-aluminum-garnet (Nd:YAG). Penetration can be achieved in almost 100% of cases using current techniques with either laser.

Argon Laser Iridectomy

Technique

Pilocarpine 2% is instilled one hour before operation to stretch the iris radial fibers if the pupil is more than 2 mm in diameter. Apraclonidine 1% is also used within one hour preoperatively to prevent or reduce the pressure rise often encountered after laser surgery. In patients with high intraocular pressure (IOP), a carbonic anhydrase inhibitor or hyperosmotic agent may be necessary preoperatively. A modified Goldmann antireflective coated fundus lens with a +66-diopter (D) button (1) or +103-D button (2) is applied to the cornea after the cup is filled with gonioscopic fluid (hydroxypropyl methylcellulose 2.5%) free of air bubbles (Fig. 3.1). The lens:

1. Concentrates the laser energy on the iris
2. Acts as a heat sink and defocuses the beam as it passes through the cornea, thereby minimizing corneal epithelial burns
3. Magnifies the area of iris selected for iridectomy, making it easier to place the burns precisely and to recognize progress, penetration, and completion
4. Obtains adequate exposure of peripheral iris
5. Stabilizes the eye
6. Prevents blinking

The button reduces the power density of the laser beam as it passes through the cornea to one fourth and increases it at the point of photocoagulation on the iris to four times. The beam diameter is doubled at the cornea and is one half that seen at the iris outside the button, thus minimizing corneal burns and anterior chamber reaction. Precision of placement of burns and recognition of the end point—namely, a clear opening through the iris—are aided by the magnification. The lens also stabilizes the eye and acts as a lid speculum.

The procedure is performed under high power (25×). The laser beam is focused to a clear, smallest possible spot. The oculars are adjusted to view the spot parfocally. An optimal site is between 10 and 2 o'clock, about three quarters of the distance from the pupil margin to the iris root, avoiding the 12 o'clock position where obstructive gas bubbles tend to collect. The iridectomy, when completed, should be covered by the upper eyelid. An iris crypt or site of thin stroma is selected. In a blue or lightly pigmented iris, a suitably located iris freckle is sought. We recommend an initial single contraction burn of 250 μm with 0.5 W power setting of 0.2 sec duration, which often facilitates the procedure. This initial burn is referred to as a "hinge."

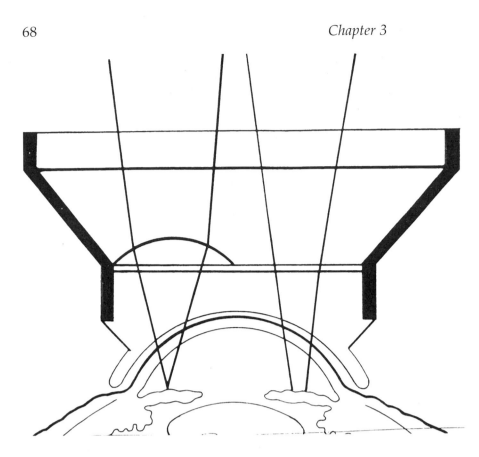

Fig. 3.1 A line drawing of the Abraham lens applied to the cornea for argon laser peripheral iridectomy. The lens concentrates the laser energy on the iris, allows adequate exposure of the peripheral iris, and acts as a lid speculum. The [+]66-D button reduces the power density of the laser beam as it passes through the cornea, thus minimizing corneal burns and anterior chamber reaction. Precision of placement of burns and recognition of the end point—namely, a clear opening through the iris—are aided by the magnification produced by the button.

The spot size is then reduced to 100 or 50 μm and energy levels are increased to 0.75 to 1.5 W for 0.1 to 0.2 sec, depending on iris thickness and color. A rapid sequence of burns is made at the center of the iris crypt or the center of the initial burn. The surgeon should use the lowest energy levels that achieve iris penetration. (This depends on experience with the technique.) It is advisable to aim the laser beam away from the fovea when penetration is achieved. An experienced surgeon burning a lightly pigmented iris may produce an iridectomy using 0.5 W and 0.1 sec duration. Another useful technique is to place a short line of circumferential burns in a "linear incision." The iris dilator muscle assists in separating the pigment lamina. This is applicable with higher power settings in the light iris.

Further application of burns should be stopped if:
1. No visible response occurs
2. The corneal epithelium shows burns (multiple, milky spots on the cornea)
3. Endothelial burns (opacities) are noted
4. The anterior chamber becomes turbid from pigment dispersion
5. 150 burns have been applied at one session

In all these circumstances, a second session is necessary. In most cases (about 80% to 90%), an iridectomy is achieved at the first session.

As penetration of the iris stroma reaches the pigmented epithelium of the iris, bursts of pigment appear in the anterior chamber ("smoke signals"). Power should then be reduced by about 50% because the pigment epithelium is more easily penetrated. With actual penetration, a mushroom cloud of aqueous and pigment ("smoke signal") slowly balloons through the iridectomy site and the peripheral anterior chamber deepens. Gonioscopy at this point reveals a more open angle than apparent prior to iridectomy.

At this time, the iridectomy should be enlarged by treating the pigment epithelium ("chipping away") at the margins of the opening with the same settings, or the spot size may be increased to 100 μm. Loose pigment inside the iridectomy and residual strands of iris stroma running across the center of the iridectomy should be eliminated if possible.

Confirmation of a Patent Iridectomy

Patency of the iridectomy is checked at the end of the procedure by noting a red reflex in the iridectomy on retroillumination and by viewing lens capsule on direct slit-lamp examination. A considerable amount of pigment may be seen in the anterior chamber at the end of the procedure. This absorbs rapidly and rarely causes any problems.

Postoperative Care

Apraclonidine 1% is instilled again at the end of the procedure. The patient should be detained in the office for at least 2 hours postoperatively to check the IOP; and gonioscopy is done to ensure that the angle is open. If the pressure is elevated, appropriate medication is given to reduce the pressure before the patient is released. In addition, prednisolone 1%, one drop q2h, is given until bedtime. The patient is examined the following morning, when visual activity is measured and examination by slit-lamp biomicroscopy and tonometry are performed.

Complications

Complications are few and usually not serious. A mild iritis rarely lasts beyond the day of surgery. Topical steroid drops (prednisolone 1%) given q2h until bedtime usually suffices. Cycloplegics are rarely necessary but posterior synechiae may develop if the iritis is unusually severe. Pupil distortion is insignificant, and pigment dispersion is transitory. Localized subcapsular opacification of the lens at the site of iridectomy does not spread. Cataract progression after laser iridectomy is seen very occasionally in elderly patients. Corneal epithelial burns resolve in one to two days. Endothelial cell damage is not reversible but usually remains localized and corneal decompensation is rare. Epithelial and endothelial burns reduce the clarity of the cornea and prevent the laser beam from reaching the iris. Oblique angling of the beam to avoid the corneal burns may enable the surgeon to complete the procedure. A new site may have to be chosen using reduced power and duration settings. Pigment proliferation can close the iridectomy in one to 6 weeks and occasionally after a much longer period. This is much less likely to occur if the original iridectomy is large enough, preferably at least 200 μm. Reopening the iridectomy is usually readily accomplished with relatively few burns. Retinal burns have been reported but are only serious if the macular area is involved. This complication can be avoided by appropriate aiming of the laser beam. The chief postoperative problem is a common transient rise of IOP within hours. Pressure levels may reach 40 mm Hg or more. Appropriate preventive measures and timely medical therapy almost always suffice to abort this elevated IOP.

Neodymium: YAG Laser Iridectomy

The Nd:YAG laser may be used in either the Q-switched short-pulsed (3) or mode-locked (4) forms. The infrared beam acts as a photodisruptor and is effective with extremely high energy and very short pulse duration. The iris pigmentation is not a relevant factor. Careful focusing of the microexplosion is critical. The laser beam should be precisely focused just within the iris stromal surface. A peripheral site is selected to minimize the risk of lens damage. Initially 2 to 4 pulses per burst at 2 to 4 mJ is suggested for multiple bursts. With a single burst, 8 mJ is usually adequate. A minor iris hemorrhage may be seen, but this is

usually self-limited. If the iris is vascularized, pretreatment at the chosen site with argon laser will prevent bleeding. The lens capsule is not seen at the end point and transillumination is not always detected. The Nd·YAG iridectomy is usually very small, but it should not be enlarged with repeated shots because of danger to the lens. The Nd:YAG laser is preferred with a very light blue iris where argon laser is often insufficient. A very thick brown iris is also more easily penetrated. The exceedingly short time needed for delivery of the laser energy is an advantage with patients who are unable to keep still enough for argon laser treatment. The contact lens used is the "Lasag, Chi 1" iris lens or an equivalent. Preoperative preparation and postoperative care are similar to that described for argon laser iridectomy.

Argon Laser Iridoplasty Peripheral Iris Contraction

The angle can be widened by application of a ring of burns to the extreme periphery of the iris (Fig. 3.2). This procedure is particularly useful as an immediate prelude to argon laser trabeculoplasty when there is limited appositional closure or an anatomically narrow angle. In plateau iris syndrome, the angle remains closed or closable after peripheral iridectomy has eliminated any pupillary block component. Iridoplasty, either combined with the peripheral iridectomy or done later, may be valuable if not always permanently effective. Ciliolenticular block glaucoma, lens-induced glaucoma, and anterior lens displacement following ciliary body swelling due to scleral buckling or panretinal photocoagulation have all been reported to respond to iridoplasty. Nanophthalmos is a classical indication for iridoplasty because appositional closure is prone to occur despite laser peripheral iridectomy. Medically unbreakable attacks of acute angle closure glaucoma can sometimes be successfully alleviated by iridoplasty if extensive peripheral anterior synechiae have not formed (5).

Technique

Miosis is obtained with pilocarpine 2%. Proparacaine 0.5% is instilled. A Goldmann goniolens is not routinely needed but is useful for peripheral placement of burns. Settings are 300 to 500 μm spot size, 200 to 400 mW power and 0.5 sec initially for direct placement of contraction burns with an Abraham lens. Lower power is selected for darkly pigmented irides and higher power for light ones. After the first burns, the power is adjusted to obtain a stromal burn, which is just enough to open the adjacent angle. Shrinkage of tissue is seen immediately by the surgeon. Deep burns of the iris should be avoided. Approximately six to eight spots per quadrant usually suffice. The minimum number necessary are placed to obtain adequate opening of the angle (see Fig. 3.2).

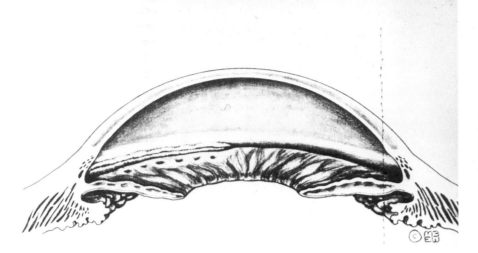

Fig. 3.2 A line drawing of the anterior chamber angle shows the effect of argon laser iridoplasty in the peripheral iris. One half of the peripheral iris has been treated with laser burns, showing shrinkage of the tissue opening the angle. In the other half of the iris periphery, the iris shows a bombe configuration, and the angle structures are obscured.

Where a Goldmann goniolens is used to facilitate placing peripheral burns, the beam strikes the iris much more tangentially and diffusely. Accordingly, higher power is required to produce stretch burns. We generally use a mirrored goniolens. Retreatment is sometimes required.

Complications

Complications are minimal. Mild iritis usually responds to topical steroids. Corneal endothelial burns, which are apt to occur when the anterior chamber is very shallow, do not usually affect corneal integrity. A transient rise of IOP is usually not severe, if it does occur.

Open Angle Glaucoma

Argon Laser Trabeculoplasty

Treatment of open angle glaucoma has been greatly improved by the widespread adoption of argon laser trabeculoplasty (ALT) in the past decade following the convincing work of Wise and colleagues (2). They applied 100 burns of 50 μm aperture at 1000 mW power for 0.1 sec to the trabecular meshwork for 360°. The theory was postulated that the focal superficial burns caused shrinkage of collagen, thereby tightening the ring of trabecular meshwork and opening up drainage spaces. The exact mechanism may be less simplistic. Tonographic studies have shown an increase in outflow facility following ALT. In open angle glaucoma, 70% to 80% of eyes respond favorably. Medical therapy is not usually reduced as a result of ALT. The average reduction of pressure has been estimated at 7 to 10 mm Hg. There is now extensive literature on variations of techniques and results. Successful pressure lowering is not usually permanent and fails in about 10% of eyes per annum.

Indications

When the IOP is not adequately lowered on medical therapy, ALT is performed. We generally exclude carbonic anhydrase inhibitors from this regimen in considering whether to proceed to ALT. Compliance with medical therapy is often unsatisfactory. The high prevalence of side effects and possible damage to trabecular meshwork and conjunctiva from topically administered drugs are additional reasons for a trend to earlier intervention with ALT. It is doubtful whether ALT may have a deleterious effect on the results of subsequent trabeculectomy surgery. The trend is toward less than maximum tolerated topical medical therapy and earlier intervention with ALT. Its use as primary therapy is not established, but it is being more widely accepted.

Technique

Clear media and a cooperative patient are prerequisites for performing ALT. The usual medical regimen is administered. One drop of 1% apraclonidine is administered one hour before ALT is carried out. In patients who have advanced visual field loss, a hyperosmotic agent may also be given beforehand to minimize or prevent a postoperative IOP rise. A Goldmann three-mirror antireflective coated goniolens is used. The 59° angled dome-shaped mirror is selected. Alternatively, the Ritch lens provides two sets of mirrors, one inclined at 59° for viewing the inferior angle and one at 64° for the superior angle. One mirror of each set has a magnifying button to produce ×14 magnification and reduce the spot size from 50 to 35 μm (5). Precise binocular focusing is essential. Comfortable elbow supports for the surgeon facilitate accuracy in performing the procedure. Blue-green wavelengths are chosen.

Laser burns are placed at equal intervals on the anterior portion of the trabecular meshwork including the anterior edge of the adjacent pigment line (Fig. 3.3). The laser is set at 50 μm, 750 mW, and 0.1 sec. Power is adjusted upward to produce blanching of the pigment zone. The power should not exceed 1200 mW. Very small gas bubbles are acceptable, but it is better to slightly reduce power (Fig. 3.4). Large bubbles indicate excessive treatment power. More power is needed for lightly pigmented angles and less power for heavily pigmented angles. With the mirror at the 12 o'clock position, the inferior angle is visualized, moving clockwise to treat the inferotemporal quadrant of the right eye and counterclockwise for the left eye. The temporal 180° may be treated or the inferior 180° may be treated if the superior angle is not accessible. Fifty spots are evenly placed. Limiting one session of treatment to 180° reduces the postoperative reaction and IOP rise. It is probably not necessary to proceed to treat the remaining 180° if the initial response is entirely satisfactory at 6 weeks. Untreated angle is thus held in reserve and may not need to be exploited for months or years. Apraclonidine 1% is again instilled at the end of the procedure. Pressures are taken at one and 2 hours and if there has been no IOP elevation at 2 hours, the patient may be allowed to leave. Postoperative treatment is with topical prednisolone 1% one drop q.i.d. for 5 days. The patient is reexamined the morning after ALT, again after one week, 3 weeks, and 6 weeks. The response may take 3 to 6 weeks to become established. A second session of 180° may be necessary at that time.

Results are less favorable in aphakic eyes, and posterior pseudophakic eyes tend to react less well than phakic eyes. It is advisable whenever possible to carry out ALT before cataract surgery, rather than afterward, unless a combined trabeculectomy with cataract extraction is the procedure of choice. Eyes with pre-ALT pressures above 35 to 40 mm Hg are not usually controlled. The fall of pressure is optimal when pre-ALT pressures are 22 to 35 mm Hg. With pressures below the high teens, ALT has little pressure-lowering effect. Older patients generally respond better than young patients. Congenital/infantile/juvenile glaucoma, secondary glaucoma due to uveitis, and Iridocorneal Endothelial (ICE) syndrome do not respond well. Pseudoexfoliation glaucoma is very responsive but prone to late sudden loss of control. Pigmentary glaucoma also does as well initially as primary open angle glaucoma, but the failure rate is higher after several years.

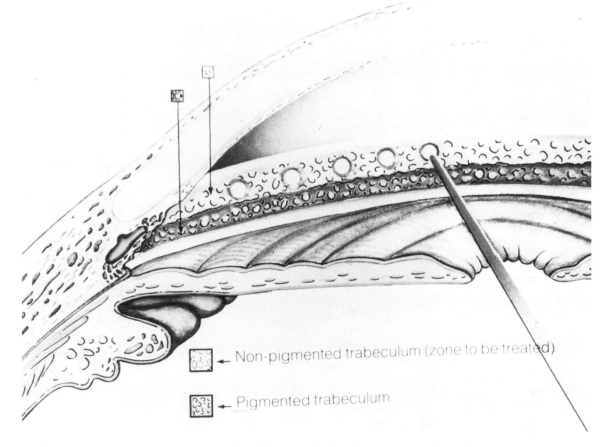

← Non-pigmented trabeculum (zone to be treated)

← Pigmented trabeculum

Fig. 3.3 The sapphire-tipped probe of the CW contact Nd:YAG laser (Surgical Laser Technologies, Inc.) is applied to the conjunctival surface 1mm from the limbus. The HeNe beam is visible in the photograph.

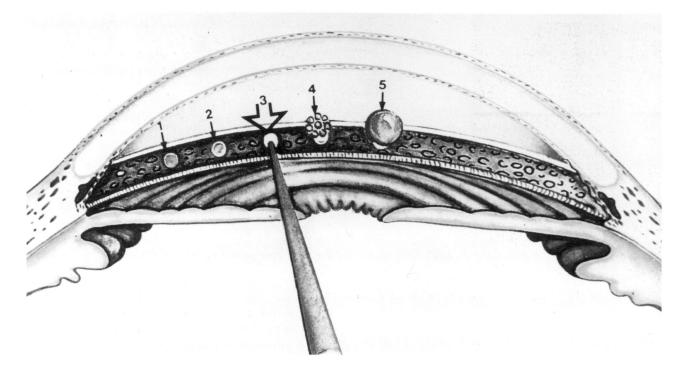

Fig. 3.4 The laser probe is advanced subconjunctivally and placed tangential to the limbus before the laser is activated. The HeNe beam is visible in the photograph.

Complications

The chief complication of ALT is a postoperative pressure rise that is manifested in 2 to 3 hours and is usually transient. The rise is frequently less than 10 mm Hg but may be over 20 mm Hg. Apraclonidine 1% usually prevents this complication. The postoperative pressure spike is much less likely when prophylactic medical measures are taken as well as treating only 180° of angle with accurate placement of burns on the pigment line and immediately adjacent anterior trabecular meshwork. Iritis is usually mild and rapidly resolves. It is rarely seen when topical steroids are used routinely. Localized bleeding at the site of a burn in the trabecular meshwork or into Schlemm's canal sometimes occurs. It is rapidly self-limited and requires no treatment, or simple photocoagulation if the source is identifiable. Burns that are misplaced posteriorly can result in peripheral anterior synechiae (see Fig. 3.4). A sustained rise has been estimated to occur in 1.5% to 2% of ALT procedures, sometimes necessitating a trabeculectomy. A precariously vulnerable visual field may show sudden deterioration unless the postoperative IOP rise is prevented. Corneal epithelial burns, often forming a semicircle, disappear overnight. Endothelial damage is rare.

An alarming though infrequent complication is syncope. This should be anticipated so that quick action can be taken to prevent the patient from falling to the floor and sustaining head or bodily injury.

Other Anterior Segment Laser Procedures for Glaucoma

Transpupillary Argon Laser Ciliophotocoagulation

Transpupillary argon laser ciliophotocoagulation is useful in aphakic eyes that have a sector iridectomy or give access to at least 18 ciliary processes when the pupil is fully dilated. The laser settings are 100 to 200 μm, 0.2 sec, and 750 to 1000 mW. The power is adjusted to create whitening and shriveling of the ciliary processes (Fig. 3.5). Postoperative steroids are used as with ALT. The results are not always sufficient to control the glaucoma, but some pressure lowering is often achieved. This procedure may be combined with ALT when less than 180° of angle is available.

Laser Pupilloplasty (Photomydriasis)

Extreme miotic pupils may sometimes be enlarged by argon laser burns applied around the pupil border to contract the iris. Two concentric circles of burns are placed on the sphincter. Settings are 200 μm for the inner ring and 500 μm for the outer ring at 250 to 750 mW for 0.2 sec. An

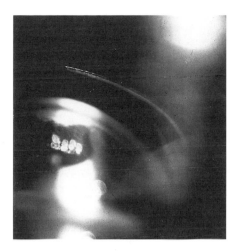

Fig. 3.5 Photograph of an eye shows the effects of transpupillary argon laser ciliophotocoagulation, which has created whitening and shriveling of the ciliary processes within the iridectomy.

alternative technique is to apply radially placed burns at similar settings, overlying the sphincter. We have found the latter method to be more effective.

Goniophotocoagulation

Neovascularization of the angle has been treated with some success by direct argon laser photocoagulation of blood vessels (6). This technique is applicable when discrete vessels are found bridging the angle and running onto the iris. Recurrent bleeding into the anterior chamber from trabeculectomy sites can also be effectively stopped by goniophotocoagulation. The settings are 100 μm spot size, 200 to 600 mW for 0.2 sec.

Reopening for Failing Drainage Sites

Pigmented tissue, such as an iris pillar that is blocking a trabeculectomy cleft, can be photocoagulated with the argon laser. A Goldmann three-mirror lens is used. Settings are 50 to 100 μm, 800 to 1200 mW at 0.1 sec.

An obstructed filtering site in which nonpigmented tissue is visible can be treated transcamerally with the Nd:YAG laser. A reactive pressure rise may be pronounced and last for days or even one to 2 weeks. Settings are 5 to 10 mJ. Successful results are sometimes obtained, but this procedure has not proven gratifying in our experience. The roles of the Nd:YAG laser and the excimer laser have not yet been defined in trabeculectomy and sclerostomy for outflow blockage.

Suture Lysis

Trabeculectomy scleral flap sutures can be severed by argon laser burns. Settings are 50 to 100 μm spot size, 600 to 1000 mW for 0.1 to 0.2 sec. This maneuver is useful within one week of filtering surgery to release a tightly sutured scleral flap and allow freer drainage from the anterior chamber to the subconjunctival space. The procedure is facilitated by compressing the overlying conjunctiva with a Hoskins laser lens designed for this purpose or by using the periphery of the cup of Zeiss goniolens. Preliminary instillation of a drop of 2.5% phenylephrine will constrict the overlying conjunctival vessels. By such means, the underlying suture is visualized. Multiple sutures should not be severed at one session. No definitive evidence indicates that the long-term results of trabeculectomy are significantly improved by suture lysis.

Laser Cyclophotocoagulation

Since its introduction by Bietti in 1950 (7), cyclocryotherapy (CCT) has been a mainstay in the treatment of refractory glaucomas. IOP is lowered by thermal destruction of aqueous-producing ciliary body tissue across an intact sclera. However, significant postoperative complication rates including phthisis and visual loss have generally limited use of CCT to eyes that have failed or are considered likely to fail standard filtration surgery.

The use of laser as an alternative means of performing ciliablative surgery was introduced by Beckman and colleagues in 1972 (8,9). Compared to freezing, focused laser energy applied transsclerally would theoretically reduce adjacent tissue destruction and minimize inflammatory sequelae. After initial work with the ruby laser, the more readily available Nd:YAG laser soon attracted the interest of investigators. The infrared (1064 nm) Nd:YAG laser operating in the thermal mode has much better scleral transmission than do lasers emitting shorter wavelengths (10–12). Early rabbit studies using Nd:YAG transscleral cyclophotocoagulation (CPC) showed effective reduction of IOP (10,11).

Histologic studies on rabbit (10,11) and human enucleated eyes (13,14) show selective destruction of ciliary processes sparing the overlying ciliary muscle, sclera, and conjunctiva. Compared to CCT, Nd:YAG CPC shows less ciliary body necrosis and less postoperative inflammation in rabbits (15). Two methods have been developed for performing Nd:YAG CPC: noncontact and contact.

Noncontact Nd:YAG laser (Lasag Microruptor 2, Thun, Switzerland) operating in the pulsed free-running thermal modes uses a slit-lamp delivery system. Retrobulbar anesthesia is required. Optimum focus of the helium-neon (HeNe) aiming beam is 1.5 mm from the limbus (16). The offset dial on the laser is set at 9, serving to defocus laser energy 3.6 mm behind the sclera into the ciliary body. Using a short 20-msec pulse and high energy 1.8 to 8.2 J, 32 to 40 shots are placed circumferentially around the eye (17–20). Raised white conjunctival lesions appear at the laser burn sites. Clinical studies of noncontact Nd:YAG CPC show success rates, including retreatments, of 48% to 86% (17–20). However, risk of serious complications is high, including a 40% incidence of moderate to severe pain (19), a 10.7% incidence of phthisis, a 30% incidence of visual loss (18), intense inflammation with hypopyon, cataract, vitreous hemorrhage (20), flat anterior chamber with choroidal detachment (21), focal scleral thinning (22), and one reported case of sympathetic ophthalmia (23).

The continuous wave (CW) contact Nd:YAG laser (Surgical Laser Technologies, Inc., Malverin, PA) introduced by Federman and colleagues (24) in 1987 uses a fiber-optic delivery system with a 600-μm quartz optical cable attached to a 2.2-mm diameter synthetic sapphire-tipped hand-held probe. By eliminating laser transmission through air, the efficiency of energy delivery is increased because of diminished backscatter of radiation (25). Investigators hoped that by possibly reducing the total energy required for cilioablation, there would be less adjacent tissue damage and fewer postoperative complications. Compared to noncontact Nd:YAG CPC, the contact laser uses a much longer exposure time, resulting in much less power delivered per pulse. Each pulse of noncontact laser delivers 90 to 400 W of power (1.8 to 8.2 J over 20 msec) compared to 5 to 9 W (3.5 to 6.3 J over 0.7 sec) with the contact laser. In rabbits, longer laser exposure resulted in less explosion effects on ocular tissue (26).

Technique

Preoperatively, all glaucoma medications are continued. Very high IOP is reduced with topical Iopidine or intravenous mannitol. Retrobulbar anesthesia is required. Protective eyewear is worn by all operating room personnel.

The fiberoptic quartz cable is calibrated and checked for transmission greater than 70%. The synthetic sapphire tip is attached to the hand-held probe. With the patient in the supine position, a lid speculum is inserted and the fellow eye is patched. Laser parameters, established by Gina Gladstein, MD (personal communication), are 5 W power, 0.7 sec, air blow, pulse mode. Allingham and coworkers (25) established that optimum probe placement is 2 mm from the limbus, so the anterior edge of the probe tip (2.2 mm diameter) should be placed 1 mm from the limbus. The probe is applied perpendicular to the scleral surface, with gentle compression of the overlying conjunctiva (Fig. 3.6). The 3 and 9 o'clock positions are spared to avoid the long posterior ciliary arteries. The number of laser applications is titrated according to the preoperative IOP level. For first laser treatment, 55 burns are applied for IOP less than 30 mm Hg, 75 burns for IOP 30 to 40 mm Hg, and 90 burns for IOP greater than 40 mm Hg. For retreatments, 15 fewer burns are applied for each different preoperative IOP level (Gina Gladstein, MD, personal communication). Postoperatively, all glaucoma medications are continued. Prednisolone acetate 1% is added q2h for the first day, and then q.i.d. for several weeks until inflammation subsides. IOP should be checked at one hour, one day, one week. Laser treatment may be repeated more than once if no clinical response is seen after 1 to 4 weeks.

Midterm success rates of contact Nd:YAG CPC, including retreatments, are similar to CCT and noncontact Nd:YAG CPC. Schuman and colleagues (27) report a 65% success (3 to 22 mm) in 116 eyes after a minimum of one year follow-up. Gladstein and coworkers (personal communication) report a 70% success (5 to 22 mm Hg drop in IOP) in 72 eyes followed for a mean of 12.5 months. Complication rates with contact Nd:YAG CPC are, however,

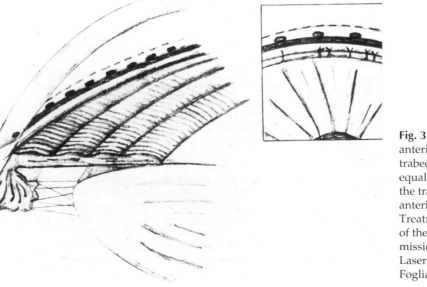

Fig. 3.6 A line drawing representing the anterior chamber angle shows argon laser trabeculoplasty. Laser burns are placed at equal intervals on the anterior portion of the trabecular meshwork, including the anterior edge of the adjacent pigment line. Treatment is usually performed over 180° of the inferior angle. (Reproduced by permission from Buratto L, Ricci A, Vitali D. Laser microsurgery of glaucoma. Milan: Fogliazza.)

far less than with the other modalities of ciliodestructive surgery. In the immediate postoperative period, there is significantly less pain and inflammation (21). There is also a decreased incidence of complications in the late postoperative period. Gladstein and coworkers report a 1% incidence of hypotony and a 7% rate of visual loss of more than two lines of Snellen acuity. Schuman and colleagues report an 8.5% incidence of hypotony, and a 41% loss of vision; however, much higher laser power of 7 to 9 W was used in their study group (28).

In conclusion, Nd:YAG CPC is an effective alternative to CCT. The contact method is preferred because of the decreased rate of serious complications compared to both CCT and noncontact Nd:YAG CPC. Current indications for treatments are eyes with refractory glaucoma on maximal tolerated medical therapy that have failed or are considered likely to fail standard filtration surgery. Included are eyes with neovascular glaucoma, aphakia, pseudophakia, uveitis, congenital or juvenile glaucoma, scleral buckle, penetrating keratoplasty, and blind eyes with intractable pain. Recently, indications for performing contact Nd:YAG CPC are expanding as complication rates continue to remain very low. Although CCT has usually been reserved as the treatment of last resort, contact Nd:YAG CPC can be used to treat selected eyes that would otherwise undergo invasive filtration surgery.

Holmium Laser Sclerostomy

The formation of a scleral fistula using laser energy is presently being investigated as an alternative to the trabeculectomy procedure. Some of the advantages of laser sclerostomy include a decreased risk of complications from surgery—in particular, a decreased risk of postoperative flat chamber or suprachoroidal hemorrhage because of the smaller ostium formed by the laser, and a decreased risk of bleb failure from conjunctival scarring by minimizing or eliminating conjunctival dissection. The procedure is easy to perform more than once in the same eye.

Laser sclerostomy can be performed *ab externo* or *ab interno*. The authors prefer the *ab externo* approach because it can be performed with minimal instrumentation and invasion of the anterior chamber. Laser *ab interno* sclerostomy requires passing a laser probe across the anterior chamber into contact with the angle structures through a small corneal or limbal incision. Laser energy is then delivered within the anterior chamber using either CW Nd:YAG (32–34), YAG (32-34) excimer (35), or high-powered argon lasers. An alternative method of delivery is by channeling laser energy through a gonioscopy lens to the anterior chamber. Enhancement of the laser energy is achieved by staining the sclera at the intended sclerostomy site with 1% methylene blue by iontophoresis while the laser is tuned to emit close to the 668-nm absorption peak of the dye (31).

In the *ab externo* procedure, the fistula is created from the subconjunctival side by means of a fiberoptic probe in contact with the sclera or cornea, which is introduced through a small conjunctival incision in the fornix. Currently, the holmium:YAG, erbium:YAG, and excimer lasers are being used for this technique. The holmium laser is the only one presently approved by the Food and Drug Administration for this purpose, clinical experience has been greatest with the chromium-sensitized thulium, holmium-doped yttrium, argon, and garnet lasers (THC-YAG), coupled to a quartz fiberoptic probe. The most widely used holmium laser is the Model gLASE 210, manufactured by Sunrise Technologies, Inc., Fremont, CA. The laser emits at 2100 nm, a wavelength highly absorbed by water, has a 200-μm spot size, pulses at 5 Hz, and has a maximal output of 350 mJ. The fiberoptic probe is so designed that the laser energy is delivered at approximately 90° to the fiber axis. Thus, with the probe applied to the sclera, laser energy is emitted into the anterior chamber. A HeNe beam is used to focus. The laser unit is compact and portable and operates on standard household current (Fig. 3.7).

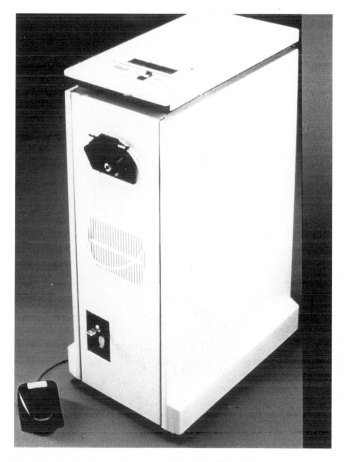

Fig. 3.7 The holmium laser, model gLASE 210 (Sunrise Technologies, Inc., Fremont, CA). The laser is compact and easily portable.

Surgical Technique

Retrobulbar anesthesia is necessary. A 19-gauge hyperdermic needle is introduced through the conjunctiva into the subconjunctival space approximately 8 to 10 mm from the site of laser sclerostomy. The needle is attached to a syringe filled with 2% Xylocaine local anesthetic. The needle is advanced under the conjunctiva toward the limbus, injecting Xylocaine ahead of it to form a track, until the limbus is reached. At that point, a crescent-shaped dissecting knife (Alcon) is introduced along the track to the limbus, and the dissection is commenced at the limbus into the cornea, fashioning a corneal pocket approximately one third of the thickness through the cornea and extending about 1 mm into the cornea. The probe is then inserted through the conjunctival opening into the conjunctival track and advanced to the limbus and into the corneal pocket, so that the probe straddles the cornea and adjacent limbus (Fig. 3.8). With the probe applied to the deep surface of the corneal pocket, the HeNe beam should be aimed into the anterior chamber well anterior to the iris root. The laser is set at 140 mJ for 40 burns. During the procedure, bubbles will be seen entering the anterior chamber as the sclerostomy is completed. Such penetration is usually achieved after about 15 pulses. Additional pulses are delivered until a total of 25-40 pulses is achieved. During the procedure, the conjunctival surface overlying the probe is constantly bathed in salt solution to diminish any heat produced by the probe. At the end of the procedure, the anterior chamber will shallow considerably, corneal striae are visible, and the eye is hypotonic. The probe is then removed and an air syringe with cannula is used to introduce Healon into the anterior chamber through a previously performed paracentesis opening in the cornea. The chamber is deepened with Healon, and the conjunctival opening can then be closed with a single 10-0 nylon suture. In high-risk eyes, adjunctive 5-fluorouracil (5-FU) or mitomycin C is given. This creates a white, diffuse bleb (Fig. 3.9). The internal osteum is visible on gonioscopy (Fig. 3.10).

The major complications of holmium sclerostomy—conjunctival burns at the limbus (avoided by copious conjunctival irrigation with salt solution), flat anterior chamber, iris incarceration in the fistula, and choroidal hemorrhage—are avoided by the insufflation of Healon into the anterior chamber at the end of the procedure, and by ensuring that the sclerostomy is performed well anterior to the iris root.

Hoskins and colleagues (29) reported a 60% success rate after 6 months in a pilot study of 21 eyes. The authors have operated on 17 eyes followed for 2 years, with a success rate of 52%. These eyes all had severe glaucoma, and at least one and, in most patients, two filtering procedures had failed to control IOP.

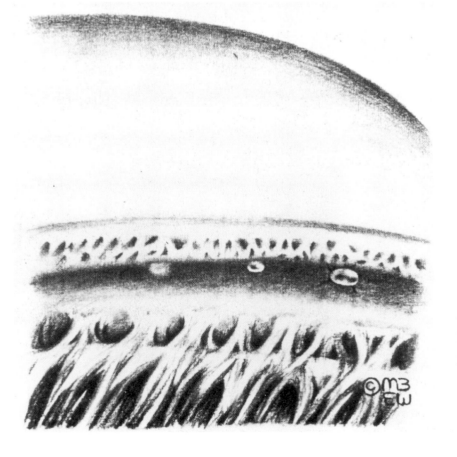

Fig. 3.8 A line drawing of the anterior chamber angle shows incorrect placement of laser burns on the pigmented ciliary band. Burns placed in this manner may result in peripheral anterior synechiae, hemorrhage, and uveitis. The laser burns are excessive, and large gas bubbles have formed. (Reproduced by permission from Buratto L, Ricci A, Vitali D. Laser microsurgery of glaucoma. Milan: Fogliazzo.)

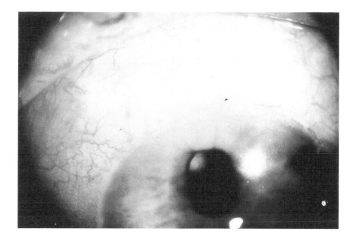

Fig. 3.9 Postlaser sclerostomy bleb following adjunctive 5-FU injections, creating a white, diffuse bleb.

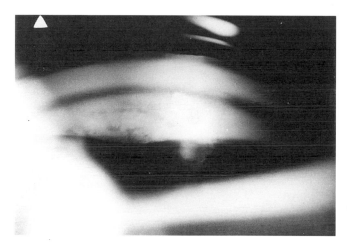

Fig. 3.10 The internal ostium is visible on gonioscopy, surrounded by iris pigment and indentation of the peripheral iris surface at the site of the sclerostomy (Holmium laser sclerostomy).

In the *ab interno* approach to laser sclerostomy, the fistula is created from within the anterior chamber. Either a noncontact slit-lamp/gonioscopy lens delivery system or a fiberoptic delivery system with contact probe can be used. In 1986, Latina and coworkers (30) introduced dye-enhanced scleral ablation using a microsecond pulsed-dye laser. Laser energy is delivered by slit lamp. The sclera is stained at the intended sclerostomy site with 1% methylene blue noninvasively by iontophoresis. The laser is tuned to emit close to the 668-nm absorption peak of the dye, allowing for scleral perforation at reduced energy levels. In rabbits, full-thickness sclerostomies were achieved in 50% of eyes after an average of 12 laser pulses with 20-msec pulse, 100 to 150 mJ, and 200 μm spot size (31). Pilot clinical trials are currently underway. It appears that complete staining of the sclera is critical to successful laser treatment. Because of uneven uptake of methylene

blue, there is currently investigation into using alternative dyes for scleral enhancement.

Fiberoptic *ab interno* sclerostomy is performed by passing a laser probe across the anterior chamber into contact with angle structures, through a small corneal or limbal incision. Investigation using the continuous wave Nd:YAG, excimer, and high-powered Nd:YAG lasers are underway. The infrared-emitting contact Nd:YAG laser creates thermal sclerostomies by hemostatic cutting. Higginbotham and colleagues (33) showed a statistically increased bleb survival in rabbits with laser sclerostomy performed with a synthetic sapphire-tipped Nd:YAG laser compared to standard external thermal sclerostomy. Human trials are still in early phases.

Diode Lasers

The infrared-emitting (810 nm) semiconductor diode laser has several appealing characteristics that have attracted its use in ophthalmology. The laser is compact, portable, and air cooled; it uses standard household current, and has a long operational life with low cost maintenance. Recent models have been developed with high-power output enabling its use for performing iridotomy, trabeculoplasty, and transcleral CPC (Fig. 3.11).

The diode laser produces iridotomies by photocoagulation with absorption of energy by melanin resulting in local thermal damage (36). The technique is similar to that used with the argon laser, with slit-lamp delivery system and Wise or Abraham contact lens. Laser parameters for the penetrating burns are 75 to 100 μm spot size, 700 to

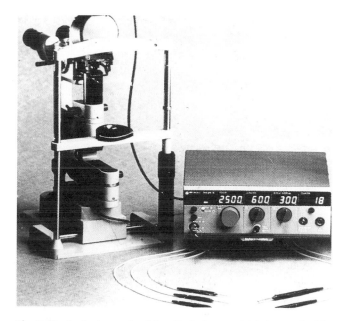

Fig. 3.11 A photograph of the diode laser, which is attached by a fiberoptic cable to a slit lamp. The various probes can be attached to the laser, as shown. The laser body is small, lightweight, and easily portable.

1000 mW of power, and 0.05 to 0.2 sec exposure (37,38). Complications include transient corneal endothelial and focal lens burns, as well as pupillary distortion (38). Diode laser trabeculoplasty (DL T) is performed with a slit-lamp delivery system and gonioscopy lens. A pilot study by McHugh and colleagues (39) on 20 human eyes achieved a mean 9.5 mm Hg IOP reduction at 6 months with no significant complications, using 100 μm spot size, 800 to 1200 mW of power, 0.2 sec exposure. Another study by Brancato and coworkers (40) comparing the efficacy of DLT to ALT showed no significant differences.

The use of the diode laser for transscleral CPC is under current investigation. The laser has good scleral transmission and better melanin absorption compared to the longer wavelength Nd:YAG laser (41). Similar ciliary body lesions are produced by both diode and Nd:YAG CPC (42–44), and similar IOP reduction is achieved in rabbits (44). Results from human clinical trials using a noncontact slit-lamp delivery system as well as a contact fiberoptic system are still preliminary.

References

1. Abraham RK, Munnerlyn C. Laser iridotomy. Improved methodology with a new iridotomy lens. Ophthalmology 1979;86(suppl):126.
2. Wise JB, Munnerlyn C, Erickson MS. A high-efficiency laser iridotomysphincterotomy lens. AJO 1986;101:533–546.
3. Fankhauser F, Kwasniewska S. Nd:yttrium; garnet laser. In: L'Esperance F, ed. Ophthalmic Lasers, 3d ed. St. Louis: CV Mosby, 1986:781–886.
4. Aron-Rosa D, Aron JJ, Grieseman M, Thuzel R. Use of the neodymium YAG laser to open the posterior capsule after lens implant surgery: a preliminary report. Am Intraocular Implant Soc J 1980;6:352.
5. Ritch R. Nd:YAG laser treatment for medically unresponsive attacks of angle-closure glaucoma. Am J Ophthalmol 1966; 62:507–509.
6. Simmons RJ, Depperman SR, Ducker DK. The role of goniophotocoagulation of the anterior chamber angle. Ophthalmology 1980;87:79.
7. Bietti G. Surgical intervention on the ciliary body: new trends for the relief of glaucoma. JAMA 1950;142:889.
8. Beckman H, Kinoshita A, Rota A. Transscleral ruby laser irradiation of the ciliary body in the treatment of intractable glaucoma. Trans Am Acad Ophthalmol Otolaryngol 1972;76:423.
9. Beckman H, Sugar HS. Neodymium laser cyclophotocoagulation. Arch Ophthalmol 1973;90:27.
10. Wilensky JT, Welch D, Mirolovich M. Transcleral cyclophotocoagulation using a Nd:YAG laser. Ophthalmic Surg 1985;16:95.
11. Devenyi RG, Trope GE, Hunter WH. Nd:YAG transscleral cyclocoagulation in rabbit eyes. Br J Ophthalmol 1987;71:441.
12. Fankhauser F, Van der Zypen E, Kwasniewska S, Roe P, England C. Transsceleral cyclophotocoagulation using an Nd:YAG laser. Ophthalmic Surg 1986;17:94.
13. Shields SM, Stevens JL, Rass MA, Smith ME. Histopathologic findings after Nd:YAG transscleral cyclophotocoagulation. Am J Ophthalmol 1988;106:100.
14. Blasini M, Simmons R, Shields MO. Early tissue response to transscleral Nd:YAG cyclophotocoagulation. Invest Ophthalmol Vis Sci 1990;31:1114.
15. Harrison M, Higginbotham EJ, Zou X, et al. A comparative study of contact transscleral Nd:YAG laser cyclophotocoagulation versus cyclocryotherapy in rabbits. Invest Ophthalmol Vis Sci 1989;30(suppl):30–34.
16. Hampton C, Shields MB. Transscleral Nd:YAG cyclophotocoagulation. A histologic study of human eyes. Arch Ophthalmol 1988;106:1121.
17. Klapper RM, Wandel T, Donnenfeld E, Perry HD. Transscleral Nd:YAG thermal cyclophotocoagulation in refractory glaucoma: a preliminary report. Ophthalmology 1988; 95:719.
18. Trope GE. Mid-term effects of Nd:YAG transscleral cyclo-photocogulation in glaucoma. Ophthalmology 1990; 97:73.
19. Kalenak JW, Parkinson JM, Rass MA, Kolker AE. Transscleral Nd:YAG laser cyclophotocoagulation for uncontrolled glaucoma. Ophthalmic Surg 1990;21:346.
20. Badeeb O, Trope GE, Mortimer C. Short-term effects of Nd:YAG transscleral cyclophotocoagulation in patients with uncontrolled glaucoma. Br J Ophthalmol 1988;72:615.
21. Maus M, Katz LJ. Choroidal detachment, flat anterior chamber, and hypotony as complications of Nd:YAG laser cyclophotocoagulation. Ophthalmology 1990;97:69.
22. Fiore PM, Melamed S, Krug JH. Focal scleral thinning after Nd:YAG cyclophotocoagulation. Ophthalmic Surg 1987; 20:215.
23. Edward DP, Brown SJ, Higginbotham E, Jennings T, Tessler HH. Sympathetic ophthalmia following Nd:YAG cyclotherapy. Ophthalmic Surg 1989;20:544.
24. Federman JL, Ando F, Schubert HD, Eagle RC. Contact laser for transscleral photocoagulation. Ophthalmic Surg 1987; 18:183.
25. Allingham RR, Dekater AW, Bellows AR, Hsu J. Probe placement and power levels in contact transscleral Nd:YAG cyclophotocoagulation. Arch Ophthalmol 1990;108:738.
26. Schubert HD, Svan EP, Federman JL. Tissue effects related to exposure time in CW Nd:YAG transscleral photocoagulation and photofiltration. Invest Ophthalmol Vis Sci 1989; 30(suppl):281.
27. Schuman JS, Puliafito CA, Allingham RR, et al. Contact transscleral continuous wave Nd:YAG laser cyclophotocoagulation. Ophthalmology 1990;97:571.
28. Schuman JS, Bellows AR, Shingleton BJ, et al. Contact transscleral Nd:YAG laser cyclophotocoagulation. Ophthalmology 1992;99:1089.
29. Hoskins HD, Iwach AG, Vassiliadis A, Drake MV, Hennings DR. Subconjunctival THC:YAG laser thermal sclerostomy. Ophthalmology 1991;90:1394.
30. Latina M, Long F, Deutsch T, Puliafito CA, Epstein DL, Oseroff A. Dye-enhanced ablation of sclera using a pulsed dye laser. Invest Ophthalmol Vis Sci 1986;27(suppl):254.
31. Latina MA, Dobrogowski M, March WF. Laser sclerostomy using a goniolens and pulsed dye-laser. Invest Ophthalmol Vis Sci 1989;30(suppl):281.
32. Federman JL, Wilson RP, Ando F, Peyman G. Contact laser: thermal sclerostomy ab interno. Ophthalmic Surg 1987; 18:726.
33. Higginbotham EJ, Rao G, Peyman G. Internal sclerostomy with the Nd:YAG contact laser versus thermal sclerostomy in rabbits. Ophthalmology 1988;95:385.

34. Javitt SC, O'Connor SS, Wilson RP, Federman JL. Laser sclerostomy *ab interno* using a continuous wave Nd:YAG laser. Ophthalmic Surg 1989;20:552.
35. Berlin MS, Rajacion G, Duffy M, Grundfest W, Goldenberg T. Excimer laser photoablation in glaucoma filtering surgery. Am J Ophthalmol 1987;103:713.
36. Jacobson JJ, Schuman JS, Al Roumy H, Puliafito CA. Diode laser peripheral iridectomy. Int Ophthalmol Clin 1990; 30:120.
37. Schuman JS, Puliafito CA, Jacobson JJ. Semiconductor diode laser peripheral iridotomy. Arch Ophthalmol 1990;108:1207.
38. Emoto I, Okisaka S, Nakajima A. Diode laser iridotomy in rabbit and human eyes. Am J Ophthalmol 1992;113:321.
39. McHugh D, Marshall J, Ffytche TJ, Hamilton PA, Raven A. Diode laser trabeculoplasty (DLT) for primary open-angle glaucoma and ocular hypertension. Br J Ophthalmol 1990,76:743.
40. Brancato R, Carassa R, Trabucchi G. Diode laser compared with Nd:YAG laser for trabeculoplasty. Am J Ophthalmol 1991;112:50.
41. Brancato R, Pratesi R. Applications of diode laser in ophthalmology. Laser Ophthalmol 1987;3:119.
42. Assia CI, Hennis HL, Stewart WC, Legler UFC, Carlson AN, Arple DJ. A comparison of Nd:YAG and diode laser transscleral cyclophotocoagulation and cyclotherapy. Invest Ophthalmol Vis Sci 1991;32:2774.
43. Brancato R, Leoni G, Trabucchi G, Campellini A. Histopathology of continuous wave Nd:YAG and diode laser contact transscleral lesions in rabbit ciliary body. Invest Ophthalmol Vis Sci 1991;32:1586.
44. Schuman JS, Jacobson JJ, Puliafito CA, Noecker RJ, Reidy WT. Experimental use of semiconductor diode laser in contact transscleral cyclophotocoagulation in rabbits. Arch Ophthalmol 1990;108:1152.

4

Lasers in Cataract Surgery

Stephen A. Obstbaum
King W. To
Ezra L. Galler

Only a decade ago the pioneering work of Aron-Rosa and Fankhauser made the neodymium:yttrium-aluminum-garnet (Nd:YAG) laser a practical and desirable ophthalmic instrument (1–6). In this short period of time the Nd:YAG (or YAG) laser has been widely applied in ophthalmology.

Unlike the argon, krypton, dye, ruby, and CO_2 lasers, the Nd:YAG laser does not rely on photocoagulation to achieve its effect. This laser produces photodisruption by using high-power laser pulses to disrupt tissue. Optical breakdown is the basis of the laser's mechanism of action. Ionization of atoms occurs as a result of the high electromagnetic fields generated when light energy is focused and delivered in an extremely short period of time. Optical breakdown develops when light energy is concentrated in both time and space. The Q-switched Nd:YAG laser is capable of delivering focused energy over extremely short pulses that are on the order of nanoseconds (10^{-9} sec). The ionized tissue with its sheared-off electrons is referred to as a *plasma*. In this state of matter, neutral atoms, positive ions, and its free electrons are moving at a high velocity and colliding with one another. Temperatures of up to 10,000°C are reached in the space undergoing optical breakdown. The spark produced by the Nd:YAG laser is the result of the release of light as the electrons recombine with their atoms in a lower energy state; an example of this in nature is the lightning bolt. The microsurgical capability of the Nd:YAG laser is primarily the result of the acoustic and shock waves produced at the site of the plasma formation. Thermal energy appears to also play a role in the cutting action of the Nd:YAG laser. Tissues in the area of optical breakdown are subjected to very high temperatures and are vaporized. As a result, the mechanical cutting action of the Nd:YAG laser occurs at the point of focus of the laser beam. Beyond its focus, the light generated by the Nd:YAG laser diverges and minimizes the chances of inadvertent damage to the retina or other intraocular structures (7).

The widespread acceptance of the Nd:YAG laser in such a short period of time is testimony to its usefulness in a variety of anterior segment conditions. This chapter reviews the applications of the Nd:YAG laser in cataract surgery.

Nd:YAG Posterior Capsulotomy

Posterior capsule opacification is the prime consequence of extracapsular cataract extraction. Surgical discission of the opacified posterior capsule was the accepted method of treating this condition. With the introduction of the Nd:YAG laser, eye surgeons were able to open opacified capsules and significantly reduce the dreaded complication of endophthalmitis associated with surgical discission. The Nd:YAG laser influenced the method of cataract surgery and prompted many surgeons to abandon the practice of primary posterior capsulotomy. There is increasing evidence of the benefit derived from an intact posterior capsule (8,9). It is therefore desirable to maintain the integrity of the posterior capsule intraoperatively. Should postoperative opacification occur, a controlled Nd:YAG laser capsulotomy is performed.

Posterior capsule opacification following extracapsular cataract surgery occurs because of proliferation and migration of anterior lens epithelium (10). These cells display myofibroblastic differentiation and their contraction results in wrinkling of the posterior capsule producing visual distortion. The proliferating anterior epithelial cells originate at the site of apposition of the anterior capsular flaps to the posterior capsule. As a result, some authors have suggested that a wide anterior capsulectomy may reduce the risk of developing posterior capsule opacification (10). The incidence of postoperative capsular opacification is nearly 30% after 2 to 3 years (11,12) and approximately 50% after 3 to 5 years of follow-up (13,14). In the pediatric population, all postoperative eyes will eventually develop an opacified capsule.

The incidence of cystoid macular edema (CME) and retinal detachment is lower with extracapsular cataract extraction than intracapsular cataract extraction (15–20). CME is also reduced when the posterior capsule is left intact at the time of surgery when compared to cases that undergo a primary surgical capsulotomy (8,9). There is therefore a strong motivation to retain an intact posterior capsule. With the knowledge that the posterior capsule will opacify in many cases with the passage of time, posterior capsulotomy with the Nd:YAG laser has become a prominent procedure.

Indications

The most common indication for Nd:YAG posterior capsul-otomy is reduced vision with impairment of life-style because of opacification of the posterior capsule. Determining how much the capsular opacification contributes to the reduction in vision is not always a simple task. Direct ophthalmoscopy is helpful because the view of the fundus obtained by the observer is similar to that of the patient's view of the world. Indirect ophthalmoscopy, because of the intense illumination, can penetrate significant media opacities and, therefore, is not as reliable as the direct ophthalmoscope. Slit-lamp examination with retroillumination is helpful in evaluating the surface characteristics of the capsule (Fig. 4.1). Other useful methods include retinoscopy and the use of the potential acuity meter (PAM). Although the PAM is an aid in assessing the visual acuity, it may give a falsely good acuity reading in patients with CME (21). Because CME may also cause reduced vision after cataract extraction, its potential role should be considered. Other potential causes of impaired vision postoperatively, such as uncorrected astigmatism, corneal decompensation, intraocular lens (IOL) malposition, and retinal detachment, also require consideration before Nd:YAG capsulotomy.

The Nd:YAG capsulotomy is also indicated in patients who require regular and frequent evaluations of the retina. Such patients include those with diabetic retinopathy, age-related macular degeneration, or risk factors for retinal detachment. Although these patients may not have significantly reduced postoperative visual acuity, the presence of the opacified capsule can make visualization of the retina and interpretation of fluorescein angiograms difficult. A larger than normal Nd:YAG laser posterior capsulotomy may be indicated in situations where visualization of the peripheral retina is necessary.

Contraindications

Optimal visualization of the target is essential for precise laser focusing so that unless a clear view of the posterior capsule is obtained, Nd:YAG laser capsulotomy should not be performed. This can occur in cases with corneal irregularity, scars, or decompensation. In addition, any optical aberration can prevent adequate focusing on the posterior capsule that may result in use of higher energy levels, thereby increasing the risk of damage to the intraocular lens and neighboring ocular structures. Nd:YAG laser posterior capsulotomy is also contraindicated in patients who cannot or are unwilling to cooperate. Relative contraindications include CME, active uveitis, and risk factors for retinal detachment.

Technique

The goal of Nd:YAG laser posterior capsulotomy is to create an adequate opening in the posterior capsule using the minimum amount of energy and fewest number of applications. Although no studies confirm a relationship between an increase in complications and these parameters, we believe that using the least amount of energy that will complete the task is desirable. In general, the size of the capsulotomy is dictated by the pupillary diameter under

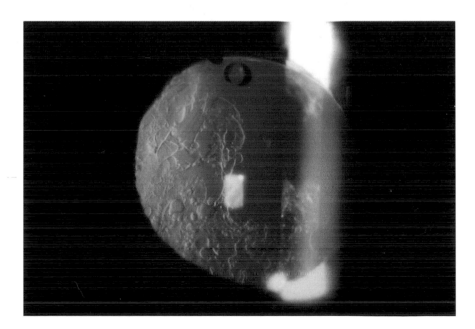

Fig. 4.1   Retroillumination of lens capsule—Elschnig pearl formation.

scotopic conditions, which usually varies between 3.9 and 5.0 mm (22). When the size of the capsulotomy is as large as the pupil in dark conditions, glare and other undesirable optical aberrations are significantly reduced (22). Spontaneous enlargement of a capsulotomy can occur, (Figs. 4.2 and 4.3), although it is a rare complication of Nd:YAG laser posterior capsulotomy (23).

A pupil that is pharmacologically dilated before the capsulotomy will alter its accurate location and size. This may result in an eccentrically placed capsulotomy or one that is too large. Several options exist to obviate this potential problem:

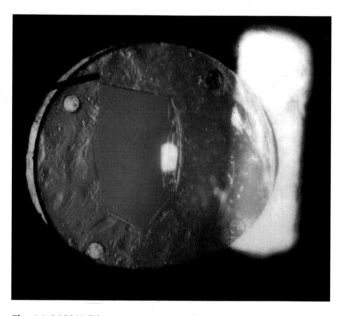

Fig. 4.2 Nd:YAG laser posterior capsulotomy.

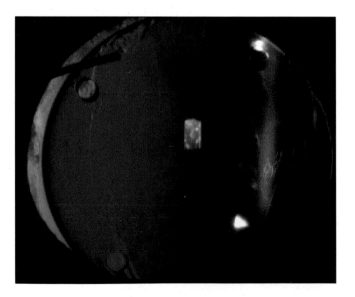

Fig. 4.3 Same eye as in Fig. 4.2, 3 years later. Posterior capsulotomy has significantly increased in size.

1. Place a laser burst in the center of the pupillary opening prior to dilating the pupil.
2. Measure the horizontal and vertical aperture before dilating the pupil.
3. Perform the capsulotomy with an undilated pupil.

Each of these techniques has its advantages. The selection of any one of these methods if done in an appropriate manner can yield good results. It should be mentioned, however, that some ophthalmologists prefer to place the initial laser applications peripherally in the pupillary area. The first option is therefore not as widely accepted as the other two.

An often overlooked step is the adjustment of the oculars of the slit lamp prior to treatment. To gain the maximal benefit, the slit-lamp beam and the aiming beam of the helium-neon (He Ne) laser are adjusted to become parfocal. Test shots on a target, such as a piece of scotch tape, are helpful in ensuring that the oculars have been accurately adjusted.

The space between the IOL and the posterior capsule is observed by slit-lamp examination. We prefer to begin photodisruption of the posterior capsule away from the visual axis and in an area where there is maximum separation from the IOL. With this technique, the risk of damaging the IOL is reduced and if the IOL is marked, it is not in the visual axis. One should avoid focusing directly on the posterior surface of the IOL. In areas where there is not much space between an IOL and the posterior capsule, one may consider focusing behind the capsule rather than directly on the posterior capsule. The optical breakdown produces a shock wave that is generated in an anterior direction so that focusing in the anterior vitreous allows for capsular disruption while reducing the likelihood of IOL damage.

Our goal is to minimize the amount of energy delivered to the eye and still obtain an adequate capsulotomy. This may be accomplished by starting with low energy levels such as 1 to 2 mJ per pulse and placing the shots across tension lines so that the largest opening per pulse is achieved (Fig. 4.4). Most posterior capsulotomies can be performed with single pulses of between 1 to 3 mJ. Thick, fibrotic capsules will usually require higher energy levels.

The use of a contact lens is optional. In many cases with a cooperative patient, a contact lens is not needed. It is helpful, however, in controlling the lids and stabilizing the globe. The use of a contact lens also reduces the energy needed for the posterior capsulotomy by focusing the laser energy in a more precise point of optical breakdown.

These guidelines have been effective in our hands. Each ophthalmologist will develop the skills that are suited for the perfection of his or her technique. The suggestions we have offered have been successful for us. Specific techniques are tailored to the particular case and may be

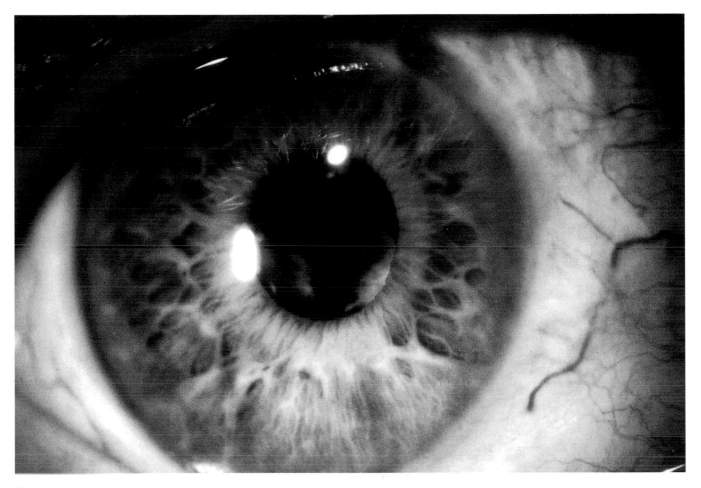

Fig. 4.4 Several laser spots placed across lines of tension produce retraction.

dictated by the behavior of the capsule during the course of the procedure.

Complications

Compared to surgical capsulotomies, the Nd:YAG laser is a safer method of restoring vision in patients with opacified posterior capsules (24–26). However, Nd:YAG laser capsulotomies are not entirely risk free. Increased intraocular pressure (IOP) is a well-recognized complication following Nd:YAG capsulotomy (25–56). A rise in the IOP after Nd:YAG capsulotomy is a common, but fortunately, transient side effect. In most cases the IOP returns to pretreatment levels after a week; however, persistent IOP elevations may rarely occur. The pressure peak usually occurs 3 hours after treatment. Patients with open angle glaucoma are at a higher risk for developing pressure spikes after treatment. This is not unexpected because the proposed mechanism of the IOP rise is related to blockage of the trabecular meshwork by cellular debris (30). Therefore, the IOP response in patients with a preexisting compromised outflow system should be monitored closely. Prophylactic therapy with pilocarpine or aqueous sup-

pressants to blunt the pressure spike has been studied (38,48,54,56) and may be considered on patients with glaucoma or ocular hypertension. Aproclonidine is effective in controlling the IOP rise after Nd:YAG capsulotomy.

Retinal detachments may occur after Nd:YAG laser capsulotomy (26,28,31,32,53,57–62). The incidence of this relatively rare complication has been reported as low as 0.1% in an earlier report and as high as 3.6% in a more recent study (28,61). The incidence of retinal detachment after primary or secondary knife discission of the posterior capsule is estimated to be 2.3% to 6.1% (63–66). The estimated time period between the Nd:YAG capsulotomy and the development of retinal detachment is usually between 5 to 7 months (58–61). However, this complication may occur as early as the first 2 months after capsulotomy. The exact role the laser plays in the development of retinal detachment is unclear. One theory suggests that the retinal detachment is related to a physical change in the vitreous, which is the result of loss of the physical barrier provided by the posterior capsule (58). It has been proposed that without an intact posterior capsule, hyaluronic acid from the vitreous diffuses forward and through the trabecular meshwork, resulting in vitreous instability and possible vitreous detachment with its associated complications such as retinal tear, retinal detachment, and macular hole formation (58). Whether the retinal complications following Nd:YAG laser capsulotomy are because of the loss of an intact posterior capsule that normally acts as a diffusion barrier or a result of the Nd:YAG laser photodisruptive burst itself causing a change in the vitreous is unclear (61). A risk factor for retinal detachment is present in almost one third of cases of retinal detachment after Nd:YAG laser posterior capsulotomy (60). Such risk factors include axial myopia, vitreoretinal disease such as lattice degeneration, and a history of retinal detachment in the fellow eye (60,62). These factors should be considered when evaluating such a patient for Nd:YAG capsulotomy. If Nd:YAG laser capsulotomy is performed in these cases, periodic fundus examinations are essential in the first year after capsulotomy, although retinal tears and detachments can occur at a later time as well.

Intraocular lens damage in association with Nd:YAG posterior capsulotomy was first noted by Aron-Rosa in 1981. Since then, extensive research has been done in this area (67–86). Nd:YAG capsulotomy in the presence of adjacent posterior chamber IOLs can result in damage to the IOL in up to 40% of cases (27; Fig. 4.5). Damage can range from small surface chips to edge-to-edge full-thickness cracks, which have been known to occur with glass IOLs (87). Fortunately the laser damage of most IOLs results in minimal visual impairment. Polymethylmethacrylate (PMMA) and hydroxyethylmethacrylate (HEMA) IOLs are more resistant to damage than glass or silicone IOLs (73,81). Cast-molded PMMA IOLs appear to be the most resistant to Nd:YAG laser damage (73). Injection-molded PMMA IOLs are more susceptible to damage than lathe-cut PMMA IOLs (83). The damage threshold, which is defined as that power density producing damage 50% of the time, of PMMA appears to decrease after four successive Nd:YAG applications (88); as a result, the use of bursts of Nd:YAG shots may be associated with an increased tendency for inadvertent damage to the IOL. Irregularities on the surface of IOLs, whether due to grasping and insertion of the IOL or inadequate polishing of the surface of the IOL in the manufacturing process, may increase the chances of IOL damage by the laser. Damage to IOLs may result in the release of substances, such as plastic monomers, which may be toxic to intraocular tissues. The release of toxic substances following Nd:YAG IOL damage does not appear to result in significant intraocular

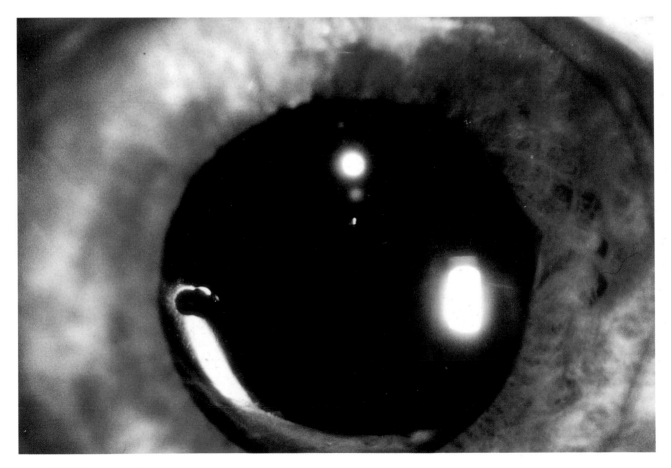

Fig. 4.5 Nd:YAG-induced lens pitting.

toxicity (69,82) and may only occur at laser energy levels above 5 mJ which is more than the usual range of 1 to 2 mJ used for most routine Nd:YAG capsulotomies (71).

The exact relationship of the damage threshold of IOLs with laser wavelength is unclear. The erbium:yttrium-lithium-fluoride (Er:YLF) laser, which produces a wavelength of 1228 nm, has been reported to have a higher threshold for IOL damage and a lower threshold for capsulotomy than the Nd:YAG laser, which operates at 1064 nm (89). IOLs designed with laser ridges are effective in maintaining a distance between the posterior surface of the IOL and the posterior capsule (76) thereby facilitating Nd:YAG laser capsulotomy. However, evidence is accumulating that the laser ridge does not inhibit posterior capsule opacification related to Elshnig pearl formation as effectively as a biconvex or posterior convex optic (12,64,90,91).

The incidence of CME following Nd:YAG capsulotomy has been estimated to be 2.3% (32). If the anterior hyaloid is disrupted during the procedure, there is an increased likelihood that CME will develop (92). Another study that prospectively evaluated CME after Nd:YAG capsulotomy suggests that the risk of this complication is minimal (93).

Other less common complications of YAG capsulotomy include damage to the corneal endothelium, iritis, neovascular glaucoma in diabetic patients, pupillary block, hyphema, macular hole, peripheral retinal hemorrhage, and endophthalmitis (42,46,58,94–102). Endophthalmitis, as a complication of posterior capsulotomy, was thought to have been completely eliminated when the surgical discission of the posterior capsule was replaced by the Nd:YAG laser capsulotomy. However, it appears that endophthalmitis can be a rare complication, presumably due to the release of previously sequestered microorganisms (100–102).

Potential Clinical Applications of the Nd:YAG Laser

Preoperative anterior capsulotomy with the Nd:YAG laser (Fig. 4.6) was originally described by Aron-Rosa (2). She suggested that this technique would facilitate extracapsular cataract extraction by reducing both surgical manipulations in the anterior chamber and shortening operative time. Modifications on her technique of preoperative anterior capsulotomy have been used by other surgeons (103–106). Although this technique has only been

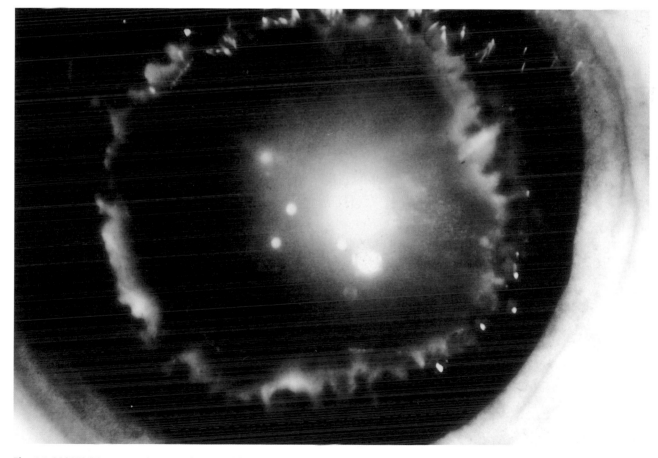

Fig. 4.6 Nd:YAG laser anterior capsulotomy. (Courtesy of Daniele Aron-Rosa, MD.)

adopted by a minority of ophthalmologists for routine cataract surgery, it may be useful in patients with subluxated lenses requiring cataract extraction, especially in young patients where intracapsular technique of removal could often result in vitreous loss (107). In the presence of abnormal zonular integrity, operative anterior capsulotomy may result in further loss of zonular support and complete dislocation of the lens. Preoperative Nd:YAG anterior capsulotomy could minimize the stress on the zonules and provide a precise capsulotomy.

Postoperative anterior capsule fragmentation has been used to treat remnants of the anterior capsule after extracapsular surgery that have become visually impairing. The retained anterior capsule can often be severed using energy levels of 1 to 3 mJ. Because of the proximity of the cornea in the treatment of the anterior capsule, it is important to minimize the amount of energy used and avoid treating portions of capsular fragments that are adjacent or adherent to the corneal endothelium.

To decrease the time required for phacoemulsification and thereby increase the efficiency of phacoemulsification, preoperative Nd:YAG laser application of the lens nucleus has been attempted (108–111). The objective of Nd:YAG pretreatment of the lens nucleus without opening the anterior capsule is to ease phacoemulsification of the nucleus. Preliminary studies of this technique known as Nd:YAG phacofracture or photophacofragmentation has been shown to decrease the ultrasound time necessary and subjectively ease the emulsification process (110,111).

The removal of an anterior chamber IOL can be complicated by the presence of fibrosis in the angle that involves the haptic. In such situations, the Nd:YAG laser may facilitate the removal of the IOL by preoperatively severing the inferior haptics that are fibrosed into the angle (112). Pretreatment with the Nd:YAG may minimize the surgical manipulation of the eye. Energy settings between 6 to 12 mJ and 25 to 100 shots are necessary to sever PMMA or polypropylene haptics (112).

The shock wave produced by Nd:YAG photodisruption has been used to treat iris capture of posterior chamber IOLs (112). By focusing the laser light just anterior to the IOL, the implant can be "pushed" back behind the iris. This technique should be considered only after medical therapy, patient positioning, and external pressure on the globe have failed to reposition the IOL. Care must be taken not to focus on or too closely to the IOL because inadvertent damage to the implant would result.

Postoperative iridocapsular adhesions can be lysed by the Nd:YAG laser. When iridocapsular adhesions result in visual symptoms such as in a case where there is exposure of a positioning hole, the Nd:YAG laser may be useful in its treatment (113). Another rather uncommon use of the Nd:YAG laser is in the treatment of lens subluxation in patients with visual disturbance (114). The procedure known as Nd:YAG zonulysis is an alternative to surgical removal of the lens, which is associated with a high complication rate. Nd:YAG zonulysis involves severing specific zonules so that a clear aphakic visual axis can be obtained.

Lasers for Cataract Extraction

The current technology of ultrasonic phacoemulsification has potential problems, including concern about the safety of unused energy released at the tip possibly affecting nontarget tissues, such as the iris, posterior capsule, and corneal endothelium. Laser technology has many uses in ophthalmology and is generally known to be safe and effective. These and other reasons have prompted investigators to study laser energy sources for the removal of the cataractous lens.

Aron-Rosa did extensive research in the early 1980s in preoperative anterior capsulotomy with the Nd:YAG laser. Due to its questionable benefits and frequent complications, it has largely been abandoned by the majority of ophthalmologists. A logical growth of this research, however, was the idea to use the Nd:YAG laser for photodisruption/photofragmentation of the lens nucleus prior to standard ultrasonic phacoemulsification while leaving the anterior capsule intact. In 1987, Zelman reported 300 cases (110) and in 1988, Chambless reported 1000 cases (111). They both stated that by softening the nucleus with the laser treatment, they were able to perform phacoemulsification on darker, harder nuclei than previously possible. Chambless noted a 58.7% decrease in emulsification time after laser nucleolysis in vitro using cataractous human lens nuclei that were obtained through extracapsular extraction (111).

The series reported by Zelman and Chambless, however, were not randomized, prospective studies. Levin and Wyatt compared 32 subjects randomly assigned to have Nd:YAG laser photophacofragmentation approximately one week prior to phacoemulsification to a group of 37 patients who had phacoemulsification without pretreatment. The visual acuity of all the patients in the former group was significantly decreased immediately after photofragmentation. Otherwise, the procedure was without adverse effect. None of the eyes had a posterior capsule rupture, an increased intraocular pressure, or uveitis. One patient inadvertently had a small rupture of the anterior capsule, but it was plugged by an air bubble and there was no leakage of lens material. The authors did find a statistically significant decrease in the amount of ultrasonic time required (0.81 min versus 0.92 min at 70% power), but this did not alter the total surgical time nor the outcome of surgery and was therefore felt to be of little, if any, clinical significance. Four other patients had photophacofragmentation prior to planned extracapsular extraction. The surgeon reported difficulty removing the nuclear material by nucleus expression in these cases.

Considering the significant decrease in visual acuity in the period between phacofragmentation and extraction, the difficulty with nucleus removal if an extracapsular extraction becomes necessary, and the significant albeit small risks of anterior and posterior capsular rupture and their complications, the authors felt that it is not a worthwhile procedure and recommended against doing it (115). In response to this article, Chambless acknowledged their criticisms but felt that the usefulness of the procedure should not be judged only by decrease in ultrasound time, but also by the subjective ease of the phacoemulsification in the hands of a surgeon experienced in the technique. He claimed that he has not had capsular rupture over the last six to seven years and stood firm that laser phacofracture significantly aids in the case of emulsification of harder nuclei (116).

Dardenne and colleagues used the 1053-nm picosecond pulsed Nd:YLF laser for photophacofragmentation. The lenses of 10 rabbit eyes were treated with linear patterns delivered from a posterior to an anterior orientation. None of the eyes had a capsular perforation, elevated IOP, or inflammation and were followed for 2 weeks. All lenses were liquefied and appeared to contain only a fraction of their original material. A portion of the lens of five patients was treated in an identical manner prior to cataract extraction and could be aspirated without any phacoemulsification at the time of surgery (117).

Research has been done to harness laser technology for the actual removal of cataractous lenses. Trokel and coworkers first reported using a UV laser (193 nm excimer) in ophthalmic surgery in 1983 (118). In 1985, Puliafito and collaborators studied the interaction of 193 nm and 248 nm excimer laser energy with human cadaver and bovine corneal and lens tissue. Light and electron microscopic analysis revealed perforation of the lens capsule and a smooth-edged zone of lens ablation without charring. The 248-nm laser caused more damage adjacent to the ablation zone compared with the 193-nm ArF laser (119). In 1986, Nanevicz compared the interaction of four excimer lasers (193 nm ArF, 248 nm KrF, 308 nm XeCl, 351 nm XeF) with bovine lenses. Ablation of lens tissue was accomplished with all but the 351-nm laser. The 248-nm laser had the highest ablation rate but the least precision. The 193-nm laser had the lowest ablation threshold and was the most precise. The 308-nm laser was intermediate in both its ablation rate and its precision (120). The 193-nm laser seems ideal, but currently cannot be transmitted by a fiberoptic delivery system, and it is therefore impractical with regard to cataract extraction. Fiberoptic transmission is also difficult with 248 nm laser energy, but is possible with the 308-nm laser, thereby making it the most promising. In 1987, Bath and colleagues reported using a 308-nm excimer laser to deliver up to 20 mJ through a 600 μm quartz fiberoptic. Clean drill holes were produced in freshly enucleated human cadaver lenses and based on

their depth, the ablation threshold was calculated to be $0.5 J/cm^2$. They have shown that "laserphaco" can be accomplished through a 1-mm corneal/capsular incision with a laser delivery/irrigation-aspiration prototype device of their own design (121,122). This optimizes the benefits of small incision surgery and may also allow implantation of injectable/malleable IOL materials, the theoretical advantage of which is the preservation of accommodative function in the pseudophakic eye.

Maguen and coworkers demonstrated the ability of the 308-nm excimer laser with a 600-μm fiberoptic delivery system to ablate eight human cadaver lenses. Total delivered energy to ablate one lens ranged from 35 to 63 J. They showed that at a distance of only 1 mm separation between fiberoptic and tissue, a dramatic decrease in fluence occurred, and decreased further with increasing distance until 5 mm when no laser–tissue interaction could be observed. They also showed that ablation of the lens capsule, especially the posterior capsule, was relatively difficult at the fluences used to ablate cortex and nucleus, and required an exceedingly larger number of pulses to perforate even with no separation between fiberoptic and capsule. They proposed that this laser system coupled to an effective irrigation/aspiration (I/A) device may be useful in endocapsular lens extraction. A photoacoustic effect was observed by the authors, but its significance was not known (123).

The safety of using UV laser energy is a concern because there is potential for mutagenesis, carcinogenesis, retinotoxicity, and cataractogenesis (124,125). The latter two have been well documented when the laser energy is generated in the air. It is unknown if ablation in a fluid medium will decrease the risks, although Maguen speculated that it will (123). Further study of these risks is needed and proper shielding of both patients' and surgeons' eyes will be required before human trials can be performed.

Tsubota demonstrated the ability of the pulsed Er:YAG laser to ablate the lens in freshly enucleated rabbit eyes. The laser energy was delivered through a 200-μm fiberoptic and measured 50 mJ at its end. With minimal power, the surface tissue of the lens was coagulated. At energy levels greater than $636 mJ/mm^2$ tissue loss was observed, and the periphery was covered with the powder of the ablated tissue. The tissue around the ablated area showed a thermal effect of the laser (126).

Dodick has developed a device for removal of the cataractous lens using a pulsed 1064-nm Nd:YAG laser delivered by a 300-μm fiberoptic and coupled to an I/A system in a handpiece similar in size and shape to current I/A probes used in extracapsular surgery. Instead of the laser energy interacting directly with the lens tissue, however, the beam is directed inside the device to strike against a titanium target near the aspiration port (Fig. 4.7). This facilitates plasma formation and optical breakdown

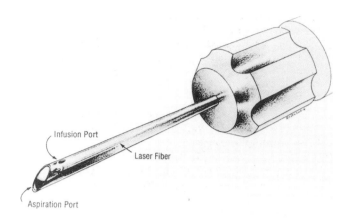

Fig. 4.7 Nd:YAG laser phacolysis probe. (Reproduced by permission from Jack M. Dodick and Arch Ophthalmol 1993;111:903.)

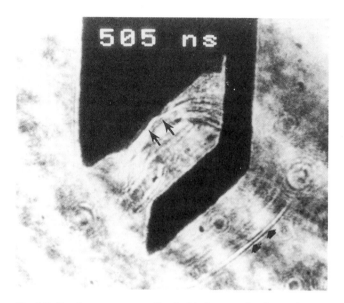

Fig. 4.8 Shock wave propagation inside laser probe shown in Fig. 7. (Reproduced by permission from Benson W, Marshall J, Spaeth G, eds. Annual of Ophthalmic Laser Surgery. Philadelphia: Current Medicine, Inc., 1992:27.)

at lower laser energy because metals have low ionization potentials. The resultant shock wave propagates toward the mouth of the probe and causes disruption of nuclear material held there. Dodick refers to this process as Nd:YAG laser phacolysis. Dodick and Christiansen have designed a high-speed photographic system to record and analyze the formation and propagation of shock waves that occur at the tip of the probe. The speed of the shock wave was calculated to be 1790 m/sec inside the probe tip. This is faster than the speed of sound and is accelerated to this velocity by the explosion that results from plasma formation. By 505 nsec after the laser pulse, the shock wave reached the mouth of the probe and slowed to 1446 m/sec (Fig. 4.8). The pressure of the shock wave was calculated

to be 2.4 kBar. The authors propose that this photographic method will be useful in developing the ideal target shape and configuration to produce the maximum shock wave up to but not beyond a certain focal point, as well as to study the shock wave patterns of current ultrasound phacoemulsification devices for comparison. The device has been used on human cadaver lenses as well as in animal studies and has been shown to cause no apparent damage to the corneal endothelium, trabecular meshwork, or retina (presented at the American Society of Cataract and Refractive Surgery [ASCRS] Annual Meeting, Los Angeles, March 4–7, 1990). Dodick has been granted an Investigational Device Exemption for Nd:YAG laser phacolysis on 10 human subjects and reported no complications and a good outcome in the first procedure done on a 60-year-old man with a nuclear cataract (127–129).

References

1. Aron-Rosa D, Aron JJ, Griesemann M, et al. Use of neodymium-YAG laser to open the posterior capsule after lens implant surgery: a preliminary report. Am Intraocular Implant Soc J 1980;6:352–354.
2. Aron-Rosa D. Use of a pulsed neodymium:YAG laser for anterior capsulotomy before extracapsular cataract extraction. Am Intraocular Implant Soc J 1981;7:332–333.
3. Aron-Rosa D, Griesemann JC, Aron JJ. Use of a pulsed neodymium-YAG laser (picosecond) to open the posterior lens capsule in traumatic cataract: a preliminary report. Ophthalmic Surg 1981;12:496–499.
4. Fankhauser F, Roussel P, Steffen J, et al. Clinical studies on the efficiency of high power laser radiation upon some structures of the anterior segment of the eye. Int Ophthalmol 1981;3:129–139.
5. Fankhauser F, Lortscher H, Van der Zypen E. Clinical studies on high and low power laser radiation upon some structures of the anterior and posterior segment of the eye. Int Ophthalmol 1982;5:15–32.
6. Fankhauser F, Van der Zypen E. Future of the laser in ophthalmology. Trans Ophthalmol Soc UK 1982;102:159–163.
7. Mainster MA, Sliney DH, Belcher CD, et al. Laser photodisruptors: damage mechanisms, instrument design and safety. Ophthalmology 1983;90:973–991.
8. Chambless WS. Phacoemulsification and the retina: cystoid macular edema. Ophthalmology 1979;86:2019-2022.
9. Kraff MC, Sanders DR, Jampol LM, et al. Effect of primary capsulotomy with extracapsular surgery on the incidence of pseudophakic cystoid macular edema. Am J Ophthalmol 1984;98:166–170.
10. McDonnell PJ, Zarbin MA, Green WR. Posterior capsule opacification in pseudophakic eyes. Ophthalmology 1983;90:1548–1553.
11. Emery JM, Wilhelmus KR, Rosenberg S. Complications of phacoemulsification. Ophthalmology 1978;85:141–150.
12. Sterling S, Wood TO. Effect of intraocular lens convexity on posterior capsule opacification. J Cataract Refract Surg 1986;12:655–657.
13. Kraff MC, Sanders DR, Lieberman HL. Total cataract extraction through a 3 mm incision: a report of 650 cases. Ophthalmic Surg 1979;10:46–54.

14. Wilhelmus KR, Emery JM. Posterior capsule opacification. Ophthalmic Surg 1980;11:264–267.

15. The Miami Study Group. Cystoid macular edema in aphakic and pseudophakic eyes. Am J Ophthalmol 1979;88:45–48.

16. Wetzig PC, Thatcher DB, Christiansen JM, et al. The intracapsular versus the extracapsular technique in relationship to retinal problems. Trans Am Ophthalmol Soc 1979;77: 339–347.

17. Jaffe NS, Luscombe SM, Clayman HM, et al. A fluorescein angiographic study of cystoid macular edema. Am J Ophthalmol 1981;92:775–777.

18. Binkhorst CD, Kato A, Tjan TT. Retinal accidents in pseudophakia. Intracapsular versus extracapsular surgery. Trans Am Acad Ophthalmol Otolaryngol 1976;81:120–127.

19. Hurite F, Sorr EM, Everett WG. The incidence of retinal detachment following phacoemulsification. Ophthalmology 1979;86:2004–2006.

20. Moses L. Cystoid macular edema and retinal detachment following cataract surgery. Am Intraocular Implant Soc J 1979; 5:326–329.

21. Faulkner W. Laser interferometric prediction of postoperative visual acuity in patients with cataracts. Am J Ophthalmol 1983;95:626–636.

22. Holladay JT, Bishop JE, Lewis JW. The optimal size of a posterior capsulotomy. Am Intraocular Implant Soc J 1985; 11:18–20.

23. Clayman HM, Jaffe NS. Spontaneous enlargement of neodymium:YAG posterior capsulotomy in aphakic and pseudophakic patients. J Cataract Refract Surg 1988; 14: 667–669.

24. Liesegang TJ, Bourne WM, Ilstrup DM. Secondary surgical and neodymium-YAG laser discissions. Am J Ophthalmol 1985;100:510–519.

25. Durham DG, Gills JP. Three thousand YAG lasers in posterior capsulotomies: an analysis of complications and comparison to polishing and surgical discissions. Trans Am Ophthalmol Soc 1985;83:218–235.

26. Shah GR, Gills JP, Durham DG, et al. Three thousand YAG lasers in posterior capsulotomies: an analysis of complications and comparison to polishing and surgical discission. Ophthalmic Surg 1986;17:473–477.

27. Terry AC, Stark WJ, Maumenee AE, et al. Neodymium-YAG laser for posterior capsulotomy. Am J Ophthalmol 1983;96:716–720.

28. Aron-Rosa DS, Aron JJ, Cohn HC. Use of a pulsed picosecond Nd:YAG laser in 6664 cases. Am Intraocular Implant Soc J 1984;10:35–39.

29. Blackwell C, Hirst LW, Kinnas SJ. Neodymium-YAG capsulotomy and potential blindness. Am J Ophthalmol 1984;98: 521–522.

30. Channell MM, Beckman H. Intraocular pressure changes after neodymium-YAG laser posterior capsulotomy. Arch Ophthalmol 1984;102:1024–1026.

31. Johnson SH, Kratz RP, Olson PF. Clinical experience with the Nd:YAG laser. Am Intraocular Implant Soc J 1984; 10: 452–460.

32. Keates RH, Steinert RF, Puliafito CA, et al. Long-term follow-up of Nd:YAG laser posterior capsulotomy. Am Intraocular Implant Soc J 1984;10:164–168.

33. Parker WT, Clorfeine GS, Stocklin RD. Marked intraocular pressure rise following Nd:YAG laser capsulotomy. Ophthalmic Surg 1984;15:103–104.

34. Parker WT, Clorfeine GS. YAG capsulotomy and IOP rise. Ophthalmic Surg 1984;15:787.

35. Stamm BD. Marked intraocular pressure rise following Nd:YAG laser capsulotomy. Ophthalmic Surg 1984;15:788.

36. Vine AK. Ocular hypertension following Nd:YAG laser capsulotomy: a potentially blinding complication. Ophthalmic Surg 1984;15:283–284.

37. Aron-Rosa DS. Influence of picosecond and nanosecond YAG laser capsulotomy on intraocular pressure. Am Intraocular Implant Soc J 1985;11:249–252.

38. Brown SV, Thomas JV, Belcher CD, et al. Effect of pilocarpine in treatment of intraocular elevation following neodymium:YAG laser posterior capsulotomy. Ophthalmology 1985;92:354–359.

39. Chambless WS. Neodymium:YAG laser posterior capsulotomy results and complications. Am Intraocular Implant Soc J 1985;11:31–32.

40. Deutsch TA, Goldberg MF. Neodymium:YAG laser capsulotomy. Int Ophthalmol Clin 1985;25:87–100.

41. Ficker LA, Steele AD. Complications of Nd:YAG laser posterior capsulotomy. Trans Ophthalmol Soc UK 1985; 104:529–532.

42. Flohr MJ, Robin AL, Kelley JS. Early complications following Q-switched neodymium:YAG laser posterior capsulotomy. Ophthalmology 1985;92:360–363.

43. Gabel VP, Neubauer L, Zink H, et al. Ocular side effects following neodymium:YAG laser irradiation. Int Ophthalmol Clin 1985;25:137–149.

44. Kraff MC, Sanders DR, Lieberman HL. Intraocular pressure and the corneal endothelium after neodymium-YAG laser posterior capsulotomy: relative effects of aphakia and pseudophakia. Arch Ophthalmol 1985;103:511–514.

45. Leys MJ, Pameijer JH, de Jong PT. Intermediate term changes in intraocular pressure after Nd:YAG laser posterior capsulotomy. Am J Ophthalmol 1985;100:332–333.

46. Nirankari VS, Richards RD. Complications associated with the use of the neodymium:YAG laser. Ophthalmology 1985;92:1371–1375.

47. Parrish RK, Slomovic A. Myopia and unexpected intraocular pressure elevations after neodymium-YAG laser capsulotomy. Arch Ophthalmol 1985;103:1277.

48. Richter CU, Arzeno G, Pappas HR, et al. Prevention of intraocular pressure elevation following Nd:YAG laser posterior capsulotomy. Arch Ophthalmol 1985;103:912–915.

49. Richter CU, Arzeno G, Pappas HR, et al. Intraocular pressure elevation following Nd:YAG laser posterior capsulotomy. Ophthalmology 1985;92:636–640.

50. Schubert HD, Morris WJ, Trokel SL, et al. The role of the vitreous in the intraocular pressure rise after neodymium:YAG laser capsulotomy. Arch Ophthalmol 1985;103:1538–1542.

51. Schubert HD. A history of intraocular pressure rise with reference to the Nd:YAG laser. Surv Ophthalmol 1985; 30: 168–172.

52. Slomovic AR, Parrish RK. Acute elevations of intraocular pressure following Nd:YAG laser posterior capsulotomy. Ophthalmology 1985;92:973–976.

53. Stark WJ, Worthen D, Holladay JT, et al. Neodymium:YAG lasers: an FDA report. Ophthalmology 1985;92:209–212.

54. Boen-Tan TN, Stilma JS. Prevention of IOP rise following Nd:YAG laser capsulotomy with pre-operative timolol eye drops and 1 tablet acetazolamide 250 mg. Doc Ophthalmol 1986;64:59–67.

55. Demer JL, Koch DD, Smith JA, et al. Persistent elevation in intraocular pressure after Nd:YAG laser treatment. Ophthalmic Surg 1986;17:465–466.

56. Stilma JS, Boen-Tan TN. Timolol and intraocular pressure elevation following Nd:YAG laser surgery. Doc Ophthalmol 1986;61:233–239.

57. Fastenberg DM, Schwartz PL, Lin HZ. Retinal detachment following neodymium-YAG laser posterior capsulotomy. Am J Ophthalmol 1984;97:288–291.

58. Winslow RL, Taylor BC. Retinal complications following YAG laser capsulotomy. Ophthalmology 1985;92:785–789.

59. Ober RR, Wilkinson CP, Fiore JV, et al. Rhegmatogenous retinal detachment after neodymium-YAG laser capsulotomy in phakic and pseudophakic eyes. Am J Ophthalmol 1986;101:81–89.

60. Leff SR, Welch JC, Tasman W. Rhegmatogenous retinal detachment after YAG laser posterior capsulotomy. Ophthalmology 1987;94:1222–1225.

61. Rickman-Barger L, Florine CW, Larson RS, et al. Retinal detachment after neodymium:YAG laser posterior capsulotomy. Am J Ophthalmol 1989;107:531–536.

62. Koch DD, Liu JF, Gill EP, et al. Axial myopia increases the risk of retinal complications after neodymium-YAG laser posterior capsulotomy. Arch Ophthalmol 1989;107:986–990.

63. Hurite FG, Sorr EM, Everett WG. The incidence of retinal detachment following phacoemulsification. Ophthalmology 1979;86:2004–2006.

64. Lindstrom RL, Harris WS. Management of the posterior capsule following posterior chamber lens implantation. Am Intraocular Implant Soc J 1980;6:255–258.

65. Fung WE, Coonan PC, Ho BT. Incidence of retinal detachments following extracapsular cataract extraction. A prospective study. Retina 1981;1:232–237.

66. Coonan P, Fung WE, Webster RG, et al. The incidence of retinal detachment following extracapsular cataract extraction. A ten-year study. Ophthalmology 1985;92:1096–1101.

67. Clayman HM, Karrenberg FG, Parel JM. Intraocular lens damage from the neodymium-YAG laser. Ann Ophthalmol 1984;16:551–553, 556.

68. Fallor MK, Hoft RH. Intraocular lens damage associated with posterior capsulotomy: A comparison of intraocular lens designs and four different Nd:YAG laser instruments. Am Intraocular Implant Soc J 1985;11:564–567.

69. Lindstrom RL, Skelnik DL, Mowbray SL. Neodymium:YAG laser interaction with intraocular lenses: an in vitro toxicity assay. Am Intraocular Implant Soc J 1985;11:558–563.

70. Myers WD, Myers TD, Marks RG, et al. Intraocular lens design for the neodymium:YAG laser. Am Intraocular Implant Soc J 1985;11:35–36.

71. Terry AC, Stark WJ, Newsome DA, et al. Tissue toxicity of laser-damaged intraocular lens implants. Ophthalmology 1985;92:414–418.

72. Bath PE, Dang Y, Martin WH. Comparison of glare in YAG-damaged intraocular lenses: injection-molded versus lathe-cut. J Cataract Refract Surg 1986;12:662–664.

73. Bath PE, Romberger AB, Brown P. A comparison of Nd:YAG laser damage thresholds for PMMA and silicone intraocular lenses. Invest Opthalmol Vis Sci 1986;27:795–798.

74. Bath PE, Romberger A, Brown P, et al. Quantitative concepts in avoiding intraocular lens damage from the Nd:YAG laser in posterior capsulotomy. J Cataract Refract Surg 1986;12:262–266.

75. Fechner PU. Optic damage seen with YAG laser treatment. J Cataract Refract Surg 1986;12:533–534.

76. Wohl LG, Kline OR. Effectivity of laser ridge intraocular lenses. Ophthalmic Surg 1986;17:667–669.

77. Balacco-Gabrieli C, Palmisano C, Castellano L. Preliminary research on the resistance of IOLs to a Q-switched Nd-YAG laser. Ophthalmologica 1986;193:10–13.

78. Bath PE, Boerner CF, Dang Y. Pathology and physics of YAG-laser intraocular lens damage. J Cataract Refract Surg 1987;13:47–49.

79. Bath PE, Hoffer KJ, Aron-Rosa D, et al. Glare disability secondary to YAG laser intraocular lens damage. J Cataract Refract Surg 1987;13:309–313.

80. Hansen SO, Apple DJ, Tetz MR, et al. Comparative histopathologic study of various lens biomaterials in primates after Nd:YAG laser treatment. J Cataract Refract Surg 1987;13:657–661.

81. Keates RH, Sall KN, Kreter JK. Effect of the Nd:YAG laser on polymethylmethacrylate, HEMA copolymer, and silicone intraocular materials. J Cataract Refract Surg 1987;13:401–409.

82. Skelnik DL, Lindstrom RL, Allarakhia L, et al. Neodymium:YAG laser interaction with Alcon IOGEL hydrogel intraocular lenses: an in vitro toxicity assay. J Cataract Refract Surg 1987;13:662–668.

83. Wilson SE, Brubaker RF. Neodymium:YAG laser damage threshold: a comparison of injection-molded and lathe-cut polymethylmethacrylate intraocular lenses. Ophthalmology 1987;94:7–11.

84. Capon M, Mellerio J, Docchio F. Intraocular lens damage from Nd:YAG laser pulses focused in the vitreous. Part I: Q-switched lasers. J Cataract Refract Surg 1988;14:526–529.

85. Sliney DH, Dolch BR, Rosen A, et al. Intraocular lens damage from Nd:YAG laser pulses focused in the vitreous. Part II: Mode-locked lasers. J Cataract Refract Surg 1988;14:530–532.

86. Smith SG, Snowden FM. Neodymium:YAG laser damage of intraocular lenses. J Cataract Refract Surg 1988;14:660–663.

87. Fritch CD. Nd:YAG laser damage to glass intraocular lens. Ann Ophthalmol 1984;16:1177.

88. Likhachev VA, Ryvkin SM, Salmanov VM, et al. Fatigue in the optical damage of transparent dielectrics. Sov Phys-Solid State 1967;8:2754–2755.

89. Horn GD, Johnston M, Arnell LE, et al. A new "cool" lens capsulotomy laser. Am Intraocular Implant Soc J 1982;8:337–342.

90. Downing JE. Long-term discission rate after placing posterior chamber lenses with the convex surface posterior. J Cataract Refract Surg 1986;12:651–654.

91. Sellman TR, Lindstrom RL. Effect of a plano-convex posterior chamber lens on capsular opacification from Elschnig pearl formation. J Cataract Refract Surg 1988;14:68–72.

92. Alpar JJ. Experiences with the neodymium:YAG laser: interruption of anterior hyaloid membrane of the vitreous and cystoid macular edema. Ophthalmic Surg 1986;17:157–165.

93. Lewis H, Singer TR, Hanscom TA, et al. A prospective study of cystoid macular edema after neodymium:YAG laser posterior capsulotomy. Ophthalmology 1987;94:478–482.

94. Ruderman JM, Mitchell PG, Kraff M. Pupillary block following Nd:YAG laser capsulotomy. Ophthalmic Surg 1983;14:418–419.

95. Kerr-Muir MG, Sherrard ES. Damage to the corneal endothelium during Nd/YAG photodisruption. Br J Ophthalmol 1985;69:77–85.

96. Sherrard ES, Kerr-Muir MG. Damage to the corneal endothelium by Q-switched Nd:YAG laser posterior capsulotomy. Trans Ophthalmol Soc UK 1985;104:524–528.

97. Gstalder RJ. Pupillary block with anterior chamber lens following Nd:YAG laser capsulotomy. Ophthalmic Surg 1986; 17:249–250.

98. Slomovic AR, Parrish RK, Forster RK, et al. Neodymium-YAG laser posterior capsulotomy: central corneal endothelial cell density. Arch Ophthalmol 1986;104:536–538.

99. Weinreb RN, Wasserstrom JP, Parker W. Neovascular glaucoma following neodymium-YAG laser posterior capsulotomy. Arch Ophthalmol 1986;104:730–731.

100. Tetz MR, Apple DJ, Price FW Jr, et al. A newly described complication of Nd:YAG laser capsulotomy: exacerbation of an intraocular infection. Arch Ophthalmol 1987;105:1324–1325.

101. Meisler DM, Zakov ZN, Bruner WE, et al. Endophthalmitis associated with sequestered intraocular *Propionibacterium acnes*. Am J Ophthalmol 1987;104:428-429.

102. Carlson AN, Koch DD. Endophthalmitis following Nd:YAG laser posterior capsulotomy. Ophthalmic Surg 1988;19:168–170.

103. Woodward PM. Anterior capsulotomy using a neodymium YAG laser. Ann Ophthalmol 1984;16:534,536–539.

104. Drews RC. Anterior capsulotomy with the neodymium:YAG laser: Results and opinions. Am Intraocular Implant Soc J 1985;11:240–244.

105. Manchester T. YAG laser anterior capsulotomy. CLAO J 1985;11:47–49.

106. Richburg FA. Neodymium:YAG laser for anterior capsulotomy. Am Intraocular Implant Soc J 1985;11:372–375.

107. Woodward P. Nd-YAG laser anterior capsulotomy in Marchesani syndrome. Am Intraocular Implant Soc J 1984;10:215–217.

108. Chambless WS. Neodymium:YAG laser anterior capsulotomy and a possible new application. Am Intraocular Implant Soc J 1985;11:33–34.

109. Ryan EH, Logani S. Nd:YAG laser photodisruption of the lens nucleus before phacoemulsification. Am J Ophthalmol 1987;104:382–386.

110. Zelman J. Photophaco fragmentation. J Cataract Refract Surg 1987;13:287–289.

111. Chambless WS. Neodymium:YAG laser phacofracture: an aid to phacoemulsification. J Cataract Refract Surg 1988; 14:180–181.

112. Steinert RF, Puliafito CA. The Nd-YAG laser in ophthalmology: principles and clinical applications of photodisruption. Philadelphia: WB Saunders, 1985:129–130.

113. Schechter RJ. Pupillary peaking with exposure of an intraocular lens positioning hole corrected by Nd:YAG laser treatment. J Cataract Refract Surg 1988;14:86–87.

114. Tchah H, Larson RS, Nichols BD, et al. Neodymium:YAG laser zonulysis for treatment of lens subluxation. Ophthalmology 1989;96:230–235.

115. Levin ML, Wyatt KD. Prospective analysis of laser photophaco fragmentation. J Cataract Refract Surg 1990; 16:96–98.

116. Chambless WS. Laser photophaco fragmentation. J Cataract Refract Surg 1990;16:386–387. Letter.

117. Dardenne CM, Frueh BE, Klancnik EG, et al. Lens liquefaction using a picosecond IR laser. Invest Ophthalmol Vis Sci 1991;32(suppl):797.

118. Trokel SL, Srinivasan R, Braren B. Excimer laser surgery of the cornea. Am J Ophthalmol 1983;96:710–715.

119. Puliafito CA, Steinert RF, Deutsch RF, Hillenkamp F, Dehm EJ, Adler CM. Excimer laser ablation of the cornea and lens: experimental studies. Ophthalmology 1985;95: 741–748.

120. Nanevicz TM, Prince MR, Gawande AA, Puliafito CA. Excimer laser ablation of the cornea and lens. Arch Ophthalmol 1986;104:1825–1829.

121. Bath PE, Kar H, Apple DJ, et al. Endocapsular excimer laser phakoablation through a 1-mm incision. Ophthalmic Laser Ther 1987;2:245–248.

122. Bath PE, Mueller G, Apple DJ, Brems R. Excimer laser lens. Arch Ophthalmol 1987;105:1164–1165. Letter.

123. Maguen E, Martinez M, Grundfest W, Papaioannout T, Berlin M, Nesburn AB. Excimer laser ablation of the human lens at 308 nm with a fiber delivery system. J Cataract Refract Surg 1989;15:409–414.

124. Zuclich JA. Ultraviolet-induced photochemical damage in ocular tissues. Health Phys 1989;56.671–682.

125. Kochevar IE. Cytotoxity and mutagenicity of excimer laser radiation. Lasers Surg Med 1989;9:440–445.

126. Tsubota K. Application of erbium:YAG laser in ocular ablation. Ophthalmologica 1990;200:117-122.

127. Dodick JM, Sperber LTD. Can cataracts be removed using laser technology? Ophthalmol Clin North Am 1991;4: 355–364.

128. Dodick JM, Christiansen J. Experimental studies on the development and propagation of shock waves created by interaction of short Nd:YAG laser pulses with a titanium target. J Cataract Refract Surg 1991;17:794–797.

129. Dodick JM, Sperber LTD, Lally JM, Kazlas M. Neodymium-YAG laser phacolysis of the human cataractous lens. Arch Ophthalmol 1993;111:903–904.

5

Laser Surgery in Diabetic Retinopathy

David B. Karlin

The use of laser photocoagulation in the treatment of diabetic retinopathy is probably one of the best examples in which laser energy has revolutionized the treatment of a serious disease. In the case of diabetic maculopathy with macular edema, the use of laser surgery has frequently meant the difference between conserving useful vision or facing the eventual loss of sight.

Diabetic retinopathy is the leading cause of blindness in the United States for persons between the ages of 20 and 70 years. There are approximately 11 million diabetic individuals in the United States today, and 600,000 new cases of diabetes mellitus are diagnosed each year.

Diabetic retinopathy is characterized as a microangiopathy in which compromised capillaries demonstrate increased vascular permeability, resulting in retinal edema. The condition develops following long-standing elevated blood glucose levels, as measured by glycosylated hemoglobin. Hypertension, renal disease, and obesity comprise systemic risk factors in the creation of diabetic retinopathy. The development of portable home blood glucose monitoring and perhaps pancreatic islet cell transplantation may improve metabolic control and may reduce the incidence of diabetic retinopathy.

Classification

Diabetic retinopathy has been divided into two forms. Juvenile diabetic retinopathy (type I) usually occurs at an early age and is frequently insulin dependent. Adult-onset diabetic retinopathy (type II) usually occurs later in life and frequently responds to medication without the patient having to undergo insulin therapy. A further division of diabetic retinopathy is made between nonproliferative or background (Fig. 5.1) diabetic retinopathy (BDR) and proliferative (Fig. 5.2) diabetic retinopathy (PDR). Juvenile-onset diabetes has a higher risk of PDR but since there are more adult-onset diabetics, the latter group has a higher incidence of blinding sequelae.

Nonproliferative diabetic retinopathy is defined as retinal pathology limited within the retina. Ophthalmoscopic signs include dot and blot deep hemorrhages, microaneurysms, hard exudates, and macular edema (see Fig. 5.1).

The intermediate term of preproliferative diabetic retinopathy (PPDR) is also useful in this classification because it designates a bridging stage between BDR and PDR. Its characteristic ophthalmoscopic signs include intraretinal microvascular abnormalities (IRMA), cotton wool spots, venous beading, small vessel closure, moderately severe retinal hemorrhages, or microaneurysms (Fig. 5.3). The greater the number of preproliferative changes, the greater the tendency for the development of PDR. In fact, the Diabetic Retinopathy Study demonstrated that 50% of eyes harboring at least three preproliferative factors will develop proliferative retinopathy resulting in visual loss within 2 years, if no treatment is performed.

In the diabetic individual, occlusions begin on the venous side of the capillary network. This leads to vascular permeability that results in retinal edema. Vascular closure causes retinal ischemia. It is retinal ischemia secondary to vascular occlusion that provides the stimulus for preretinal proliferation of neovascular and fibrovascular tissue. The danger signs of retinal ischemia that lead to PDR are cotton wool exudates, venous beading, hemorrhagic infarcts, and white-sheathed or occluded retinal vessels. In advanced cases, neovascularization will develop in an attempt to nourish the ischemic retina. This results in neovascularization of the disc (NVD; Fig. 5.4) and neovascularization of the retina (NVE; Fig. 5.5). If NVD and NVE are not treated by laser, vitreous hemorrhage, retinal detachment, rubeosis irides, and neovascular glaucoma frequently develop, contributing to the rapid demise of the eye.

In cases of PDR, the pathologic changes have broken through the retinal internal limiting membrane and have extended into the vitreous body. PDR can be divided into two stages. The first stage is a *proliferation* of new vessels and fibrous tissue. Later, a *contraction* element is added in which shrinkage of tissue develops, leading to preretinal macular gliosis and traction retinal detachment (Fig. 5.6). Ophthalmoscopic signs in these patients include NVD, NVE, preretinal and vitreous hemorrhage, glial proliferation, and retinal detachment. Visual acuity remains good in the diabetic eye provided little macular edema is

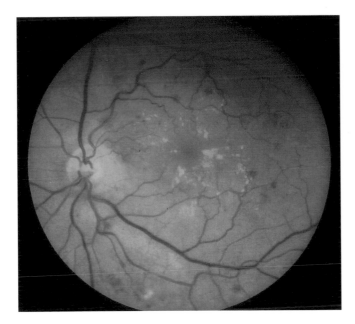

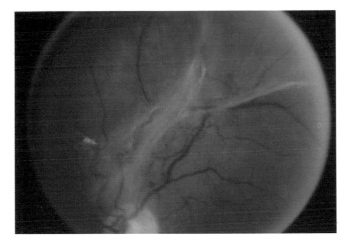

Fig. 5.2 Fundus photo of a left eye showing proliferative diabetic retinopathy with glial proliferation and neovascularization of the retina (NVE) along the distribution of the superior temporal vascular arcade.

Fig. 5.1 Fundus photo of a left eye showing background diabetic retinopathy with microaneurysms, dot and blot hemorrhages, and deep, hard exudates.

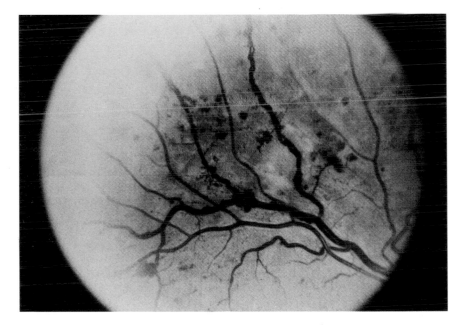

Fig. 5.3 Black and white fundus photo of the superior temporal vascular arcade of the right eye shows the preproliferative stage of diabetic retinopathy with prominent venous beading, intraretinal microvascular abnormalities (IRMA), cotton wool spots, retinal hemorrhages, and microaneurysms (MA).

present. Once significant macular edema develops, however, the patient is at great risk for loss of central vision.

The natural history and eventual course of cases of BDR, PPDR, and PDR are frequently inconsistent. This is true among patients having the same degree of diabetic retinopathy as well as between the two eyes of a single patient exhibiting the same degree of retinopathy. Some eyes develop rapid, progressive changes; others progress slowly. A minority of eyes can even regress spontaneously, remaining free of symptomatology. Ophthalmic research is still being directed toward the identifica-

tion of those signs pointing to a progression of diabetic retinopathy.

There are 11,000 new cases of diabetic macular edema occurring each year in the United States. Javitt (1) states there are 22,000 new cases of PDR per year. It is estimated that 5000 new cases of blindness are caused by the above mentioned complications. Kahn and Hiller (2) and Palmberg (3) found blindness to be 25 times more common in diabetics than in nondiabetic persons. The use of external laser photocoagulation via slit-lamp delivery, the use of indirect laser photocoagulation, and the use of endolaser

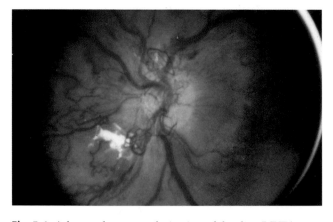

Fig. 5.4 Advanced neovascularization of the disc (NVD) in a case of advanced proliferative diabetic retinopathy. If not treated with laser photocoagulation, retinal and vitreous hemorrhage will eventually result in loss of visual acuity.

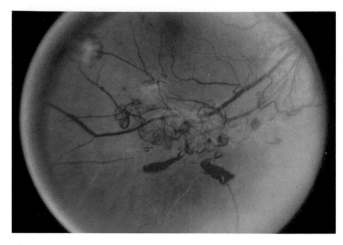

Fig. 5.5 Advanced neovascularization of the retina (NVE) in a case of advanced proliferative diabetic retinopathy. Similar to the case in Fig. 5.4, if not treated with laser photocoagulation, retinal and vitreous hemorrhage will ultimately result in loss of visual acuity.

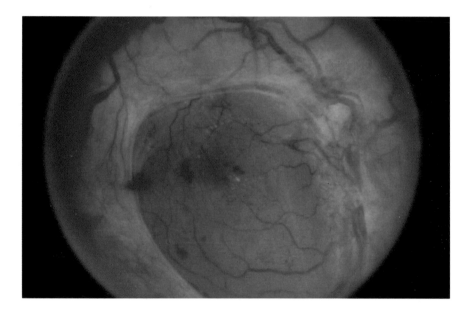

Fig. 5.6 Fundus photo of a case of advanced proliferative diabetic retinopathy demonstrating macular gliosis 360° completely enveloping the posterior pole, with a traction retinal detachment.

photocoagulation as an ancillary procedure in trans pars plana vitrectomy, have all resulted in rehabilitating eyes for useful vision and rehabilitating many diabetic patients as productive members of society. It has been largely through the use of laser photocoagulation that the American Academy of Ophthalmology has been able to make the statement that it is the goal of ophthalmology to eradicate the devastating visual complications of diabetic retinopathy by the advent of the twenty-first century.

Clinical Trials

The National Institutes of Health have been conducting clinical trials to determine which course of therapy is most beneficial in treating certain diseases. Clinical trials are warranted when the risks and benefits of treatment are

considered so equal that a randomized trial is indicated to determine which course of action is most beneficial. Perhaps the earliest and greatest use of clinical trials has been in the field of ophthalmology. Certainly, clinical trials have reached their highest level in the three National Eye Institute-sponsored Diabetic Retinopathy Study, Diabetic Retinopathy Vitrectomy Study, and the Early Treatment Diabetic Retinopathy Study. Laser photocoagulation of the retina has played a key role in each of these studies.

Diabetic Retinopathy Study

The Diabetic Retinopathy Study (4) demonstrated the value of argon laser and xenon arc photocoagulation in reducing severe visual loss in patients with diabetic retinopathy. The comparison of treated and untreated eyes demonstrated a 50% reduction in the degree of visual loss in those eyes that have had laser photocoagulation.

Diabetic Retinopathy Vitrectomy Study

The Diabetic Retinopathy Vitrectomy Study (5,6) demonstrated the value of early vitrectomy with the ancillary procedure of endolaser photocoagulation as the treatment of choice for patients with severe PDR. Eyes were randomized to either photocoagulation but no vitrectomy within one year, or to early vitrectomy with or without preoperative laser photocoagulation. The rationale behind early vitrectomy is that removal of the vitreous body destroys the scaffold for fibrovascular growth. This subsequently causes regression of neovascularization and therefore prevents traction retinal detachment and neovascular glaucoma. Results indicated that after 4 years, 35% of eyes having undergone early vitrectomy retained visual acuity of 20/40, whereas only 10% of those eyes randomized to late vitrectomy could achieve vision of 20/40.

Early Treatment Diabetic Retinopathy Study

The third clinical trial entitled Early Treatment Diabetic Retinopathy Study (7) clearly showed the value of laser photocoagulation for patients with nonproliferative, mild, or proliferative diabetic retinopathy and clinically significant macular edema. The study was designed to determine whether laser photocoagulation in the formative stages of diabetic retinopathy could prevent the late, more advanced complications of diabetic retinopathy. Initially, one eye was randomly assigned to either focal or scatter laser photocoagulation after fulfilling the enrollment criteria. In the focal approach, laser photocoagulation is aimed at sealing discrete retinal vessels producing macular edema, as demonstrated by prior fundus fluorescein angiography. In scatter treatment, laser photocoagulation is used to produce 1500 to 2000 laser lesions of 500 to 1000 μm size, scattered throughout the entire retina, sparing the macula. The results showed that panretinal (scatter) or focal laser photocoagulation (or both) slows the growth of neovascularization and the development of retinal and vitreous hemorrhage, while preserving central visual acuity.

Another aspect to this study was the role of aspirin in the treatment of diabetic retinopathy. It is well documented that abnormal clumping and adhesions of platelets occur in the diabetic patient. Because these platelet abnormalities contribute to microvascular occlusions in retinal vessels, it was thought that aspirin therapy might reduce retinal ischemia and therefore prevent neovascularization of both the optic disc and the retina. Unfortunately, results showed no evidence of a beneficial or a harmful effect from the administration of aspirin on the course of diabetic retinopathy.

General Indications for Laser Treatment

Treatment using laser photocoagulation should be performed for patients with PDR, BDR showing marked advancement, diabetics exhibiting leakage into the macular area, and patients with macular edema. It has been shown that patients with PDR treated with panretinal (scatter) photocoagulation (PRP; usually in three divided sessions) have had a 50% reduction in visual loss.

Because many older type I diabetic patients demonstrate both posterior subcapsular cataract formation as well as PDR, the question is frequently asked whether cataract surgery or PRP should be performed first. Certainly, it is hard to apportion what percent of visual loss is due to the cataract and what percent is due to the retinopathy. This is especially true when macular edema plays a significant role in the loss of central visual acuity. There is a fourfold increase in the incidence of rubeosis irides and an increase in hemorrhagic glaucoma once cataract extraction is performed in an eye having uncontrolled PDR. PRP prior to cataract surgery markedly decreases the incidence of both rubeosis irides and hemorrhagic glaucoma. It is therefore important to remember that PRP should always be performed before cataract surgery if there is adequate visualization of the underlying retina through the cataractous lens. Frequently, I would recommend krypton instead of argon green laser photocoagulation because the higher krypton wavelength penetrates better through the dense cataractous lens. If the cataract is too opaque and precludes an adequate view of the retina, I would suggest a planned extracapsular cataract extraction or phacoemulsification with an intraocular lens (IOL) implantation prior to laser photocoagulation. Naturally, the ideal procedure here is that the posterior lens capsule is left intact and a posterior chamber intraocular lens is inserted. Retinal laser therapy is then carried out either at the time of surgery or following cataract surgery.

If the retina can be clearly visualized through a noncataractous lens and clear vitreous, then laser photocoagulation is performed through either a slit-lamp delivery system or via indirect ophthalmoscopy in which the laser energy has been incorporated into the headscope. If the media is clouded as a result of a cataractous lens or the vitreous exhibits massive hemorrhage preventing adequate visualization of the underlying retina, lensectomy coupled with trans pars plana vitrectomy must be performed before adequate laser photocoagulation can be attempted.

In the latter case, endolaser photocoagulation is performed in the operating room as an ancillary procedure to vitrectomy. Similarly, in cases of clear media vitrectomy where traction retinal detachment is present threatening the macular area, endolaser photocoagulation is frequently performed as part of the vitrectomy procedure. Lastly, in cases of advanced proliferative

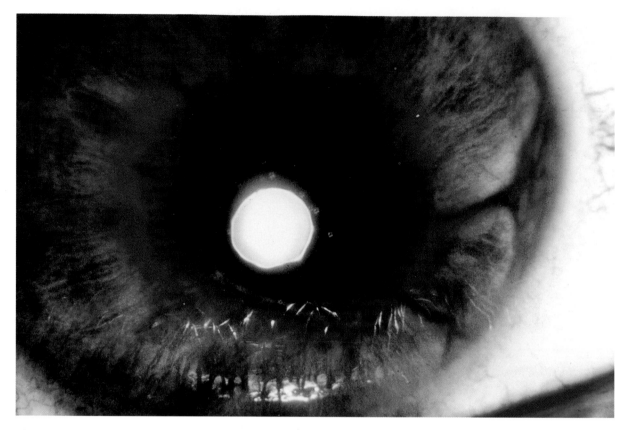

Fig. 5.7 Advanced rubeosis irides in a case of advanced proliferative diabetic retinopathy. Laser photocoagulation is the treatment of choice.

vitreoretinopathy (PVR) with massive vitreoretinal membranes, the intraoperative use of laser photocoagulation with the resultant formation of a good chorioretinal adhesion has frequently meant the difference between success and failure.

It is unfortunate that many patients with diabetes mellitus are never examined by an ophthalmologist. Klein and colleagues (8) report that 55% of diabetic persons with high risk of visual loss have never had laser photocoagulation. In an earlier report by Witkins and Klein (9), in their same Wisconsin Epidemiologic Study, the authors have shown that 11% of juvenile-onset and 7% of adult-onset diabetic patients with high-risk characteristics have not been seen by an ophthalmologist within the past 2 years.

The presence of rubeosis irides (Fig. 5.7) or early neovascularization of the angle presents another indication for the use of laser photocoagulation. Usually, PRP is the treatment of choice. Gonioscopy is therefore essential in determining the presence of angle neovascularization. Murphy and Egbert (10) found that prompt laser treatment can frequently prevent occurrence of neovascular glaucoma and phthisis bulbae, two conditions that frequently contribute to the demise of the eye. The earliest indication of anterior segment neovascularization as shown by new blood vessels located at or near the pupillary mar-

gin of the iris or the sudden elevation of intraocular pressure, frequently indicates the urgency of PRP. The local occurrence of NVE usually calls for focal laser photocoagulation. Widespread areas of NVE or evidence of NVD should be treated by PRP, usually in divided sessions. A fundus fluorescein angiogram is, of course, essential prior to laser application, because it will pinpoint areas of leakage from microaneurysms (Fig. 5.8) as well as leakage from areas of neovascularization.

Management Recommendations

Argon and krypton laser photocoagulation are the most widely used modalities for treating diabetic retinopathy. Laser photocoagulation is indicated for patients with high-risk proliferative disease, patients with clinically significant macular edema, and iris or angle neovascularization.

Table 5.1 indicates the management recommendations for diabetic retinopathy as set forth by Wilkinson and colleagues (11) for the American Academy of Ophthalmology in its preferred practice pattern entitled Diabetic Retinopathy. The following text description corresponds to each of the nine listings in the table. Note that each of the nine categories is designed to establish a framework of classification and that individual and specific needs for

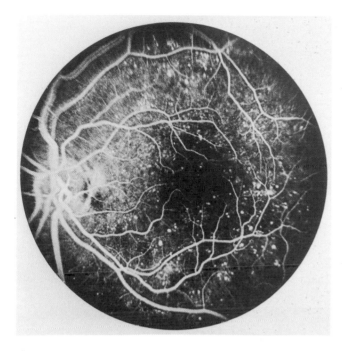

Fig. 5.8 The venous phase of a fundus fluorescein angiogram of the right eye. Note the myriad number of microaneurysms in the posterior pole.

laser surgery may sometimes vary from patient to patient within an individual subset.

1. Normal or Minimal Nonproliferative Diabetic Retinopathy

Patients with normal or minimal nonproliferative (background) diabetic retinopathy (i.e., with rare microaneurysms) should have annual examinations because 5% to 10% of patients who are initially normal will develop diabetic retinopathy within one year. Similarly, 5% to 10% of patients with minimal BDR will have an increase in their disease within one year. Fluorescein angiography and laser surgery are infrequently indicated for patients within this category.

2. Nonproliferative Diabetic Retinopathy Without Macular Edema

Patients with retinal microaneurysms and occasional blot hemorrhages or hard exudates should have repeat examinations within 6 months because disease progression is common. Fluorescein angiography and laser therapy are usually not indicated.

3. Nonproliferative Diabetic Retinopathy with Macular Edema That is Not Clinically Significant

Patients with macular edema that is not clinically significant should have repeat examinations within four to six months because they are at risk of developing clinically significant macular edema. While laser surgery may not be indicated for this category, fluorescein angiography may be of value in establishing the cause of the visual loss.

4. Nonproliferative Diabetic Retinopathy with Clinically Significant Macular Edema

The Early Treatment Diabetic Retinopathy Study defines any of the following features of macular edema as clinically significant.

  a. Thickening of the retina at or within 500 μm of the center of the macula.

  b. Hard exudates at or within 500 μm of the center of the macula if associated with thickening of the adjacent retina (not residual hard exudates remaining after the disappearance of retinal thickening).

  c. A zone or zones of retinal thickening one disc area or larger, any part of which is within one disc diameter of the center of the macula.

Patients having the above criteria should have laser photocoagulation to substantially reduce the risk of visual loss. Fluorescein angiography should be performed before laser treatment to identify the leaking areas and pinpoint the treatable lesions. The patient should be well controlled medically before the ophthalmologist considers photocoagulation for diabetic macular edema. The diastolic blood pressure should be reduced below 100 mm Hg. The hemoglobin A_1 level should be equal to or less than 10 mg/dl. Lastly there should be little to no evidence of renal failure.

5. Preproliferative Diabetic Retinopathy

In preproliferative diabetic retinopathy, the risk of progression to proliferative disease is very high. PPDR is characterized by the presence of venous beading or large retinal blot hemorrhages, multiple cotton wool spots or multiple IRMA. Klein and colleagues (12,13) have shown that between 10% and 40% of patients with preproliferative changes will develop PDR within one year.

Many diabetic retinologists recommend PRP in at least one eye for patients with bilateral PPDR because the incidence of progression to proliferative retinopathy is so high. Fundus fluorescein angiography is certainly indicated to determine the presence or absence of areas of nonperfusion and leakage from neovascularization.

6. Non–High-Risk Proliferative Diabetic Retinopathy

The Diabetic Retinopathy Study Research Group (14) states that the treatment with laser photocoagulation for non–high-risk PDR is controversial, with many retinologists electing to treat these cases, especially if involvement is bilateral. If laser treatment is delayed, follow-up within 2 to 3 months is mandatory because a significant percentage of these patients will ultimately develop high-risk characteristics requiring treatment. Fluorescein angiography is required before treatment to determine the areas of retinal nonperfusion, to provide a good differential diagnosis between hemorrhage and neovascularization, and to establish the cause of visual loss.

Table 5.1 Management recommendations for various types and stages of diabetic retinopathy.

Diabetic Status of Retina	Follow-up (mo)	Laser	Fluorescein Angiography	Color Fundus Photography
1. Normal or minimal nonproliferative diabetic retinopathy	12	No	No	No
2. Nonproliferative diabetic retinopathy without macular edema	6-12	No	No	Rarely
3. Nonproliferative diabetic retinopathy with macular edema that is not clinically significant	4-6	No	Occasionally	Occasionally
4. Nonproliferative diabetic retinopathy with clinically significant macular edema	2-4	Yes*	Yes	Yes
5. Preproliferative diabetic retinopathy	3-4	Uncertain†	Occasionally	Occasionally
6. Non–high-risk proliferative diabetic retinopathy	2-3‡	Uncertain†	Occasionally	Occasionally
7. Non–high-risk proliferative diabetic retinopathy with clinically significant macular edema	2-3‡	Yes†	Yes	Yes
8. High-risk proliferative diabetic retinopathy	3-4	Yes	Occasionally	Yes
9. High-risk proliferative diabetic retinopathy not amenable to photocoagulation	1-6	Not Possible§	No	Occasionally (if possible)

*For exceptions, see Int Ophthalmol Clin 1987;27:332.
†Treatment indicated in some cases. Photocoagulation indicated for clinically significant macular edema.
‡If treatment is deferred. If treated, follow-up in 3-4 mo.
§Vitrectomy indicated in highly selected cases.
SOURCE: Reproduced by permission from Wilkinson, Benson WE, Blumenkranz M. Diabetic Retinopathy—Preferred Practice Pattern. American Academy of Ophthalmology Retinal and Quality of Care Panels, November 1993.

7. Non–High-Risk Proliferative Diabetic Retinopathy with Clinically Significant Macular Edema

Many investigators favor focal laser photocoagulation treatment for macular edema in this situation according to the Early Treatment Diabetic Retinopathy Study Research Group (15). Indications for angiography and fundus photography are similar to those for patients with non–high-risk PDR.

8. High-Risk Proliferative Diabetic Retinopathy

The Diabetic Retinopathy Study Group's high-risk characteristics for profound visual loss include:
a. NVD greater than one-quarter to one-third disc area.

b. Vitreous or preretinal hemorrhage associated with less extensive NVD, or with NVE one-half disc area or more in size.

The risk of profound visual loss among patients with high-risk PDR can be substantially reduced by means of PRP delivered in a scatter pattern throughout the fundus. PRP leads to regression of neovascularization. This proven technique has been fully described in the literature by the Diabetic Retinopathy Study Research Group in their DRS report No. 14 (16).

Indications for retreatment may include:
a. Increasing neovascularization

b. New areas of neovascularization
c. New vitreous hemorrhage
d. Failure of the neovascularization to regress

Technique of Panretinal Laser Photocoagulation

Three types of laser delivery systems are used in the release of laser energy to the retina. The oldest method emits laser energy via a slit-lamp delivery system. Intraoperative endophotocoagulation was added during the late 1970s as an effective alternate invasive technique for laser application at the time of vitrectomy surgery. Laser delivery via a binocular indirect ophthalmoscope is the latest method of delivering laser energy to the retina. Like slit-lamp delivery, it is noninvasive.

Treatment is performed using either the argon blue-green, argon green, krypton, or diode laser. Argon blue-green is less frequently used today because of the chance of phototoxicity to both the patient's retina as well as to the macula of the operating surgeon. The krypton or diode laser is preferred when cataractous changes or vitreous hemorrhage prevents adequate retinal visualization.

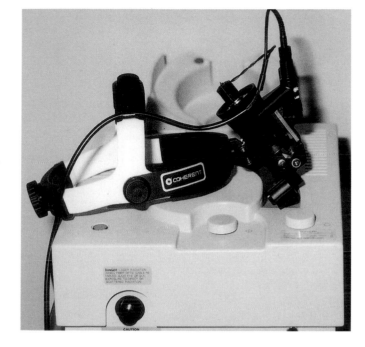

Fig. 5.9 The argon laser incorporated into the binocular indirect ophthalmoscope.

Non-Contact Lenses

Lenses for retinal photocoagulation consist of contact and non-contact varieties. There are many fewer indications for the non-contact photocoagulation lenses. The most commonly used method for non-contact viewing and treatment is the use of a +20 and a +30 diopter (D) condensing lens to deliver laser energy that has been incorporated into the binocular indirect ophthalmoscope (Fig. 5.9). Other non-contact delivery lenses include the Hruby lens as well as the +60, +78, and +90 D lenses (Fig. 5.10). Producing laser photocoagulation through a +60 or +90 D non-contact lens provides a larger spot size of the retinal lesion than would be created with a Goldmann three-mirror lens of the same micron setting. In this case, the size of the lesion resembles that created with the Rodenstock lens.

The non-contact lenses are used primarily in cases where there is a relative contraindication to the placement of a lens directly in contact with the corneal surface. Such situations may occur when edema of the cornea is present directly following surgical vitrectomy or recent trauma. Recurrent epithelial corneal erosions from basement membrane disease secondary to diabetes mellitus comprise a second group of cases. Lastly, photocoagulation through the +20 D lens via indirect ophthalmoscopy may become necessary in the presence of vitreous hemorrhage or cataract formation where this means becomes the only way to view the fundus.

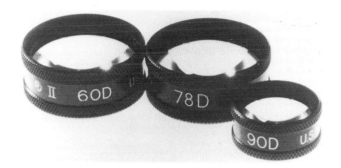

Fig. 5.10 Photograph showing the +60, +78, and +90 D lenses used to visualize the fundus and occasionally used in the non-contact mode for laser photocoagulation.

The Hruby lens is a high −58 D lens attached to the slit lamp. It gives an upright image of high resolution but with a small field. It should be used for diagnostic purposes only and not for laser treatment. The +90 D lens differs from the Hruby lens in providing an inverted image of the retina, similar to the view obtained with indirect ophthalmoscopy. Its learning curve is longer than with the Hruby lens because of this. Its advantage is that it provides a wider field than the Hruby lens. However, like the Hruby lens, it should be used mainly for observation and diagnostic purposes and only infrequently for treatment.

Contact Corneal Lenses

The pupil is dilated with Mydfrin 2.5% and Mydriacyl 1% to achieve full dilatation. Ophthaine is used for topical anesthesia. A retrobulbar anesthetic may be given when working directly in the macular area to decrease photophobia as well as to prevent ocular motility.

All the following corneal contact lenses described below make use of methylcellulose 2.0% to act as the coupling agent and to provide some protection to the underlying corneal epithelium. All lenses used in the contact mode should have antireflection coating. The coating serves two purposes—it decreases the amount of scattering of light, and it protects the operating surgeon from reflected laser light.

Corneal contact lenses used today are the Goldmann lens (17), the Rodenstock panfunduscopic lens (18), the Mainster lens (19), the Yannuzzi lens (20), and the Vogt quadraspheric fundus lens (21).

The oldest and best known contact lens used for retinal laser photocoagulation is the Goldmann (17) triple-mirror lens (Fig. 5.11). It has a dioptric power of −64 and has become the standard lens for macular photocoagulation. It is used for peripheral as well as for central macular laser treatment. Its three peripheral mirrors have various angles allowing for laser application from the posterior pole (via the central mirror) to the equator, from the equator to the ora serrata, and for the ora as well as for gonioscopy. Thus, the entire retina from the optic nerve to the ora serrata can be visualized and treated by rotating the lens so that the slit beam of the microscope can impinge on the central mirror as well as on the three peripheral mirrors. The advantage of the Goldmann lens is that it gives a di-

rect view with great magnification. Its disadvantage is that it provides only a small field with the potential hazard of inadvertent foveal laser photocoagulation if certain precautions are not followed. If the patient does not fixate centrally or if the lens is tilted toward the center, the danger of foveal coagulation becomes very real.

The Rodenstock panfunduscopic lens (Fig. 5.12) was developed to eliminate the use of mirrors to perform laser photocoagulation from the posterior pole to a point anterior to the equator. It gives a wide angle view, thus providing a greater field of vision than the Goldmann lens. Hence, photocoagulation can be accomplished at a much more rapid rate. There is a greater safety factor in using the Rodenstock lens because the large panoramic view enables the surgeon to see the optic nerve, the macula, and the periphery in one simultaneous view. The single inconvenience of the Rodenstock lens is the longer learning curve because the surgeon obtains an inverted image similar to that found with indirect ophthalmoscopy. In addition, the size of the laser lesion is 40% larger than that obtained with the Goldmann lens, a factor that must be kept in mind when working in the parafoveal region of the eye.

The author prefers the Rodenstock lens because one can obtain a better simultaneous overall view of both the posterior pole as well as the retinal periphery. The advantage is that the larger area seen with the Rodenstock lens helps to prevent inadvertent photocoagulation of the parafoveal and foveal areas. The Rodenstock panfunduscopic lens is a high plus lens, producing an inverted real image of the fundus similar to that seen with indirect ophthalmoscopy. By minifying the fundus view, one obtains a wider field. Since the actual spot size on the

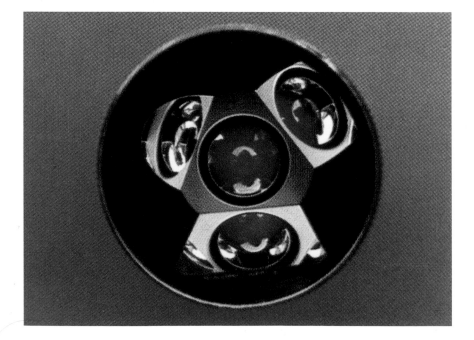

Fig. 5.11 The Goldmann triple-mirror lens. The central mirror is used for fundus visualization and laser photocoagulation in the area of the posterior pole. The peripheral mirrors are used for equatorial and anterior fundus laser photocoagulation as well as for gonioscopy.

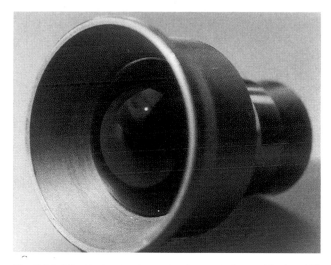

Fig. 5.12 The Rodenstock panfunduscopic lens with the ability to achieve laser photocoagulation of the posterior pole and the equatorial area with visualization through a single lens.

Guidelines in Laser Treatment

The question is frequently raised as to whether retrobulbar anesthesia should be used. In the vast majority of photocoagulation, no retrobulbar anesthesia is required. However, if one is working in the posterior pole where photophobia may be intense, a retrobulbar anesthetic is important to reduce light sensitivity and eliminate ocular movement. It should be noted that the temporal retina is more sensitive than the nasal retina and that the horizontal meridians in the areas of the long posterior ciliary nerves are the most sensitive. Increasing the power level (in watts) and time duration (in tenths of a second) also increases the pain reflex, at times requiring retrobulbar anesthesia. Lastly, single session PRP requires more frequent retrobulbar injections than when PRP is performed in three or more divided sessions.

Argon blue photocoagulation, operating at 488 nm, is mentioned only to be condemned. The blue wavelength is absorbed by both the yellow nucleus of the senile cataractous lens as well as by macular xanthophyll. Scattering of light is also greater with the blue laser, making treatment potentially hazardous to the lens and retina of the operating surgeon. For these reasons, the green argon laser, operating at 514 nm, should be used. In the face of a cataractous lens or where an early vitreous hemorrhage is present, the krypton red laser or the diode laser may prove successful if argon green is unable to produce adequate retinal laser lesions. The krypton (647 nm) and diode (810 nm) lasers cause deeper burns in the retina and inner choroid and therefore may be more painful, necessitating the use of retrobulbar anesthesia. Occasionally, choroidal detachments and chorioretinal hemorrhages may result when using krypton or diode lasers because of the increased tendency to ruptures in Bruch's membrane.

A few precautions should be exercised when performing photocoagulation in the posterior pole. Firstly, if using a Goldmann contact lens, a double row of laser spots should be placed temporal to the fovea. This acts as a demarcation line, minimizing any tendency to foveal photocoagulation. Secondly, the inferior retina should be treated first so that if vitreous hemorrhage develops, the superior retina can still be adequately treated at a subsequent session. Lastly, when treating retinal tissue directly below the fovea, one should be aware that Bell's phenomenon can cause an upward rotation of the globe, leading to possible foveal coagulation. This tendency can be minimized through the use of a retrobulbar anesthetic.

Treatment is usually performed in three divided sessions. Some surgeons accomplish the entire PRP in only one session. However, as shown by Doft and Blankenship (22), single session PRP is more prone to the development of exudative retinal detachment, choroidal detachment, and angle closure glaucoma than multiple session laser treatments. In the three session technique, session one

retina is magnified approximately 40% with the Rodenstock lens, using the laser set at a spot size of 500 μm produces approximately a 750-μm diameter lesion in the retina. The Rodenstock lens has also gained popularity in performing laser photocoagulation on eyes with small, undilatable pupils. Since the Rodenstock lens magnifies the entrance pupil while the Goldmann lens minifies it, the Rodenstock lens makes it easier to successfully perform a PRP in glaucomatous eyes previously subjected to miotic therapy or in eyes with small pupils due to posterior synechiae from previous bouts of iridocyclitis.

The Mainster (19) corneal contact lens was developed to improve on the main deficiency of both the Goldmann lens and the Rodenstock lens. It was designed to increase the small field of the Goldmann lens and to increase the magnification of the Rodenstock lens. The Mainster lens acts like the Rodenstock lens in providing an inverted, real image.

The Yannuzzi (20) lens was designed for macular photocoagulation to treat lesions in the parafoveal area. It is a modification of the Krieger widefield fundus lens. Yannuzzi's modifications allow positive pressure to be applied against the sclera while minimizing corneal pressure. This technique may aid in the control of hemorrhage that may complicate laser photocoagulation in the treatment of subretinal neovascularization when using the deeper penetrating krypton laser.

The Volk quadraspheric lens (21) is of recent development. One of the reasons for fabricating the Volk quadraspheric lens was to improve visualization through a miotic pupil. The Volk lens, like the Rodenstock and Mainster lenses, also provides an inverted mirror image of the retinal target tissue.

usually consists of treating the inferior parafoveal, inferior temporal, and temporal areas. Session two treats the superior parafoveal, superior temporal, and far-out temporal periphery. Session three treats the superior and inferior nasal quadrants. Fig. 5.13 shows a typical case of retinal photocoagulation after laser application. The two main advantages of multiple treatments are fewer operative and postoperative complications and less tendency in having to perform retrobulbar anesthesia.

The goal of therapy is to produce at least 1500 to 2000 laser lesions per eye. If one is working within the temporal arcades, one uses 50 to 100 μm size lesions. Five hundred to 1000 μm spot sizes are used outside the temporal arcades as well as in the nasal quadrants. The energy duration is usually set at 0.2 sec. The power level usually is set at a threshold level of 0.2 to 0.3 W and the power is then turned up in 25 mW increments until a white lesion is seen in the retina. Lesions are placed approximately one-half to one lesion apart to prevent scotomata and serious night blindness. Confluent treatment is introduced to retinal areas harboring NVE. If a retinal hemorrhage occurs, increasing the pressure on the contact lens will usually cause it to stop. Retinal hemorrhages are more prevalent with krypton and diode laser photocoagulation than with argon because the energy absorption with krypton and diode lasers occurs deeper within the retina, sometimes affecting the choriocapillaris. In the occasional case where a vitreous hemorrhage may occur in the postoperative period of the first session, instruct the patient to elevate the head and sit with bilateral patches. This frequently allows the hemorrhage to settle inferiorly, enabling subsequent laser to be placed superiorly in Session II.

The object of PRP for PDR is to place a total of 1500 to 2000 laser burns within an eye, using either 500 μm size lesions with the Goldmann lens or 250 to 350 μm size burns with the Rodenstock lens. The lesions are placed one burn diameter apart from a point immediately outside the temporal arcades to the equatorial area. The posterior pole between the arcades and the fovea as well as the area immediately surrounding the optic disc are spared. If NVD is present, laser burns should come within one half of a burn diameter inferior, nasal, and superior to the disc.

The intensity of the laser burn should be either light or medium and of gray to white in color. A higher powered laser burn will be intensely white. Naturally, the higher powered burns will encompass a greater area than the less intense burns and if higher power is used, fewer laser burns become necessary.

The question arises as to whether to treat directly over abnormal areas or whether to surround these areas with laser burns. NVD and neovascularization in the foveal area (posterior pole NVE) should never be treated directly. Likewise, fibrovascular fronds emanating from the optic disc or located within the macular area are also not photocoagulated directly. A good tight PRP will usually result in less neovascularization of these areas. Flat NVE outside the macula as well as microaneurysms and IRMA are treated directly overlying these areas with confluent laser burns. It is important to remember that the size of the laser lesion should be larger than the diameter of the vessel to be treated to minimize the possibility of a retinal or vitreous hemorrhage. Finally, one should not treat drectly over areas of gliosis or areas of traction retinal detachment because contraction of the laser scars may increase the area of the traction detachment. In such cases, laser marks are used to wall off the traction areas by surrounding these abnormalities with tight laser applications.

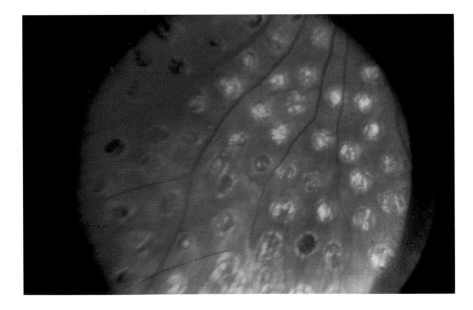

Fig. 5.13 Partial fundus view of an area of panretinal photocoagulation of the retina demonstrating the recent acute white chorioretinal laser lesions coupled with the old pigmented chorioretinal laser lesions as shown in the left side of the photograph.

9. High-Risk Proliferative Diabetic Retinopathy Not Amenable to Photocoagulation

It may be impossible to perform argon laser photocoagulation on some patients with severe vitreous or preretinal hemorrhage (Fig. 5.14). In other cases, advanced, active PDR may persist despite extensive PRP.

Alternatives to Argon Laser Photocoagulation

The following four modalities of treatment have frequently provided beneficial results when argon green laser photocoagulation has proven to be ineffective.

- Krypton or diode laser photocoagulation
- Xenon arc photocoagulation
- Panretinal cryoablation
- Early vitrectomy

Krypton or diode laser photocoagulation has frequently been used when the argon laser has been unable to produce a good chorioretinal reaction in the face of an advancing diabetic posterior subcapsular cataract or when vitreous hemorrhage is present. The krypton and diode lasers have the advantage of penetrating through a cataractous lens and vitreous hemorrhage to a greater extent than argon radiation. Krypton laser photocoagulation produces a deeper burn at the chorioretinal interface. Its disadvantage, however, is that the unwanted complication of a retinal hemorrhage is more frequent than with argon. Therefore, lower intensities and lower size lesions (250 μm as compared with 500 μm size lesions with argon) have to be used to achieve the desired effect. A clinical trial comparing argon to krypton laser photocoagulation demonstrated that the chorioretinal response to either laser was equally sufficient in impeding the progression of PDR.

Xenon arc photocoagulation was the earliest method of using a light source to produce a good chorioretinal seal.

However, a rather cumbersome instrument is used. It also has a larger incidence of iatrogenic retinal hemorrhage than argon and is not able to provide the more efficient slit-lamp delivery system. Its advantage of not requiring a corneal contact lens is largely offset by its requirement of retrobulbar anesthesia because photophobia and ocular movement are undesirable features of its delivery system.

Panretinal cryoablation is frequently used when a fairly dense cataract or vitreous hemorrhage prevents the energy of laser photocoagulation from penetrating the media to provide adequate reaction in the retina and choroid. The disadvantage of cryoablation is that the postoperative eye exhibits much inflammatory reaction and discomfort. With the recent advent of using laser energy through an indirect ophthalmoscope as a delivery system, the need for resorting to a panretinal cryoablation has largely been reduced.

Early vitrectomy is seldom required if high-risk PDR does not have much lenticular opacity or vitreous hemorrhage associated with it. If photocoagulation cannot be performed through a hazy media via either slit-lamp or indirect ophthalmoscopy delivery systems or if cryoablation is not feasible, then early vitrectomy with or without lensectomy becomes the treatment of choice. Once the vitreous hemorrhage has been cleared via vitrectomy, laser endophotocoagulation is then carried out at the time of surgery.

Early vitrectomy is beneficial in patients with extensive, active, neovascular, or fibrovascular proliferation. The Diabetic Retinopathy Vitrectomy Study (5,6) has shown the value of early vitrectomy in cases of more advanced neovascularization and severe PDR. It should be noted, however, that retinal cryoablation and early vitrectomy are indicated only in the above very special conditions where lentricular or vitreous opacification prevents the use of laser photocoagulation through standard delivery systems.

Often vitreous surgery is primarily indicated in patients with traction-macular detachment or combined traction-rhegmatogenous retinal detachment. Early vitrectomy for juvenile-onset diabetic patients with severe vitreous hemorrhage is beneficial. Intraoperative laser treatment may also be indicated for patients in this category. When the fundus cannot be visualized, ultrasonography should usually be used to search for retinal detachment.

Vitreous surgery is not a benign procedure and has the potential for serious complications, including retinal detachment, glaucoma, profound visual loss, and permanent pain and blindness. It should not be undertaken without careful consideration of the potential risks and benefits. In many instances where there is only a low risk of the spread of traction retinal detachment into the macula, vitreous surgery may best be deferred. Deferral is particularly appropriate when new vessels have regressed substantially and retinopathy appears to be inactive.

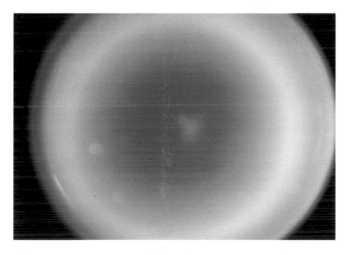

Fig. 5.14 Massive vitreous hemorrhage in which no fundus detail of the optic disc or the retina can be visualized.

The relationship between the degree of glycemic control and the severity of complications, including diabetic retinopathy with its need for laser photocoagulation, has been actively discussed within the medical community. Blood sugar levels of 200 mg% or higher are associated with an increased frequency of microvascular complications, including PDR. In addition, Klein and colleagues have shown that a positive relationship exists between the progression of diabetic retinopathy and glycosylated hemoglobin. It is therefore strongly suggested that poor levels of blood glucose control contribute to microangiopathy, including retinopathy, with the subsequent need for laser photocoagulation, as stated by Ross and coworkers (24). It is therefore recommended that the diabetic patient maintain tight control of the blood sugar level and serum A_1 level, in an attempt to prevent the devastating sequelae of PDR.

Diabetic Maculopathy

The most common cause of loss of central visual acuity in diabetic retinopathy is the presence of macular edema. Although PDR is also responsible for a great loss of vision, it is the high proportion of macular changes resulting from severe central retinopathy and edema that is most visually disabling. Diabetic macular edema occurs more frequently in adult-onset diabetes rather than in juvenile diabetes mellitus. Approximately 10% of all diabetic patients will exhibit macular edema. The fovea will be involved in almost 50% of these cases.

Diabetic macular edema can be divided into two categories, focal and diffuse. The more visually disabling diffuse form can be further divided into two groups depending on the presence or absence of cystoid macular edema (CME) as shown in the fundus fluorescein angiography of Fig. 5.15. Naturally, the presence of CME carries with it a lower prognosis for the return of good central visual acuity. The definition of diffuse macular edema is the presence of two or more disc areas of retinal thickening involving the center of the macula. Naturally, a good fluorescein angiogram is essential prior to any laser treatment.

There are three significant components to the diagnosis of macular edema in diabetic maculopathy. Firstly, there is the presence of retinal thickening at or within 500 μm of the center of the macula. Secondly, deep, hard exudates are present. These are also located at or within 500 μm of the foveal area. Thirdly, at least one disc area of retinal thickening should be present, part of which is within one disc diameter of the fovea. It has also been shown by Klein and coworkers (25) that the prevalence of macular edema increased as the severity of the diabetic retinopathy worsened. Thus, 2% to 6% of patients exhibiting BDR exhibited macular edema, whereas 70% to 74% of cases demonstrating PDR showed clinical evidence of macular edema. It has also been shown that the incidence of macular edema correlates well with the longer duration of diabetes mellitus as well as with a higher level of glycosylated hemoglobin. Sinclair and coworkers (26) have also shown that pregnancy has an adverse effect on macular edema, resulting in greater diffuse maculopathy. There is also fluorescein angiographic evidence that significant capillary macular nonperfusion (Fig. 5.16) results as the pregnancy progresses. It has also been shown that in the postpartum phase of pregnancy, macular edema resolves, leading toward improvement of central visual acuity.

Treatment of Diabetic Maculopathy

The treatment of diabetic maculopathy focuses on both systemic and local ocular methods. The goal of treatment is the elimination of macular edema, the diminution of retinal thickening, and the absorption of hard exudates.

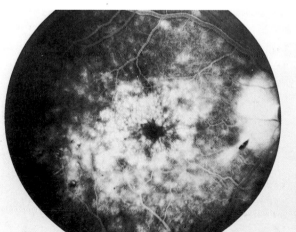

Fig. 5.15 Fundus fluorescein angiogram demonstrates marked cystoid macular edema.

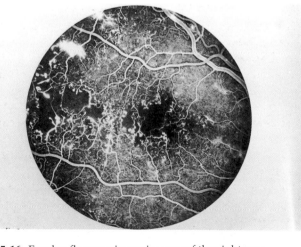

Fig. 5.16 Fundus fluorescein angiogram of the right eye demonstrates significant capillary macular nonperfusion.

Naturally, each of these objectives becomes more difficult in cases where the degree of macular edema and the number of years of diabetic retinopathy increase.

Systemic treatment consists of treating congestive heart failure and chronic renal dysfunction. Blood pressure control results in decreased retinal leakage and decreased macular edema.

Local treatment consists of laser photocoagulation for both focal and diffuse macular edema.

Focal Macular Edema

Microaneurysms are the fundamental cause of focal macular edema. They tend to be present within the areas of focal edema and are certainly the major cause of the leakage. Hard exudative circinate rings are frequently present.

Treatment of focal macular edema consists of direct photocoagulation to the microaneurysms themselves. The argon green wavelength is used because absorption by hemoglobin is desired. Because blue light is absorbed by macular xanthophyll and is phototoxic to the retina, the blue-green laser should be avoided. The goal of therapy is the photocoagulation of all microaneurysms up to 500 μm from the center of the fovea.

The argon green laser should be set at 50 μm spot size and 0.1 sec of energy duration. Milliwatt power should be set at a subthreshold level and turned up until a white lesion is produced. Treatment is directed to all microaneurysms 500 μm from the center of the macula. If macular edema persists on follow-up examination and if central visual acuity drops, focal treatment up to 300 μm of the fovea should be attempted. Grid photocoagulation could be used in treating a cluster of microaneurysms. Repeat fundus photography and repeat fundus fluorescein angiography should be performed following laser photocoagulation to document the results of treatment.

Diffuse Macular Edema

Diffuse macular edema in the diabetic patient results from a breakdown of the inner blood-retinal barrier in which capillaries and arterioles leak as well as microaneurysms. Hard exudates are usually absent in diabetics with diffuse edema. Bresnick (27) has shown that retinal pigment epithelium dysfunction also may contribute to the formation of persistence of diffuse edema in the diabetic. Candidates should have visual acuity of 20/200 or better and demonstrate no more than six clock hours of juxtafoveal capillary nonperfusion on fluorescein angiography.

Fluorescein angiography can pinpoint areas of noncapillary or decreased capillary perfusion, a condition that adds to the visual loss in the macular region (see Fig. 5.16). The observance of the fluorescein transit in the prevenous or laminar flow phase of the angiogram is the best method of determining capillary perfusion adjacent to the foveal avascular zone. If large areas of nonperfusion are present, the patient must be told that even with laser photocoagulation, the chance of restoration of good central visual acuity is somewhat guarded.

Modified Grid Laser for Diffuse Macular Edema

The treatment of diffuse diabetic macular edema is by modified grid laser photocoagulation as outlined by Olk (28). In some cases, a retrobulbar injection of Xylocaine 2% with Wydase is given. Spots of 100 μm size are applied for two to three rows around the parafoveal area up to and including the edge of the foveal avascular zone placing the lesions 100 μm apart (Fig. 5.17). The central area 500 μm from fixation is spared. Spots (200 μm) are then applied throughout all areas of diffuse leakage seen on the fluorescein angiogram, placing the lesions approximately 200 μm apart (Fig. 5.18). Additional 200 μm spots are placed confluently in areas of obvious focal leakage (Fig. 5.19). The goal of treatment is to achieve light to moderately intense burns at 0.1-sec duration. The milliwatt settings are variable depending on the density of the pigment epithelium as well as the clarity of the ocular media. The average power settings are 100 to 200 mW and the average number of spots applied range from 150 to 300 spots per treatment session (Fig. 5.20).

Modified grid laser photocoagulation does not always have to be given throughout the entire posterior pole of the eye. Treatment should be directed only to those areas of the macula demonstrating either nonprofusion or retinal thickening. These involved areas are frequently temporal to the macula. Olk (29) states that in many cases, one can treat the areas of diffuse leakage with a grid pattern and then apply additional focal treatment to those

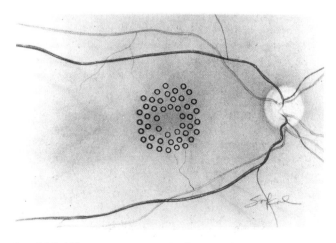

Fig. 5.17 100 μm spots are applied two to three rows around the parafoveal region. (Reproduced by permission from Olk [28].)

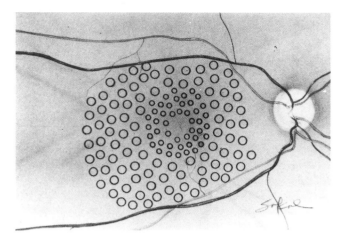

Fig. 5.18 200 μm spots are applied throughout all areas of diffuse leakage. (Reproduced by permission from Olk [28].)

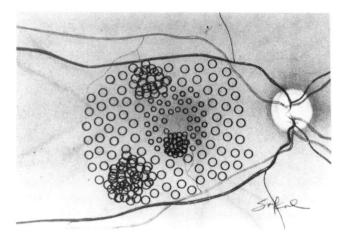

Fig. 5.19 Additional 200 μm spots are placed confluently in areas of obvious focal leakage. (Reproduced by permission from Olk [28].)

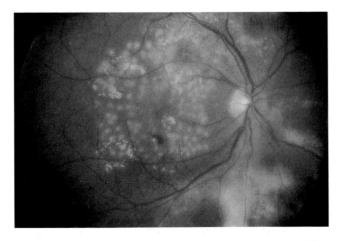

Fig. 5.20 Fundus photo of right posterior pole shows modified grid laser photocoagulation of the macula.

areas in the juxtafoveal region that require only focal treatment.

Resolution of either focal or diffuse macular edema following laser photocoagulation is frequently a slow process, sometimes taking 2 to 3 months following treatment. Therefore, repeat laser photocoagulation should not be performed earlier than 3 months postoperatively, especially if the grid pattern has been used. A fundus fluorescein angiogram should be performed prior to repeat laser therapy, to identify new areas of focal leakage as well as areas of nonperfusion. Additional treatment should be directed to placing laser burns between preexisting spots and tightening the grid pattern to within 200 μm of the foveal fixation point. Attention should also be directed to the control of renal, hypertensive, and cardiovascular abnormalities because a tight control of these factors may frequently result in improvement of macular edema.

If diffuse macular edema is coupled with PDR, it is frequently difficult to determine where the initial thrust of the treatment should be directed. I usually direct my initial photocoagulation treatment on the basis of which is the more involved area. If there is advanced PDR with fairly good visual acuity and mild diffuse diabetic retinopathy, I will frequently begin therapy with panretinal scatter photocoagulation in three divided sessions approximately one week apart. Attention will then be directed to performing the modified grid laser photocoagulation after the proliferative retinopathy has stabilized. On the other hand, if the patient exhibits advanced diffuse macular edema coupled with only one or two high-risk factors of PDR, I will start with a modified grid and focal type of laser photocoagulation before considering a PRP.

The third case scenario is where there is both advanced diffuse macular edema with advanced PDR. Fortunately, these cases are becoming less frequent because patients with diabetes mellitus are being followed more closely by ophthalmologists before the more advanced complications of diabetic retinopathy have become apparent. In the rare situations where both of these conditions coexist, I may combine modified grid laser with PRP. The modified grid applications are applied in a single session, whereas the PRP is divided into 3-5 multiple weekly sessions. There is a significant risk of at least transient post-laser chorioretinal edema following combined therapy. Consequently, the patient should be advised before laser treatment is begun, that visual acuity may decrease for a few weeks following therapy. However, with time, acuity will frequently improve to at or near the pre-laser level.

Complications of Grid Laser Photocoagulation

The main complication of modified grid laser photocoagulation is a paracentral scotoma. A haze or film is also frequently present. Both of these conditions usually decrease with time but most diabetic patients have some evidence of scotoma years after treatment. Because modified grid treatment significantly conserves central visual acuity when compared with the natural history of the disease, it is felt that the risk of paracentral scotoma is a small price to pay when faced with the irreparable loss of vision if laser treatment is not instituted. The presence of CME as well as uncontrolled systemic hypertension are both poor prognostic signs for visual improvement.

The exact mechanism for the disappearance of diabetic macular edema in laser grid treatment is unknown. However, it is felt that the combination effect on both the retinal vasculature (inner retinal barrier) as well as the retinal pigment epithelium (outer retinal barrier) open new pathways for the egress of fluid out of the retina. Furthermore, it has been shown by Olk (30) that there is no statistically significant difference of beneficial results between argon green (514 nm) or krypton red (647 nm) in the treatment of diffuse diabetic maculopathy with or without CME.

It is important to note that the use of laser photocoagulation for diffuse macular edema infrequently results in a dramatic improvement of central visual acuity. Its most important treatment effect is a reduction in the proportion of eyes that show a further loss of vision than in eyes where no laser had been used. In summary, laser treatment for diabetic maculopathy exhibiting diffuse macular edema reduces the rate of visual loss while in a minority of eyes one can obtain a modest improvement of vision.

Pregnancy and Diabetic Retinopathy

Mention must be made of the relationship of pregnancy and diabetic retinopathy. Sunness (31) provides a good summary of the incidence of diabetic retinopathy in the pregnant woman. If no diabetic retinopathy is present at the onset of pregnancy, the patient usually does not progress to proliferative retinopathy during the course of pregnancy. Therefore, the patient should be examined at each trimester. No laser treatment is required. If BDR is present at the onset of pregnancy, only 5% of women will progress to PDR during the pregnancy. Therefore, few women must be treated with laser photocoagulation. When PDR is present at the onset of pregnancy, it will usually progress during the ensuing 9 months, requiring aggressive PRP if regression of the retinopathy is to occur. In the postpartum phase, regression of the diabetic retinopathy will occur, especially if PRP was performed prior to delivery. It is advisable that patients exhibiting PDR be examined every month while pregnant.

Diagnostic Laser Evaluation for Diabetic Retinopathy

Diagnostic methods for detecting diabetic retinopathy developed at the Eye Research Institute of The Retina Foundation in Boston include the scanning laser ophthalmoscope (SLO) and the laser Doppler velocimeter (LDV).

The SLO uses a low-level scanning laser to provide a detailed image of the retina on a television monitor. The LDV is another useful tool that monitors blood flow through the retina. Results showing changes in blood flow often alert the investigator to the probability of imminent anatomic changes. Changes in circulation are often a precursor of other symptoms of diabetic retinopathy, such as edema and hemorrhage.

The LDV was developed during the 1970s by Dr. Gilbert Feke, while working at the Eye Research Institute of The Retina Foundation. The LDV studies early changes in the blood flow of the retina. A low-level laser beam is projected into the eye, where it strikes the small blood vessels in the retina. As the red blood cells move through these vessels, they scatter the laser light. By measuring differences in the frequencies of the light beam, both before it enters and as it exits the eye, the exact rate of retinal blood flow can be calculated. Laser Doppler velocimetry is a noninvasive technique that can provide objective precise measurements of retinal blood flow and monitor instantaneous changes in individual blood vessels.

Laser Doppler techniques have been used in studies that strongly suggest early diagnosis as a key to prevention or delay in visual loss. One can measure a gradual reduction in retinal blood flow during the early stages of diabetic retinopathy, in some cases even before ophthalmoscopic changes become apparent. In summary, LDV could play an important role in early detection and treatment of diabetic retinopathy, once the current experimental model of the LDV becomes less cumbersome and less time-consuming to use. It may also be possible to use LDV as a diagnostic test in evaluating the effectiveness of photocoagulation in retarding blood flow to an area of the retina that previously exhibited neovascularization.

Complications of Laser Photocoagulation

The Early Treatment Diabetic Retinopathy Study (7) demonstrated the beneficial effect of laser photocoagulation for patients with clinically significant diabetic retinopathy with and without advanced macular edema. Treatment consists of either focal or panretinal laser photocoagulation. The benefits of modified grid pattern of laser application to the macula was shown by Olk (28) to improve visual acuity through reduction of diffuse macular edema. Although laser photocoagulation is usually well tolerated and frequently results in an improvement of visual acuity, complications do arise from the procedure and can be divided into mild and severe forms.

Mild Complications of Diabetic Laser Photocoagulation

Mild complications frequently consist of some reduction in light sensitivity, resulting in some loss of peripheral visual acuity, and some loss of night vision. In doing a tight

PRP, there may also be an occasional loss of one to two lines of central visual acuity. These complications occur, at times, in patients exhibiting good vision in which PRP is the treatment of choice. Isolated paracentral scotoma may develop. Retinal edema leading to mild serous detachment of the retina may also occur, especially in those cases where a tight PRP has been accomplished in one session. Usually, there is complete resolution of the detachment. Transient loss of accommodation may arise following laser photocoagulation, and especially in the juvenile type I diabetic eye.

It is important to inform the patient prior to laser surgery that many of the above enumerated side effects will improve or disappear with time. Certainly, performing PRP in multiple divided sessions can reduce many of the mild complications. In cases of significant loss of central visual acuity due to diffuse CME that was present before laser therapy, always inform the patient that after modified grid laser therapy, significant improvement in visual acuity may not always be achieved. The modified grid pattern of laser application for diffuse macular edema has a much greater tendency to produce paracentral scotomata than PRP. These scotoma will usually diminish with time.

Severe Complications of Diabetic Laser Photocoagulation

The worst and most severe complication of PRP is inadvertent photocoagulation of the fovea, resulting in a central scotoma. The introduction of the Rodenstock panfunduscopic lens has decreased inadvertent laser treatment of the fovea. The large field of vision obtained with this lens frequently allows the retinal surgeon to see the exact position of the fovea while treating the temporal periphery. Another useful technique in preventing foveal photocoagulation is to place a double row of laser lesions about one to two disc diameters temporal to the fovea before starting panretinal treatment. These white lesions are useful demarcation lines, warning of treatment across this barrier.

Next to inadvertent foveal photocoagulation, the most severe and dangerous complication of laser photocoagulation for macular edema in the diabetic eye is choroidal neovascularization (Fig. 5.21), resulting in submacular fibrosis. This was pointed out by Varley (32) and Lewis (33) and their colleagues. Other severe macular complications include expansion of laser scars [as reported by Schatz (34)], perforation of Bruch's membrane, choroidal and retinal hemorrhage, and choriovitreal proliferation [as reported by Benson (35)]. Fortunately, choroidal neovascularization is an uncommon complication.

Han and associates (36) describe several mechanisms for fibrous proliferation after macular photocoagulation in diabetic retinopathy. The patient will frequently complain of metamorphopsia, paracentral or central scotoma, and loss of visual acuity. In such cases, choroidal neovascular membranes usually develop within 3 to 5 months of laser treatment. These membranes originate from photocoagulation scars in the macula. Fundus examination may demonstrate a gray area in the macula, localized neurosensory retinal detachment, and subretinal or intraretinal hemorrhage (see Fig. 5.21). Fluorescein angiography should be performed. Results of the fluorescein transit show early hyperfluorescence and subsequent leakage of dye (Fig. 5.22). Frequently, additional laser

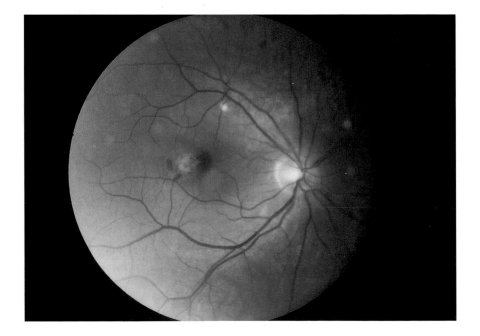

Fig. 5.21 Fundus photo demonstrates choroidal neovascularization showing a large "dirty" gray membrane in the macula, localized neurosensory elevation, and subretinal hemorrhage.

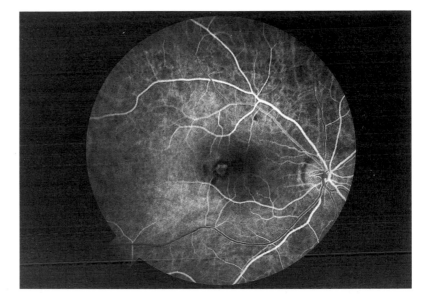

Fig. 5.22 Fundus fluorescein angiogram of the retina shown in Fig. 5.21 exhibits a subretinal neo vascular membrane (SRN) as shown in the early venous phase of the fluorescein transit.

photocoagulation to the neovascular membrane will prevent additional loss of visual acuity. However, recurrence of the neovascular membranes may result.

Investigators like Lewis (33) and Benson (35) have also suggested that small spot size, short duration, and the high intensity of the burns may be factors contributing to the formation of neovascular membranes and submacular fibrosis. As edema increases, more energy level is required to create a response in the inner retina. The increased amount of energy delivered may result in an increase in the proliferative response to laser treatment. In addition, breaks in Bruch's membrane coupled with choriocapillaris changes, may be the factors promoting neovascularization following laser application.

Laser applications should not be applied less than 300 μm from the foveal area. Despite adhering to this rule, extension of fibrous scarring into the foveal region from perifoveal laser energy can be observed in some patients. A number of reasons may account for this phenomenon. Firstly, a greater intensity of laser applications may have to be delivered in the perifoveal area because macular edema is frequently more intense in the fovea. Secondly, the foveal and perifoveal areas of the macula may have an intrinsic predilection for a proliferative response. Thirdly, most of the complications of submacular fibrosis due to laser therapy occur in the aging eye, as reported by Guyer and coworkers (37). It may be that advancing age poses a heightened tendency for fibrosis through a mechanism that thus far remains unknown.

Chronic macular edema and neurosensory retinal detachment may also be potential mechanisms for the formation of a proliferative process resulting in neovascularization and subretinal fibrotic membranes. Such a process may develop in the diabetic eye without previous laser therapy. Laser treatment may also potentiate the development of this complication.

Del Priore, Glaser, and colleagues (38) have shown that multiple layers of retinal pigment epithelial cells form in areas of laser photocoagulation. It is suggested that proliferation of these pigment epithelial cells in response to laser photocoagulation may also be responsible for fibrotic macular scarring. It is certainly known, through research of Machemer and colleagues (39), that proliferation and transformation of retinal pigment epithelial cells in the presence of retinal detachment can produce fibrotic membranes responsible for PVR.

Detection of Subretinal Neovascular Membranes with Indocyanine Green and an Infrared Scanning Laser Ophthalmoscope

Indocyanine green fluoresces in the near infrared region with a peak absorption at 790 nm. At this wavelength, only 10% of the light is absorbed by the pigment epithelium. Indocyanine green does not escape from choroidal vessels. It is, therefore, a good method for the early detection of subretinal neovascular membranes.

Webb and associates (40) introduced the Scanning Laser Ophthalmoscope (SLO). Mainster and associates (41) refined the technique for fundus imaging. The technique allows for high-quality video fluorescein angiography at low light levels. Scheider and Schroedel (42) used a modified infrared version of the SLO for indocyanine green angiography and obtained choroidal angiograms with high temporal and spatial resolution.

The detection of subretinal neovascular membranes with indocyanine green (Fig. 5.23) depends on the location of the vessels, as demonstrated by Scheider and colleagues (43). If the membranes are on the pigment epithelium, they are easily detected with fluorescein angiography. Subretinal neovascular vessels are detected with indocyanine green as in the early phase

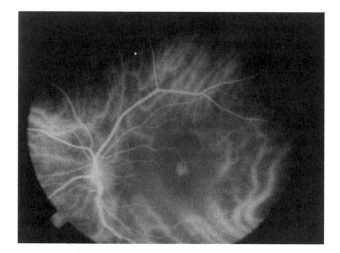

Fig. 5.23 The presence of a subretinal neovascular membrane as shown with indocyanine green dye.

of fluorescein angiography just before the dye begins to leak.

In fluorescein angiography, the membrane fluoresces before the choroid. With indocyanine green, the choroid fluoresces earlier than the membrane. Another advantage of indocyanine green is its ability to overcome the shielding effect of ocular pigments, especially when centrally located membranes are partially obscured by xanthophyll. In these cases, an exact location of the membrane is impossible with fluorescein.

In summary, indocyanine green has the advantage of bypassing the absorption of the pigment epithelium. It has the characteristic properties of lack of exudation and infrared fluorescence. Because indocyanine green does not leak regularly, this feature is most important in cases of ill-defined neovascular membranes in which exudation of fluorescein or the blockage of fluorescence by the pigment epithelium or xanthophyll prevents the diagnosis of the exact location. Indocyanine green with the infrared SLO increases the chance of early diagnosis of ill-defined subretinal neovascular membranes.

Summary

Diabetic retinopathy has presently become the leading cause of blindness in the United States today. It is also the most significant retinal vascular disease. Fortunately, through the use of laser photocoagulation, the incidence of visual disability has been greatly reduced. The efficacy and safety of laser photocoagulation as the primary treatment modality for diabetic retinopathy has become well established over the past 20 to 25 years. PRP has become the treatment of choice for PDR. Modified grid laser photocoagulation is reserved for diffuse diabetic macular edema.

Thus, laser photocoagulation has frequently succeeded in preventing the devastating complications of neovascular glaucoma and traction retinal detachment, two conditions that often lead to irrevocable blindness in the diabetic eye. The use of laser therapy has brought the goal enunciated by the American Academy of Ophthalmology of "eradicating the visual disability of diabetic retinopathy by the year 2000" a giant step forward.

References

1. Javitt JC, Canner JK, Sommer A. Cost effectiveness of current approaches to the control of retinopathy in type I diabetics. Ophthalmology 1989;96:255–264.
2. Kahn HA, Hiller R. Blindness caused by diabetic retinopathy. Am J Ophthalmol 1974;78:58–67.
3. Palmberg PF. Diabetic retinopathy. Diabetes 1977;26:703–709.
4. Diabetic Retinopathy Study Research Group. Indications for photocoagulation treatment of diabetic retinopathy. DRS Report No 14. Int Ophthalmol Clin 1987;27:239–253.
5. Diabetic Retinopathy Vitrectomy Study Research Group. Early vitrectomy for severe vitreous hemorrhage in diabetic retinopathy. Two year results of a randomized trial. DRVS Report No. 2. Arch Ophthalmol 1985;103:1644–1652.
6. Diabetic Retinopathy Vitrectomy Study Research Group. Early vitrectomy for severe proliferative diabetic retinopathy in eyes with useful vision. Results of a randomized trial. DRVS Report No. 3. Ophthalmology 1988;95:1307–1320.
7. Early Treatment Diabetic Retinopathy Study Research Group. Photocoagulation for diabetic macular edema. ETDRS Report No. 1. Arch Ophthalmol 1985;103:1796–1806.
8. Klein R, et al. The Wisconsin Epidemiologic Study of Diabetic Retinopathy. VI. Retinal photocoagulation. Ophthalmology 1987;94:747–753.
9. Witkins SR, Klein R. Ophthalmologic care for persons with diabetes. JAMA 1984;251:2534–2537.
10. Murphy PR, Egbert PR. Regression of iris neovascularization following panretinal photocoagulation. Arch Ophthalmol 1979;97:700–702.
11. Wilkinson CP, Benson WE, Blumenkranz M. Diabetic retinopathy-preferred practice pattern. American Academy of Ophthalmology Retinal and Quality of Care Panels, November, 1993. With permission.
12. Klein R, Klein BE, Moss SE. The Wisconsin Epidemiologic Study of Diabetic Retinopathy. IX. Four-year incidence and progression of diabetic retinopathy when age at diagnosis is less than 30 years. Arch Ophthalmol 1989;107:237–243.
13. Klein R, Klein BE, Moss SE. The Wisconsin Epidemiologic Study of Diabetic Retinopathy. X. Four-year incidence and progression of diabetic retinopathy when age at diagnosis is 30 years or more. Arch Ophthalmol 1989;107:244–249.
14. Diabetic Retinopathy Study Research Group. Indications for photocoagulation treatment of diabetic retinopathy. DRS Report No. 14. Int Ophthalmol Clin 1987;27:239–253.
15. Early Treatment Diabetic Retinopathy Study Research Group. Photocoagulation for diabetic macular edema. ETDRS Report No. 1. Arch Ophthalmol 1985;103:1796–1806.

16. Diabetic Retinopathy Study Research Group. Indications for photocoagulation treatment of diabetic retinopathy. DRS Report No. 14. Int Ophthalmol Clin 1987;27:239–253.

17. Goldmann H. Two Lectures on Biomicroscopy of the Eye. Berne, Switzerland: Rosch, Vogt & Co., 1954.

18. Blankenship GW. Panretinal laser photocoagulation with a wide-angle fundus contact lens. Ann Ophthalmol 1982;14: 362–363.

19. Mainster MA, Crossman JL, Erickson PJ, Heacock GL. Retinal laser lenses: magnification, spot size and field of view. Br J Ophthalmol 1990;74:177–179.

20. Yannuzzi LA, Slakter JS. Macular photocoagulation lens. Am J Ophthalmol 1986;101:619–620. Letter.

21. Barker FM, Wing JT. Ultrawide field fundus biomicroscopy with the Volk quadraspheric lens. J Am Optom Assoc 1990; 61:573–575.

22. Doft BH, Blankenship GW. Single versus multiple treatment sessions of argon laser panretinal photocoagulation for proliferative diabetic retinopathy. Ophthalmology 1982;89:772–779.

23. Klein R, Klein BE, Moss SE. Glycosylated hemoglobin predicts the incidence and progression of diabetic retinopathy. JAMA 1988;260:2864–2871.

24. Ross H, Bernstein G, Rifkin H. Relationship of metabolic control of diabetes mellitus to long-term complications. In: Ellenberg M, Rifkin H, eds. Diabetes mellitus, 3d ed. New York, Medical Examination Publishing Co., 1983, pp 907–919.

25. Klein R, Klein BE, Moss SE. The Wisconsin Epidemiologic Study of Diabetic Retinopathy. XI. The incidence of macular edema. Ophthalmology 1989;96:1501–1510.

26. Sinclair SH, Nesler C, Foxman B. Macular edema and pregnancy in insulin-dependent diabetes. Am J Ophthalmol 1984;97:154–167.

27. Bresnick GH. Diabetic maculopathy: a critical review highlighting diffuse macular edema. Ophthalmology 1983;90: 1301–1317.

28. Olk RJ. Modified grid argon laser photocoagulation for diffuse diabetic macular edema. Ophthalmology 1986;93: 938–950.

29. Olk RJ. Diabetic retinopathy. In: Yannuzzi LA, ed. Laser photocoagulation of the macula. Philadelphia: JB Lippincott, 1989:74.

30. Olk RJ. Argon green (514 nm) versus krypton red (647 nm) modified grid laser photocoagulation for diffuse diabetic macular edema. Ophthalmology 1990;97:1101–1113.

31. Sunness JS. The pregnant woman's eye. Surv Ophthalmol 1988;32:219–238.

32. Varley MP, Frank E, Purnell EW. Subretinal neovascularization after focal argon laser for diabetic macular edema. Ophthalmology 1988;95:567–573.

33. Lewis H, Schachat AP, Haimann MH, et al. Choroidal neovascularization after laser photocoagulation for diabetic macular edema. Ophthalmology 1990;97:503–511.

34. Schatz H, Madeira D, McDonald HR, Johnson RN. Progressive enlargement of laser scars following grid laser photocoagulation for diffuse diabetic macular edema. Arch Ophthalmol 1991;109:1549–1551.

35. Benson WE, Townsend RE, Pheasant TR. Choriovitreal and subretinal proliferations. Complications of photocoagulation. Ophthalmology 1979;86:283–289.

36. Han DP, Mieler WF, Burton TC. Submacular fibrosis after photocoagulation for diabetic macular edema. Am J Ophthalmol 1992;113:513–521.

37. Guyer DR, D'Amico DJ, Smith CW. Subretinal fibrosis after laser photocoagulation for diabetic macular edema. Am J Ophthalmol 1992;113:652–656.

38. DelPriore LV, Glaser BM, Quigley HA, Green WR. Response of pig retinal pigment epithelium to laser photocoagulation in organ culture. Arch Ophthalmol 1989;107:119–122.

39. Machemer R, Van Horn D, Aaberg TM. Pigment epithelial proliferation in human retinal detachment with massive periretinal proliferation. Am J Ophthalmol 1978;85: 181–191.

40. Webb RH, Hughes GW, Pomerantzeff O. Flying spot TV ophthalmoscope. Appl Opt 1980;19:2991.

41. Mainster MA, Timberlake GT, Webb RH, Hughes GW. Scanning laser ophthalmoscopy, clinical applications. Ophthalmology 1982;89:852–857.

42. Scheider A, Schroedel C. High resolution indocyanine green angiography with a scanning laser ophthalmoscope. Am J Ophthalmol 1989;108:458–459.

43. Scheider A, Kaboth A, Neuhauser L. Detection of subretinal neovascular membranes with indocyanine green and an infrared scanning laser ophthalmoscope. Am J Ophthalmol 1992;113:45–51.

6

Laser Treatment of Choroidal Neovascularization

Lawrence J. Singerman
Jeffrey C. Lamkin
Rafael Addiego
Hernando Zegarra

Age-related Macular Degeneration

Overview

It is ironic that the leading cause of blindness in most developed Western nations lacks a well-formulated and universally accepted definition. Traditionally, age-related macular degeneration (AMD) has been defined as the presence of macular pigmentary changes or drusen accounting for visual acuity of 20/30 or worse (1). One implication of this definition is that the macular findings of AMD must be causally associated with some degree of visual dysfunction. The limits of this definition are obvious because acuity is only one, incomplete measure of macular function and because many patients develop typical pigmentary changes that would compromise acuity if located more centrally. The distinction between the fundus changes associated with the normal aging process and those of early, nonexudative AMD is difficult to make (2), with the process of senescence progressing to pathologic degeneration in a continuum, driven by multiple genetic and environmental factors. Most clinicians will make the diagnosis of AMD in a patient over the age of 50 years when typical pigmentary changes develop, regardless of visual acuity.

The disorder was originally described in 1885 (3). Subsequent studies of its various manifestations and natural history have led to the widely accepted classification of atrophic ("dry") and exudative ("wet") forms of AMD (1). In the dry forms, drusen and subretinal pigmentary disturbances progress to retinal pigment epithelial (RPE) attenuation (incipient atrophy) and death (geographic atrophy), without any evidence of choroidal neovascularization (CNV). Wet forms of the disease include CNV (classic, poorly defined, or occult), pigment epithelial detachments (PEDs; serous and hemorrhagic), and subretinal fibrovascular scarring.

Atrophic and exudative AMD constitutes the leading cause of blindness in American patients over 65 years of age, accounting for 14% of all new cases of legal blindness each year. Furthermore, AMD is the second leading cause of new blindness (behind diabetes mellitus) in patients

between the ages of 45 and 64 years (4). Two large epidemiologic studies have confirmed that the exudative variety accounts for 80% to 90% of severe visual loss due to AMD (1,5). A number of potential risk factors for the development of either form of AMD have been investigated. Several factors are believed to be associated with an increased risk of visual loss secondary to AMD; these include increasing age, female sex, family history of symptomatic AMD, and light ocular pigmentation (blue irides, blond fundi). Cigarette smokers and hyperopes seem to be at higher risk, as well. The role of systemic hypertension is less clear.

Because the risk of visual loss is clearly linked to the risk of developing "wet" disease, several studies have evaluated factors associated with exudative changes. Patients with more severe disease are generally older and are more likely to have active cardiovascular disease, including hypertension. The importance of photic injury as a potential risk factor, particularly in exudative disease, is disputed (6-8).

The pigmentary alterations seen in atrophic AMD, including the various types of drusen, have also been investigated as potential risk factors for the development of exudative disease. Two independent studies have confirmed that confluent drusen and focal hyperpigmentation of the RPE are associated with exudative disease, particularly in patients under 75 years of age (4,9).

Pathology and Pathogenesis

As described above, mild cases of atrophic AMD are on a continuum with normal aging changes compatible with good vision. A number of theories regarding pathogenesis have been advanced (5), but no single hypothesis has been widely accepted. Many investigators have come to the conclusion that the disease is a primary disorder of the RPE (10). Others believe that it is a primary disturbance in Bruch's membrane leading to secondary RPE, retinal, and choroidal changes. Senescence and insufficiency of the choriocapillaris have also been suspected as a causative factor. A full discussion of the various theories of pathogenesis, as well as a review of the histopathologic findings of aging and atrophic AMD, are beyond the scope of this review, which will focus on exudative disease.

The hallmark of exudative AMD is CNV. Well-defined, classic neovascular membranes are obvious histologically as a sprout or sprouts growing under the RPE. The vascular pattern is typically described as a "cartwheel," with spokes of fragile new vessels radiating outward from a central core. Like other neovascular tissue, these membranes are abnormally permeable to most plasma constituents and leak fluid under the RPE, as well as into the subretinal and intraretinal space. Protein and lipid may deposit in any of these locations. Hemorrhage is another frequent concomitant and may also be found beneath the RPE, in the subretinal space, or intraretinally. Bruch's membrane is usually irregularly thickened in AMD but must be focally interrupted for CNV to progress. Whether the defect in Bruch's membrane results from new vessel growth or whether it is a primary event, stimulating vessel ingrowth, is disputed. Another potential stimulus for vascular ingrowth may be soft drusen. Soft drusen represent focal accumulations within a diffuse layer of membranous debris between the basement membrane of the RPE and the inner collagenous layer of Bruch's membrane. As part of a larger diffuse layer, their borders are indistinct, and they may fuse with other soft drusen to form confluent drusen (if smaller than about 300 μm) or what may be called small PEDs (if larger than 300 μm). As this confluence occurs, there seems to be a higher incidence of serous and hemorrhagic PEDs, typical CNV, and subretinal fibrovascular scarring.

Histologic review of eyes with clinical findings highly suggestive of CNV but without classic findings (so-called occult membranes) have confirmed the presence of new vessels originating in the choroid and extending into and through Bruch's membrane. This was initially reported in a case of irregular elevation of the RPE with punctate staining and leakage on angiography (11) and subsequently was confirmed in an eye with a lesion meeting the Macular Photocoagulation Study's (MPS) definition of occult CNV (12).

The end stage of either classic or occult CNV is subretinal fibrovascular organization, with secondary destruction of overlying sensory retina. Ongoing neovascularization may persist within or at the borders of subretinal scars.

Another component of exudative AMD is PED. In healthy eyes, fine filaments within the basal lamina of the RPE maintain its adherence to Bruch's membrane. The early stages of AMD include diffuse thickening beneath the basal lamina due to accumulation of membranous cellular debris extruded by RPE cells. Focal accumulations of this debris constitute soft drusen. The diffuse thickening is thought to result in deficient adherence of the RPE, with subsequent PED. Abnormal new vessels on the inner surface of Bruch's membrane, but rendered invisible by overlying fluid, may leak and account for PED. A more recent theory regarding the pathogenesis of PED holds that the primary disturbance leading to PED is excessive resistance to RPE-driven fluid transport across a Bruch's membrane that has become increasingly hydrophobic with time and accumulation of membranous debris (13). Whether avascular PED contains fluid derived from the choriocapillaris or the RPE is controversial.

Clinical Features

Most patients with exudative disease affecting the macula will be symptomatic. Blurred or distorted vision is the most frequent complaint and is typically worse at near vision. The observant patient will carefully describe metamorphopsia or micropsia; others are aware of only a vague disturbance. (A surprising number of patients, particularly older patients, fail to recognize visual loss early in the course of the disease.) Signs include reduced acuity and Amsler grid abnormalities, including distortion and scotoma.

The funduscopic manifestations of exudative AMD depend on the pathologic variant involved. The classic pattern of CNV is manifest as a grayish green retinal elevation, often accompanied by retinal thickening and localized serous detachment (Fig. 6.1). Many times, even with angiographically classic membranes, this telltale gray-green elevation is difficult to discern. Other important clues to the presence of either classic or occult CNV must be specifically sought with stereobiomicroscopy. These include exudate and hemorrhage either under or within the retina, as well as elevation of the RPE.

The second variety of exudative AMD is the retinal PED. PED tends to be circular, dome-shaped "blisters" under the RPE and retina (Fig. 6.2). They are sharply demarcated and may be associated with a larger, indistinct,

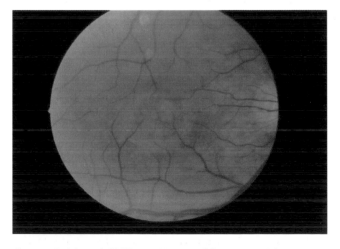

Fig. 6.1 Subfoveal CNV in a 68-year-old woman with drusen. Note the central elevation of the retina and gray-green discoloration. On stereoscopic examination, there was minimal subretinal fluid but no hemorrhage or exudate.

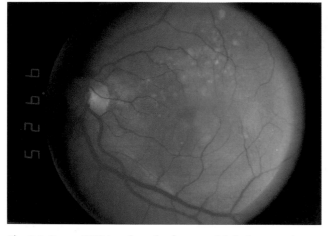

Fig. 6.2 Large PED involves the fovea and inferior macula. Note the associated drusen in the superior macula. None of the warning signs of coincident CNV are seen here (hemorrhage, exudate, fluid level, notching).

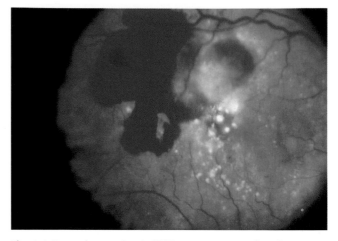

Fig. 6.4 Large hemorrhagic PED superotemporal to the fovea with hemorrhage, both under the PED as well as along its temporal margin.

superimposed serous detachment of overlying sensory retina. Associated retinal detachment may be a clue to the presence of neovascularization beneath the PED (14). Other signs of coincident neovascularization include subretinal exudate, a dark fluid level in the dependent part of the detachment, uneven elevation of the detachment, a "notch" at the border of the RPE (15), and chorioretinal folds radiating from the PED (Fig. 6.3). The most important sign, however, is associated hemorrhage. Bleeding may be confined to the perimeter of the PED or may fill the detachment, giving it a maroon or dark green appearance (hemorrhagic PED) (Fig. 6.4).

Disciform scarring represents the end stage of untreated exudative disease. There is generally elevation of atrophic retina by yellow-white, irregular thickening. The degree of elevation is variable and may reach proportions suggestive of a neoplasm or exudative retinal detachment.

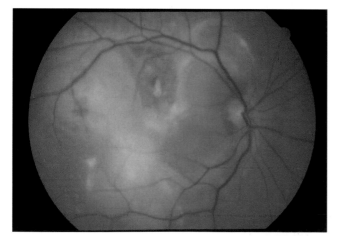

Fig. 6.3 Huge PED in a patient with AMD. Note the prominent "notch" superiorly where angiography revealed CNV.

With organization, the pigment epithelium may become hyperplastic, with subsequent pigmentation. Ongoing neovascularization at the border of scars can cause radiating folds in adjacent retina. Within the scar itself, retinal-choroidal anastamoses may develop.

Unusual findings in exudative AMD include vitreous hemorrhage, total hemorrhagic retinal detachment, and RPE tears. Bleeding may dissect through sensory retina into the vitreous cavity and obscure its source. Ultrasonography may be necessary to rule out retinal tear or detachment and may show thickening of the retina-choroid layer in the macula, suggesting AMD as the etiology. Peripheral CNV may also lead to vitreous hemorrhage with sudden visual loss. Patients with preexistent coagulopathy may have uncontrolled bleeding, with total retinal detachment and secondary angle closure glaucoma. The hazards of oral platelet inhibitors (e.g., aspirin) with active exudative AMD are unclear.

In large or long-standing PED, tractional forces may lead to tearing of the distended pigment epithelium at the edges of the detachment. This may also occur as a complication of laser treatment. The clinical appearance is distinctive, with a crescent-shaped, sharply demarcated area of exposed choriocapillaris and an adjacent mound of scrolled, retracted pigment epithelium (Fig. 6.5).

Fluorescein Angiography

Proper diagnosis and management of exudative AMD rest on combining careful stereoscopic macular examination techniques with high-quality fluorescein angiography. Any area of CNV will appear angiographically as an area of focal early hyperfluorescence, preceding retinal vascular filling, which increases in size and intensity on late views (Fig. 6.6). Two other forms of early hyper-fluorescence must be distinguished from neovascularization. RPE

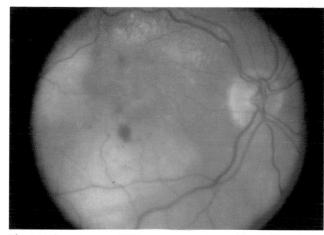

Fig. 6.5 Spontaneous RPE tear in a patient with AMD and long-standing PED. The area of exposed Bruch's membrane is hypopigmented; the retracted, scrolled RPE superiorly is hyperpigmented.

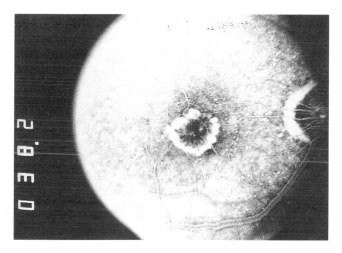

Fig. 6.6 Fluorescein angiogram, early transit view, from the patient shown in Fig. 6.1. There is classic subfoveal CNV in typical cartwheel pattern.

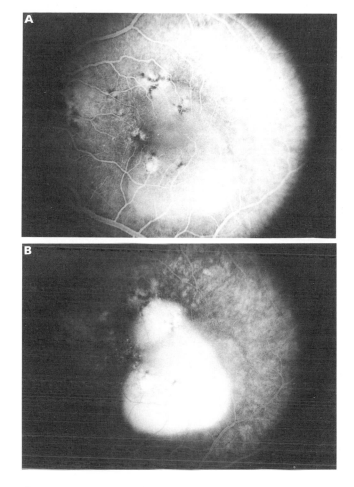

Fig. 6.7 A, Early transit fluorescein angiogram from patient shown in Fig. 6.2. The PED hyperfluoresces early in a well-demarcated oval pattern. The area of more intense hyperfluorescence inferiorly corresponded to an area of RPE atrophy and is not a "hot spot" representing CNV. B, Late transit views of the same patient. Note the late hyperfluorescence that has increased in intensity but not in size.

atrophy will appear hyperfluorescent at the same time in fluorescein transit but is differentiated from neovascularization by its fading in later views. Serous PEDs will also hyperfluoresce early (Fig. 6.7). They are usually round and sharply demarcated (unlike neovascularization) and increase in intensity in later views (like neovascularization). The size of the intense hyperfluorescence does not increase with time, distinguishing serous PED from neovascularization (although a serous retinal detachment overlying a PED may fill late and simulate enlargement). Because CNV and PED frequently coincide, a clear distinction is often easier to make in principle than in practice. Furthermore, turbid subretinal or sub-RPE fluid or blood may obscure the classic signs of neovascularization. Angiographic signs of neovascularization within PED include irregular fluorescence of the detachment, focally increased

hyperfluorescence ("hot spot"), and notching of the round PED by a small region of relative hypofluorescence (14-16).

The exact morphology of CNV varies on angiography. So-called classic disease features fan- or cartwheel-shaped networks of subretinal capillaries seen early and progressively obscured by leakage in later views. Feeding choroidal vessels are occasionally seen, more commonly in recurrent neovascularization, and present a tempting target for laser treatment. Well-defined membranes are the most amenable to treatment but, unfortunately, occur in the minority of patients (17). Classic membranes are frequently obscured by hemorrhage, exudate, or hyperpigmentation, making the diagnosis less obvious. Subretinal fluid, particularly chronic, turbid fluid, may also block the typical pattern.

Recently, "occult" neovascularization has been recognized as a variant in many patients with significant visual loss. The MPS has defined two forms of "occult" neovascularization (18). The fibrovascular PED is a region of pigment epithelial and retinal elevation with punctate early hyperfluorescence that increases on late views. The spots of hyperfluorescence do not correspond to potential window defects (drusen, RPE atrophy) and are unassociated with other signs of neovascularization. The boundaries of the hyperfluorescent elevation are indistinct, making treatment decisions difficult. The increasing hyperfluorescence is indicative of neovascularization, and clinicopathologic correlation has substantiated this definition (16).

A second variety of occult disease is termed "late-phase leakage of an undetermined source." This form features speckled or ill-defined hyperfluorescence that does not appear in the first 2 minutes of fluorescein transit, but increases steadily in late views and does not correspond to potential window defects. Frequently, dye pools in the subretinal space. The MPS defined a minimal degree of staining required to be considered occult neovascularization (19).

Angiography is rarely indicated for large disciform scars but will show irregular, mottled early hyperfluorescence with late staining. Chorioretinal anastamoses are highlighted. RPE tears have distinctive findings on angiography (Fig. 6.8). Exposed Bruch's membrane and choriocapillaris are intensely hyperfluorescent in early views but rarely leak, unless there is associated neovascularization. The heaped mound of torn epithelium causes adjacent hypofluorescence.

Prognosis

Clearly, the most important predictor of the visual impact of AMD is the type of disease, with a far more guarded prognosis for exudative disease. In one study of the disease's natural history, the cumulative risk of progression

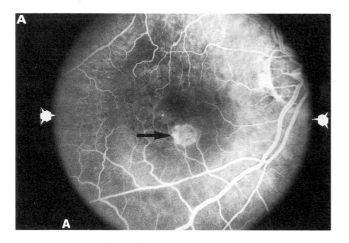

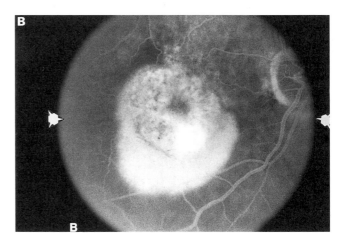

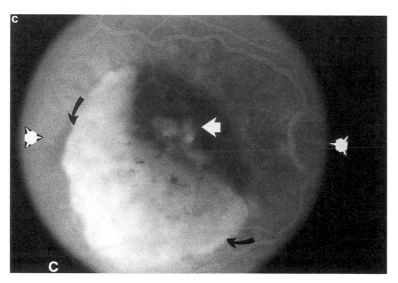

Fig. 6.8 A, Fluorescein angiogram, early transit view, of a PED with delayed hyperfluorescence and coincident CNV. The hyperfluorescent area inferior to the foveal has a fan-shaped appearance consistent with CNV. Note the minimal filling of the PED in its most dependent portion. B, Later view of the same patient. Note the delayed filling of the PED and increased hyperfluorescence from the CNV inferiorly. C, Late transit angiogram from the same patient 13 months later (also shown in Fig. 6.5). The hyperfluorescence inferiorly is secondary to a spontaneous tear of the RPE, with subsequent exposure of Bruch's membrane and choriocapillaris, intensely hyperfluorescent (*curved black arrows*). Superiorly, the retracted, scrolled RPE causes hypofluorescence (*white arrow*). (Reproduced by permission from Singerman and Stockfish [26].)

from atrophic to exudative disease approached 15% over 4.3 years of follow-up (20). Furthermore, the risk of exudative disease in a fellow eye was shown to be approximately 4% to 12% annually for the first 3 years following the onset of unilateral CNV (21).

The natural history and prognosis for exudative AMD depends on the location of disease. Neovascularization 200 μm or more from the center of the foveal avascular zone (FAZ) is termed extrafoveal, and neovascularization between 1 and 199 μm from the center of the FAZ is termed juxtafoveal (22; Fig. 6.9). CNV in AMD is more likely than CNV in other disorders to present under the center of the FAZ (subfoveal), with less than 10% presenting extrafoveally (23). Extrafoveal CNV at presentation is more likely in patients with recent onset of symptoms and good visual acuity.

In the MPS, 62% of untreated, well-defined extrafoveal membranes lost three or more lines of acuity over 3 years of follow-up (22). Another study documented that 71% of eyes with juxtafoveal disease progressed to legal blindness over less than 2 years (24). Subfoveal disease carries the poorest prognosis, with worse acuity at presentation, and more rapid, severe loss in those eyes with relatively good early acuity (25).

The natural history of PED is related to age at presentation. In patients over 50 years of age, one third to one half will develop typical CNV with severe visual loss (14). PEDs less than one disc diameter and outside the fovea are less likely to progress. A recent study of the natural history of PED associated with CNV and AMD established its poor prognosis: at 1 year follow-up, 65% had visual acuity less than 20/200, and 26% had visual acuity less than 5/200 (26). Increasing age and hemorrhage or exudate on presentation were significant risk factors for poor acuity.

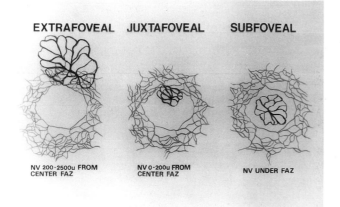

EXTRAFOVEAL   JUXTAFOVEAL   SUBFOVEAL

NV 200-2500u FROM CENTER FAZ   NV 0-200u FROM CENTER FAZ   NV UNDER FAZ

Fig. 6.9 The most important prognostic and therapeutic factor in CNV is its location in relation to the center of the FAZ. Proper assessment of location requires high-quality fluorescein angiography. (Reproduced by permission from Singerman [123].)

Treatment

In 1979, the National Institutes of Health initiated the MPS, designed to investigate the efficacy of laser photocoagulation in preventing visual loss due to CNV of various etiologies (AMD, histoplasmosis, and idiopathic). The original project enrolled patients with visual acuity of at least 20/100 and well-defined membranes with limited amounts of blood in which the entire complex was no less than 200 μm from the center of the FAZ (extrafoveal; 27). The study was stopped in 1982 after a clear treatment benefit from argon blue-green photocoagulation was established: at 18 months' follow-up, treatment reduced the incidence of severe visual loss (acuity less than 20/200) from 42% to 14%. Sixty percent of untreated eyes lost six or more lines of vision compared with 25% of treated eyes. Treatment benefit appeared to be smaller among hypertensive patients. Unfortunately, 59% of treated eyes suffered a recurrence within the first 3 years after treatment and most within the first year after treatment (28). Eyes with recurrence had a poorer long-term visual prognosis. Cigarette smoking seemed to be a risk factor for recurrence.

The second part of the MPS studied krypton red treatment of lesions less than 200 μm from, but not under, the center of the FAZ (juxtafoveal; 29). At 3 years' follow-up, 58% of untreated eyes lost six or more lines of acuity, compared with 49% of treated eyes. Among treated eyes, the average final acuity was 20/200, while that of untreated eyes was 20/250. The benefit of treatment was largest among patients without evidence of hypertension and was smaller than that in extrafoveal lesions. As with extrafoveal disease, persistence and recurrence were common following juxtafoveal treatment—32% and 22%, respectively. Higher recurrence rates were associated with certain findings in the contralateral eye, including active or previous neovascularization, the presence of more than 20 drusen, or nongeographic atrophy (30).

In 1986, the third component of the MPS began. In this trial, lesions extending under the center of the FAZ were randomized to treatment or no treatment. Treated eyes were further randomized to argon or krypton laser sources. Eligibility criteria included:

1. Recent (less than 96 hours) angiographic evidence of neovascularization, either classic or occult, under the center of the FAZ, whose total extent was clearly demarcated and less than 3.5 disc areas. (Components other than neovascularization, including elevated blocked fluorescence, thick contiguous blood, and serous elevation of the RPE, were included in estimating lesion size but were not defined as occult forms of neovascularization.) Furthermore, classic or occult neovascularization had to occupy more than one half of the entire complex (occult neovascularization was clearly defined).

2. Visual acuity from 20/40 to 20/320, inclusive

3. Age 50 years or older
4. No history of photocoagulation
5. No confounding eye disease
6. No current or past use of systemic steroids

Three months after enrollment, 20% of laser-treated eyes has lost six or more lines of acuity, compared with only 11% of untreated eyes. This apparent deleterious effect of treatment was no longer evident 1 year following treatment, and at 2 years after treatment, treated eyes had lost less vision than had untreated eyes (three and four lines, respectively). Patients in certain subgroups showed a clear treatment benefit much earlier: those with pre-treatment visual acuity less than 20/200, those with small CNV (less than one disc area), and those meeting all MPS criteria. Furthermore, treated eyes retained baseline contrast sensitivity, unlike untreated eyes. Reading speed was also faster in treated eyes. Thus, treated eyes suffered an immediate loss of acuity and then stabilized, while untreated eyes showed steady progression to greater degrees of visual compromise. Visual functions other than acuity also seemed to be better preserved in treated eyes. The MPS concluded that "treatment of subfoveal neovascular lesions that meet the eligibility criteria for this study is recommended if both the patient and the ophthalmologist are prepared for a large decrease in visual acuity immediately after treatment." Fifty-one percent of treated eyes suffered recurrence within 2 years of treatment, but this was not associated with significantly worse final acuity. There was no significant difference in outcomes based on laser source (argon versus krypton).

Patients with subfoveal recurrent neovascularization were studied separately (31). Eligibility criteria included:
1. Recent (less than 96 hours) angiographic evidence of either a leaking CNV lesion under the foveal center and contiguous with a scar from earlier treatment or CNV within 150 μm of the foveal center and contiguous with a scar from previous treatment that had expanded with subfoveal extension
2. No prior laser treatment to the foveal center
3. Total treatment area (prior plus repeat treatments) no larger than 6 disc areas and sparing some retina within 1500 μm from the foveal center (within 4 disc areas centered on the FAZ)
4. Visual acuity from 20/40 to 20/320, inclusive
5. Age 50 years or older
6. No confounding eye disease
7. No current or prior use of systemic steroids

After 2 years' follow-up, 9% of treated eyes had lost six or more lines of acuity, compared with 28% of untreated eyes. Contrast sensitivity and reading speed were also better preserved in treated eyes. Again, the MPS group recommended treatment for eyes meeting eligibility criteria. Most investigators agree that treatment of ill-defined lesions or very large lesions is not advisable. For specifics regarding treatment, see the discussion below.

The benefit of treatment of PEDs without clear evidence of neovascularization is uncertain. The first randomized, prospective study on laser treatment of PEDs suggested that treated eyes underwent more rapid visual deterioration than untreated eyes. Furthermore, multiple treatment sessions were required in the majority of cases (32). However, problems with the study included misclassification of PED with coincident CNV as avascular. A review of the original data (33), as well as longer follow-up (34), seemed to support the conclusion that treatment of PEDs did not improve visual prognosis in avascular PED.

More recent studies have produced encouraging results regarding treatment of CNV and associated PED (35). In the largest study to date, 124 consecutive eyes with neovascularization associated with PED were treated with krypton red or argon green laser (36). Neovascular membranes were considered definite in all cases, but the exact extent could not always be determined. In no case was a suspected subfoveal membrane treated. At average follow-up of 16 months, one half of treated eyes had stable or improved vision (Fig. 6.10).

Digital and Indocyanine Green Angiography

Diagnosis of AMD

The MPS has documented the benefit of treatment of CNV with specific characteristics and only for those membranes that are "well-defined." This implies that the entire extent of the neovascular complex, particularly the borders, be obvious on angiography. As described in the discussion of AMD, many cases of exudative AMD do not present this way. Overlying blood, turbid subretinal fluid, or pigment all may obscure the margins of the disease. Furthermore, fluorescein, a small molecule with limited serum protein-binding (60% to 80%), readily escapes from neovascular membranes and diffuses into surrounding fluid, scars, and sclera. Thus, fluorescein itself may make the interpretation of angiograms difficult. Indocyanine green (ICG) is a tricarbocyanine dye with a peak absorption (805 nm) and fluorescence (835 nm) in the near infrared range. Light with these longer wavelengths penetrates pigment, blood, and proteinaceous fluid more readily than do the wavelengths used to generate fluorescein images (37). Thus, ICG imaging techniques may render visible membranes that were obscured on fluorescein angiography. A second property of ICG is its rapid, high-affinity binding (98%) to serum proteins, particularly albumin. Because of its protein-binding characteristics, ICG remains within the intravascular space to a much greater degree than fluorescein does (38). Thus, membranes are not obscured with ICG dye leakage. Recurrences at the margins of previous treatment may also be more obvious because ICG will not leak and stain scars or sclera. Occult CNV and recurrences are particularly well demonstrated by ICG imaging.

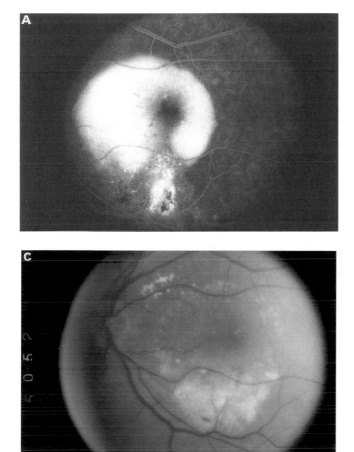

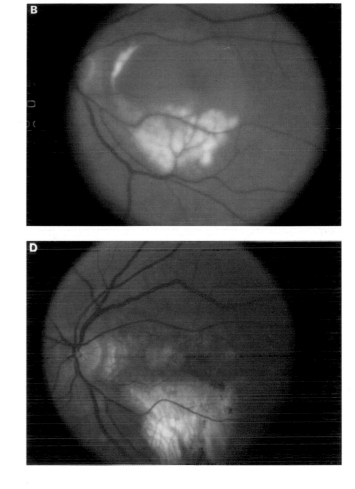

Fig. 6.10 Large PED in a patient with AMD. A, Late views from fluorescein angiogram reveal even filling of the PED superiorly with a prominent V-shaped notch inferiorly, representing displacement of leaked fluorescein by inferior sub-RPE neovascularization. Visual acuity is 20/200. B, Immediate posttreatment photographs show the clinical extent of the PED as well as the recent laser photocoagulation. C, Two months later, the PED has resolved and acuity has improved to 20/50. D, Three years later, after additional treatment for a second PED with CNV in the superior macula, visual acuity has improved to 20/20. E, The right eye of the same patient shows four discrete areas of previous treatment to CNV associated with PED in AMD. Visual acuity remains 20/20.

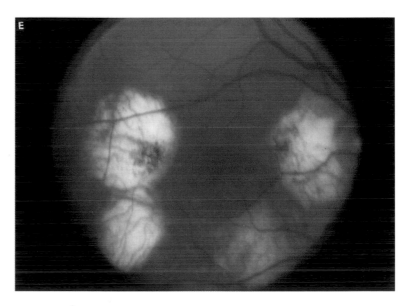

Paradoxically, ICG seems less effective than fluorescein angiography at demonstrating classic, well-defined CNV.

Historically, ICG has been used for hepatic and cardiac function studies for several decades. Its safety at standard dosages is established. Two anaphylactic deaths have been reported following intra-arterial administration, one in a patient with known hypersensitivity to penicillin and sulfa antibiotics. No deaths have been reported following intravenous administration. Regardless of the route of administration, ICG is metabolized hepatically and excreted entirely in the bile. It should be used with caution in patients with known sensitivity to iodides. The primate ocular circulation was studied with ICG for the first time in 1970, using intra-arterial administration (39). In 1971, David performed intra-arterial studies in patients (40), and in 1972, Flower and coworkers introduced less invasive and more familiar intravenous techniques (41,42). Early studies were not promising because of technologic limitations in image capturing and resolution. Technologic advances and refinements, including the use of fluorescence angiography rather than absorption angiography and new infrared-sensitive black-and-white film, led to larger clinical studies with somewhat disappointing results: ICG improved visualization of CNV relative to fluorescein angiography in only 2 of 25 cases of suspected CNV (43).

The breakthrough in ICG angiography has come with further refinements in computer-enhanced (digitized) videoangiography (44). State-of-the-art imaging systems include an interface adapter that creates video images from the fundus camera. Video images are then converted into a digital signal by a central processing unit for analysis and storage on space-efficient hard disc drives (temporary storage) or optical laser drives (archiving). The primary advantage of digitalization is computer enhancement and manipulation of the video signal. Various algorithms are available, including contrast enhancement, region mapping and comparison, area measurement, fluorescence density measurements, depth impressions, and image reversal. Digitalization also allows for more efficient image storage. Various printers can be connected for immediate generation of prints, transparencies, or slides. Computer networks can share images over long distances. The digitization process can also dramatically improve the resolution of standard fluorescein angiography and has led to the first clinical study of ICG videoangiography in human beings (45). The authors used a higher dose of ICG (3 mg/kg, compared to the traditional 0.5 mg/kg) and reported success in visualizing membranes not well seen on fluorescein images. Subsequent studies have confirmed the value of digital videoangiography with highly efficient barrier and excitation filters and intermediate ICG doses (1 to 2 mg/kg; 46,47).

Typically, ICG angiography is performed along with digitized fluorescein angiography. ICG is injected first. The diagnostic dosage is usually 50 mg or 1 to 2 mg/kg, whichever is greater. Successful studies have been achieved with lower doses, which were tried when there was a shortage of the dye. Early ICG images are taken immediately. Fluorescein is injected next. (There is no adverse interaction between the two dyes.) Early and late (15 min) fluorescein images are recorded next and are also digitalized for enhancement. Finally, late ICG images (40 min) are recorded. ICG is rapidly cleared from medium and large choroidal vessels but remains in neovascular networks, without leakage, for prolonged periods. Thus, long delays in generating late ICG images are particularly helpful in delineating CNV (leakage and diffusion render 40-min fluorescein images less valuable). In fact, these "very late" ICG studies suggest that many membranes are much larger than 15-min images (fluorescein or ICG) suggest. This may account for the high rate of "recurrence" following traditional treatment.

With the veritable explosion in interest in ICG imaging systems, two new technologic advances now constitute the frontier. First, ICG angiography combined with scanning laser ophthalmoscopy will enhance the diagnostic and therapeutic capabilities of each modality. Second, the use of semiconductor diode laser as a stimulating light source may expand the use of ICG angiography to include eyes previously unimagable due to severe media opacity.

Treatment of AMD

The absorption-fluorescence spectra of ICG has another implication of considerable importance. The semiconductor diode laser emits in the near infrared range (780 to 850 nm), the same range in which ICG absorbs light (805 nm). ICG is retained in neovascular membranes 20 to 40 minutes after intravenous injection. This fortuitous constellation of biophysical properties may permit highly efficient treatment of CNV·ICG may act as a chromophore for enhancement of laser uptake. Following pretreatment with ICG, laser energy uptake can be specifically enhanced in regions of CNV. This may permit more focal treatment at laser energies less likely to damage surrounding photoreceptors. Experimental studies show that neovascularization can be closed with 50% less energy using ICG as a chromophore (48,49). Higher doses of ICG have been used in these studies (5 mg/kg) with unknown hazards (adverse reactions have occurred with this therapeutic dose; such reactions may be rare at lower, diagnostic dosages). We will be participating in a collaborative study comparing ICG-enhanced diode laser treatment of CNV with standard treatment techniques.

Other Causes of Choroidal Neovascularization

Overview

The conditions associated with CNV include AMD, ocular histoplasmosis, idiopathic CNV, pathologic myopia, angioid streaks, multifocal choroiditis, serpiginous or helicoid choroidopathy, choroidal osteoma, choroidal rupture, hereditary dystrophies, and many others. Essentially anything that alters the RPE and Bruch's membrane can cause CNV.

Most histopathologic studies of CNV have been performed in eyes with AMD (50). The histopathologic feature common to many eyes that develop CNV is a break in Bruch's membrane. The capillary-like neovascularization originates from choroidal vessels and extends through the breaks in Bruch's membrane. In AMD, the CNV advances through a break in the outer aspect of Bruch's membrane and is located initially between the thickened inner aspect and the outer aspect of the membrane.

Because the common feature in eyes with CNV is usually a break in Bruch's membrane, and the end stage is often a disciform scar, the pathogenesis of CNV in various diseases may have similarities, irrespective of the underlying disorder.

The MPS proved the effectiveness of argon laser therapy for extrafoveal CNV associated with AMD, ocular histoplasmosis, and idiopathic CNV (27,51,52). Krypton laser therapy was also proven effective for juxtafoveal CNV in eyes with ocular histoplasmosis (53). More recently, the MPS group reported clear proof of the benefit of laser photocoagulation for subfoveal CNV in certain, carefully selected cases of AMD (18,19,31). Histoplasmic subfoveal CNV was investigated in a pilot study by some MPS investigators (54). The value of photocoagulation for subfoveal CNV in other diseases has not been studied thoroughly.

Because of the features common to the neovascularization process, regardless of etiology, we may, when necessary, cautiously extrapolate from the results of the MPS and consider laser treatment for CNV in other diseases, as long as we are mindful of the differences as well as the similarities in the various disease processes.

A major problem in the management of CNV, regardless of location or etiology, is recurrence. In the MPS, almost all the eyes that lost six or more lines of vision had recurrent CNV. The only randomized trial reporting the treatment of recurrent CNV is that by the MPS group for recurrent subfoveal CNV in AMD (31). This report and clinical experience indicate benefits of laser therapy for recurrent CNV and mandate careful follow-up of patients treated with laser for CNV of any etiology.

Ocular Histoplasmosis

Presumed ocular histoplasmosis (POH) may be the second leading cause of blindness in people under age 50 in endemic areas, such as the Ohio and Mississippi river valleys (55). The classic triad of the disease as first described by Woods and Whalen includes scars or hemorrhage with detachment of the macula associated with peripapillary chorioretinal and peripheral atrophic or punched-out chorioretinal lesions ("histo spots"; 56). It usually occurs in healthy people between 20 and 50 years of age. The multiple chorioretinal scars are probably caused by a mild or subclinical systemic infection with the fungus *Histoplasma capsulatum*. CNV may occur years later at a chorioretinal scar, and central vision may be lost (57). The end-stage disciform lesions are similar to those seen in AMD. However, the drusen characteristic of AMD are not a feature of presumed ocular histoplasmosis (50, p. 1019).

In studying the fluorescein angiograms of patients with histoplasmic CNV, it sometimes is difficult to identify and differentiate the hyperfluorescence associated with the chorioretinal scars of inactive ocular histoplasmosis or inactive laser scars from that associated with active CNV (Fig. 6.11). The hyperfluorescence from a chorioretinal scar usually begins at the periphery, the margin adjacent to normal choroid. It then spreads during the course of the

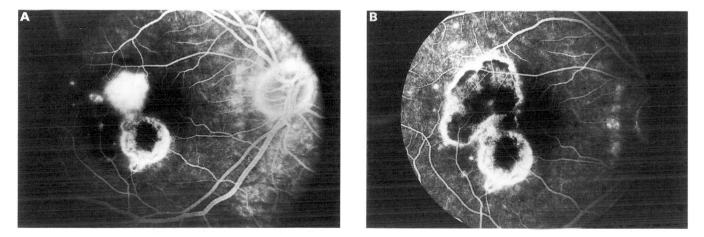

Fig. 6.11 Laser photocoagulation of CNV in presumed ocular histoplasmosis syndrome (POHS). A, Fluorescein angiogram shows late hyperfluorescence in the superior macula, consistent with CNV. Inferiorly, there is a quiescent scar from previously treated CNV. B, Angiogram from the same patient 11 days after laser treatment of the recurrent membrane. The rim of hyperfluorescence is typical of adequately treated membranes. (Reproduced by permission from Singerman LJ, Novak MA. Subretinal neovascularization. In: Yannuzzi LA, ed. Laser photocoagulation of the retina. Philadelphia: JB Lippincott, 1989: 27–46.)

angiogram toward the center of the scar. The leakage begins from the area of the scar associated with the active CNV. It then spreads out more peripherally. At the end of the fluorescein angiography, the entire area may appear hyperfluorescent in either situation. In simple chorioretinal scars, this is just staining of the scar. With active CNV, the area with serous subretinal detachment overlying the membrane shows hyperfluorescence. Recurrence must be recognized and treated promptly, before the center of the fovea is involved (Fig. 6.12).

Although it was known from natural history studies that there was a significant incidence of visual loss in patients with this disease, a substantial number, far more than in AMD, did maintain good vision (58). Spontaneous improvement after initial loss of vision has been noted (59,60). The MPS undertook to evaluate laser treatment versus no treatment in patients with CNV associated with ocular histoplasmosis syndrome (OHS).

Argon laser photocoagulation was useful in preventing severe visual loss in eyes with extrafoveal choroidal neovascular membranes (51). When the histoplasmic CNV was juxtafoveal, krypton laser was beneficial in preventing severe visual loss (53).

In the argon study of treatment of extrafoveal neovascularization, 48% of eyes in the observation group, compared with 9% in the laser treatment group, lost six or more lines of visual acuity in 3 years of follow-up (22). Thirty-nine percent of untreated eyes, compared with 5% of treated eyes, had visual acuity worse than 20/200. Whereas only 38% in the untreated group had visual acuity of 20/40 or better, 66% of treated eyes had this level of vision.

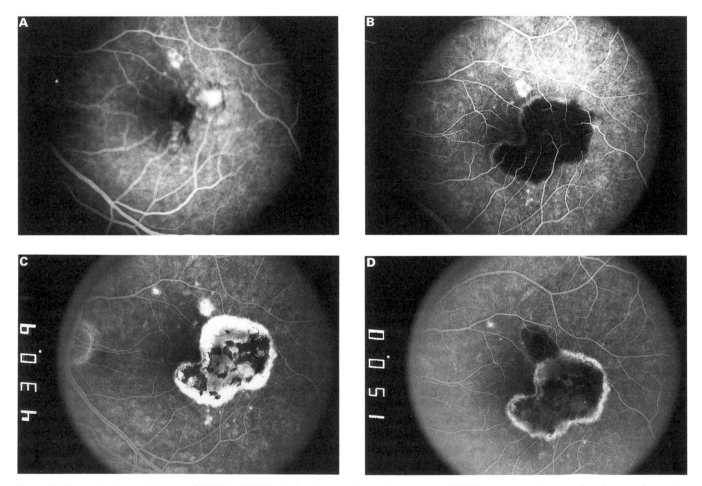

Fig. 6.12 Laser photocoagulation of CNV in POHS. A, Angiogram shows two areas of CNV, one superotemporal and one inferior to the fovea. Hypofluorescence corresponded to subretinal hemorrhage, with secondary visual loss (20/80). A small area of hyperfluorescence superiorly corresponded to an inactive chorioretinal scar. B, Five days after laser treatment, the CNV is obliterated. C, One year later, there is increased hyperfluorescence at the superonasal margin of the previous treatment, continuous with the previously inactive scar. Clinical examination revealed a small serous/hemorrhagic retinal detachment in this area (note the hypofluorescence corresponding to hemorrhage inferonasal to the upper lesion, highlighting probable CNV). D, One week following the second laser treatment to the area of reactivation, there is resolution of the detachment with no residual hyperfluorescence. Acuity improved to 20/30. (Reproduced by permission from Singerman LJ, Novak MA. Subretinal neovascularization. In Yannuzzi LA, ed. Laser photocoagulation of the retina. Philadelphia: JB Lippincott, 1989: 27–46.)

In the study of krypton laser photocoagulation for juxtafoveal neovascularization, the MPS protocol included treatment of the entire area of hyperfluorescence, in an effort to obtain complete obliteration of the CNV (53). The edge of the membrane was treated with overlapping 200-μm burns of 0.2- to 0.5-sec duration, and the remainder of the membrane was treated with 200- to 500-μm spot size, 0.5-sec duration burns. As in the argon study, substantially fewer treated eyes had large decreases in vision as compared with the no-treatment group. At 3-year follow-up, 25% of eyes in the observation group versus 5% in the treatment group lost six or more lines of vision.

Our treatment technique with either the krypton laser or the red wavelengths of the tunable dye laser is essentially the same as that in the Krypton Macular Photocoagulation Study. We will often place the burn over the choroidal neovascular membrane near its edge and allow it to *spread* over the edge of the membrane with a 0.5-sec burn. Although a retrobulbar anesthetic for akinesia was used in the study, it may not be needed in many cases (61). We have used peribulbar anesthetic and achieved effective akinesia in many cases, while minimizing the chances of some of the complications associated with retrobulbar anesthetic, including perforation of the globe.

Idiopathic Neovascularization

When CNV develops in the absence of atrophic chorioretinal scars, drusen, or other retinal abnormality, it is termed idiopathic (Fig. 6.13A). The MPS report of argon laser photocoagulation for idiopathic CNV found a substantially smaller proportion of eyes with large decreases (six or more lines) of vision in the treatment group (16%) as compared with the no-treatment group (34%; Fig. 6.13B; 22,52).

Pathologic Myopia

In pathologic myopia, linear breaks in Bruch's membrane, called lacquer cracks, may develop secondary to choroidal thinning and atrophy associated with the elongation of the globe. Choroidal new vessels can extend through these lacquer cracks and cause hemorrhage and disciform scarring (50, p. 915; 57, p. 110). The incidence of CNV in pathologic myopia is approximately 5% (62).

In pathologic myopia, the choroidal new vessels often begin very close to the fovea. This plus the frequent atrophy of RPE pose a particular challenge in laser treatment of CNV (Fig. 6.14) Furthermore, choroidal new vessels are often located along lacquer cracks, which have been occasionally seen to extend during the application of laser therapy.

The treatment of CNV complicating pathologic myopia remains controversial. Reports of the natural course have been rather contradictory, and therefore it has not been es-

tablished whether the prognosis without treatment is sufficiently severe to warrant laser therapy. Some authors have reported that eyes with CNV and pathologic myopia have a very poor visual prognosis. In Hotchkiss and Fine's series, for example, 14 of 27 such eyes lost two or more lines of vision, and 12 of the 27 became legally blind (63). Other investigators, however, have reported that the course in these eye is likely to be benign. Avila and colleagues suggested that pathologic myopia with CNV does not require laser treatment if the CNV is small with little leakage, which was the finding in the majority of their cases (64). Fried and coworkers reported that nearly two thirds of their patients with CNV and pathologic myopia had stable or improved vision without treatment (65). However, these and other previous studies all have some deficiencies in design that prevent their conclusions from being definitive.

Soubrane and Pisan described their results in a clinical trial of 38 eyes randomized to laser photocoagulation and 28 eyes randomized to observation (66). Eyes in the observation group generally had a marked deterioration in vision, with 80% showing a final acuity of less than 20/100. Eyes in the treatment group did not show any significant improvement in vision but were remarkably stable. The authors concluded that laser therapy for CNV in degenerative myopia is probably efficacious, although difficult and associated with significant risks and potential for complications.

Brancato reported that laser scars increase in size after laser therapy for CNV complicating pathologic myopia, but even if they extend to the fovea they are usually not associated with serious vision loss (67). Yannuzzi and Milch initiated a multicenter, prospective, randomized, controlled trial of CNV in pathologic myopia (68).

Angioid Streaks

Angioid streaks are breaks in a calcified Bruch's membrane. Fibrovascular tissue and choroidal new vessels may extend through the break and may lead to associated serous or hemorrhagic detachment of the retina, RPE, or both. Angioid streaks have been associated with several systemic diseases, such as pseudoxanthoma elasticum, Paget's disease of bone, Ehlers-Danlos syndrome, sickle cell disease, thalassemia, and other blood dyscrasias (Figs. 6.15 and 6.16; 50, p. 1032; 57, p. 104; 69-72). In Clarkson and Altman's series of 50 patients with angioid streaks, 25 (50%) had an identifiable systemic diagnosis (73). Histologic changes suggestive or characteristic of pseudoxanthoma elasticum have been found in skin biopsy specimens of patients who had angioid streaks but did not have clinically evident skin changes characteristic of pseudoxanthoma elasticum (74).

One of the challenges of treating angioid streaks is that most of the choroidal new vessels are located in the

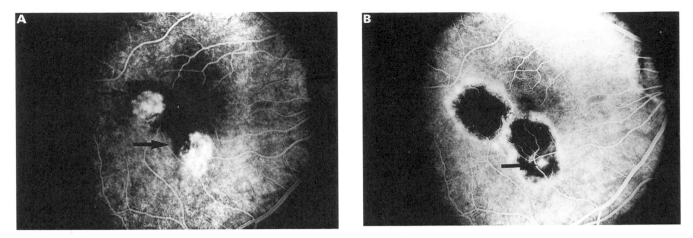

Fig 6.13 Laser photocoagulation of idiopathic CNV. A, Fluorescein angiogram shows two discrete areas of idiopathic CNV associated with hemorrhage. The arrow indicates hypofluorescence secondary to hemorrhage. B, Eight days after laser treatment, there is residual hyperfluorescence within the area that was treated (arrow). It is well surrounded by hypofluorescence and probably represents regressing CNV or thermal vasculitis. No additional treatment was necessary. (Reproduced by permission from Singerman LJ, Novak MA. Subretinal neovascularization. In: Yannuzzi LA, ed. Laser photocoagulation of the retina. Philadelphia: JB Lippincott, 1989: 27–46.)

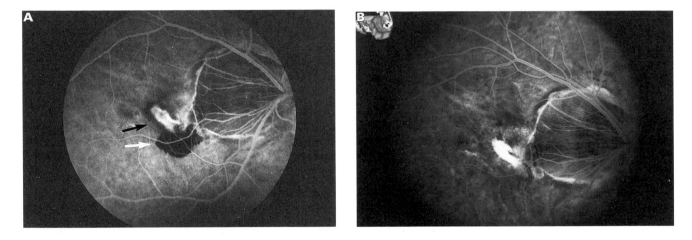

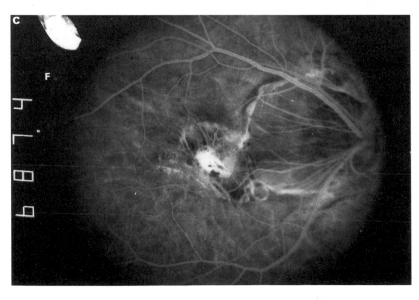

Fig. 6.14 Untreated CNV secondary to pathologic myopia. A, Fluorescein angiogram from a high myope (-20 diopter). There is a crescent of hyperfluorescence inferior to and possibly under the fovea (*black arrow*) and associated subretinal hemorrhage and fluid (*white arrow*). Visual acuity is 20/200. Treatment was not undertaken. B, Two years later, the CNV has spontaneously evolved into a fibrovascular scar. The localized detachment has resolved and acuity is 20/50. C, Six years later, there has been progressive central atrophy and scarring. Acuity has dropped to 20/200. (Reproduced by permission from Singerman LJ, Novak MA. Subretinal neovascularization. In: Yannuzzi LA, ed. Laser photocoagulation of the retina. Philadelphia: JB Lippincott, 1989: 27–46.)

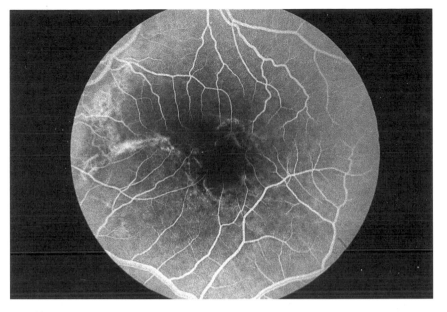

Fig. 6.15 Angioid streaks in sickle cell anemia. Angiogram reveals a streak extending toward the fovea without evidence of CNV. (Reproduced by permission from Singerman LJ, Novak MA. Subretinal neovascularization. In: Yannuzzi LA, ed. Laser photocoagulation of the macula. Philadelphia: JB Lippincott, 1989: 27–46.)

papillomacular bundle, either near the peripapillary region or just nasal to the fovea. Therefore, the laser surgeon must consider the possibility that laser treatment will cause visual field defects. In addition, in the treatment of eyes with peripapillary CNV, there is a risk of damage to the major retinal blood vessels emanating from the optic disc. Patients with Paget's disease may have particularly large CNV over the papillomacular bundle, increasing the difficulty of treatment (see Fig. 6.16).

The natural history and visual prognosis in eyes with angioid streaks complicated by CNV are very poor. Extrafoveal CNV tends to progress to subretinal disciform scarring and severe visual loss; this process often is bilateral. Both argon and krypton laser photocoagulation have been used to treat eyes with angioid streaks and CNV (72,75,76). Although the untreated eyes cannot be considered to be adequate controls in these studies, the treated

eyes clearly had a better visual outcome than did the untreated eyes.

With long-term follow-up, treated eyes may deteriorate, not necessarily due to recurrent CNV. Often there is a subtle but gradually increasing atrophic degeneration associated with substantial decline in vision, often to less than 20/200, even in the absence of marked atrophic changes in the pigment epithelium.

Gelisken, Hendrikse, and Deutman reported their findings in the long-term follow-up of patients treated with photocoagulation for CNV in angioid streaks (77). The length of follow-up ranged from 2 months to 16 years (mean 3.4 years). They concluded that treatment is beneficial and allows treated eyes to maintain useful vision longer than untreated eyes.

As with the other unusual causes of CNV, randomized trials of laser treatment for CNV with angioid streaks are

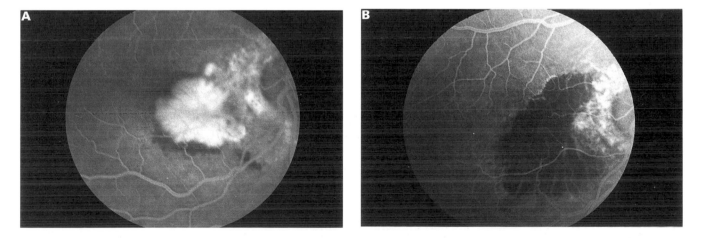

Fig. 6.16 Laser photocoagulation of CNV associated with angioid streaks in Paget's disease. A, Angiogram reveals a large area of CNV in the papillomacular bundle. Acuity is counting fingers at 3 feet. B, Three months after krypton laser photocoagulation, there is no remaining active CNV. Acuity is 20/200. (Reproduced by permission from Singerman LJ, Novak MA. Subretinal neovascularization. In: Yannuzzi LA, ed. Laser photocoagulation of the macula. Philadelphia: JB Lippincott, 1989: 27–40.)

not available and are unlikely to be performed. Thus, these retrospective data provide the best available insight into the potential of laser photocoagulation treatment to control CNV in angioid streaks. Laser therapy appears to be effective in delaying visual loss. If one can accomplish a substantial delay in visual loss, laser therapy for extrafoveal CNV in eyes with angioid streaks warrants consideration. For the best results, treatment should be as early and as complete as possible.

Multifocal Choroiditis

Several authors have reported a multifocal choroiditis not related to POHS (78-87). It is reasonable to consider that these reports describe conditions that are different points along the spectrum of the same disease (85). Although the nomenclature differs, each describes acute, multiple, discrete lesions, frequently recurrent, that involve the RPE and choriocapillaris (Table 6.1). Unlike eyes with POHS, these eyes frequently have an associated inflammation of the vitreous and anterior chamber, although this is a variable finding (87). However, they often develop choroidal new vessels similar to those seen in POH (Fig. 6.17). The final appearance of the chorioretinal scar resembles that of POH, but often the acute and subacute phases of the two diseases are quite different. Although de novo histoplasmosis scars are known to occur, this is more common in other varieties of multifocal choroiditis. Not infrequently, acute, subacute, and chronic lesions may be seen in the same eye simultaneously. The scarring can become extensive and confluent. An extensive subretinal fibrosis may occur. One report suggests that the CNV, as well as the inflammatory lesions, may respond to steroid therapy (86). Laser therapy for CNV may be effective in some cases (see Fig. 6.17; 86,88). However, in our experience, recurrent membranes, as well as de novo CNV, may occur more commonly in multifocal choroiditis than in other causes of CNV. Still, for any active inflammation threatening the macula or optic nerve we advocate treatment with oral corticosteroids. For any active CNV threatening the fovea we usually recommend laser photocoagulation. Because inflammation and CNV may coexist (see Fig. 6.17), these treatments may have to be coadministered.

Serpiginous Choroiditis

Serpiginous choroiditis is a chronic, recurring disease of unknown etiology. It most often begins in the peripapillary region and extends to the macula. It also has been called geographic choroiditis or geographic helicoid peripapillary choroidopathy. The disease usually begins unilaterally but eventually becomes bilateral, sometimes several years later (Fig. 6.18; 89). The lesions may begin in the macular region or in the peripheral fundus, rather than in the peripapillary region, but this is uncommon.

It now is well known that CNV can complicate serpiginous choroiditis (90). Affected patients often are symptomatic, with recurrent inflammation at the margin of the previous chorioretinal scarring in the absence of active CNV (see Fig. 6.18E).

In interpreting the fluorescein angiogram, the distinction must be made between the hyperfluorescence associated with recurring inflammation and that associated with CNV. The inflammatory lesion does hyperfluoresce and dye leakage accumulates in the late phases of the angiogram. However, the extent of the leakage is subtle compared with the more dramatic leakage associated with CNV. ICG angiography may be helpful in distinguishing inflammation from neovascularization. The presence of subretinal hemorrhage or lipid is an obvious clue to occult CNV (see Fig. 6.18D).

Some inflammatory lesions may respond favorably to steroid therapy (91). As with multifocal choroiditis, oral prednisone should be considered for active inflammation of the posterior pole, and laser treatment considered for active CNV. It is advisable to prescribe a systemic steroid for patients to keep and use for the first day or two after symptoms recur, until they are able to have a complete eye examination and a fluorescein angiogram. Laser photocoagulation can be beneficial in treating CNV in selected patients.

Uncommon Causes of Choroidal Neovascularization

A number of uncommon disorders occasionally are associated with CNV, including choroidal rupture, choroidal osteoma, rubella, hereditary dystrophies (e.g., choroideremia, Best's disease, fundus flavimaculatus), and many others.

Choroidal rupture is a fairly common complication of blunt ocular trauma. These are large breaks in Bruch's membrane. Occasionally CNV may develop, usually at the foveal margin of the choroidal rupture (Fig. 6.19). A patient may develop visual loss months or years after trauma because of spontaneous bleeding or serous exudation from CNV arising at a site of old rupture (57, p. 170). Neovascularization may resolve spontaneously (92,93); it also may precipitate serous or hemorrhagic detachment, in which case laser photocoagulation treatment may be useful (94).

Choroidal osteoma was first described in detail by Gass in 1978 (95). These benign tumors of cancellous bone are seen primarily in Caucasian women. The tumors are bilateral in 10% to 20% of cases. The lesions arise in the juxtapapillary and macular regions. Symptoms are associated with CNV and serous or hemorrhagic detachment of the macula. There has been little experience with the treatment of CNV in these tumors (Fig. 6.20; 96-99). Several treatments may be necessary to obliterate the CNV, but useful vision can be salvaged (Fig. 6.21; 100).

Table 6.1 Summary of Findings from Series of Patients With Multifocal Choroiditis

Author (Reference)	Diagnosis	No. of Patients	Bilateral %	Sex = F %	Age <35 y %	Vitreous Inflammation %	Anterior Chamber Inflammation %	CNV %	CME %	Positive Response to Steroids* %
Nozik, Dorsch (78)	Chorioretinopathy with anterior uveitis	2	100	50	100	100	100	NA	50	100
Dreyer, Gass (79)	Multifocal choroiditis and panuveitis	28	79	75	57	100	54	46	18	33
Watzke et al (80)	Punctate inner choroidopathy	10	80	100	90	NA	NA	40	NA	0
Palestine et al (81,82)	Progressive subretinal fibrosis and uveitis	4	75	100	100	100	50	NA	100	25
Cantrill, Folk (83)	Progressive retinal fibrosis	5	80	100	100	40	40	NA	25	40
Doran, Hamilton (84)	Multifocal choroiditis with disciform macular degeneration	4	75	75	100	NA	NA	100	NA	0
Morgan, Schatz (85)	Recurrent multifocal inner choroiditis	11	45	100	91	45	NA	35	18	89 (1 with CNV)

CNV, choroidal neovascularization; CME, cystoid macular edema.
*Percentage of patients treated with steroids who had a clearly positive response. There were other patients whose response to steroids was equivocal.
Source: Modified from Singerman LJ (87).

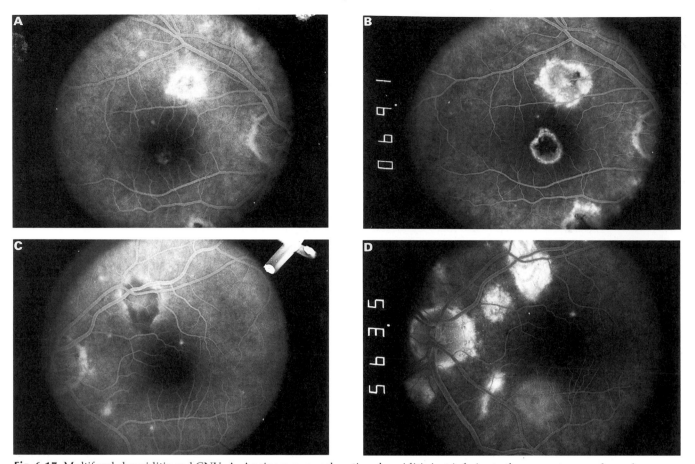

Fig. 6.17 Multifocal choroiditis and CNV. A, Angiogram reveals active choroiditis just inferior to the superotemporal arcade. The dot of hyperfluorescence in the superior macula corresponds clinically to an inactive scar. Irregular hyperfluorescence in the superior macula corresponds clinically to an inactive scar. Irregular hyperfluorescence inferior to the fovea corresponds to an area of subretinal fluid and represents active CNV. B, Following laser photocoagulation, the CNV inferiorly is quiescent. The previously active inflammation superiorly has spontaneously resolved. C, The left eye of the same patient shows multiple foci of active choroiditis without obvious CNV. The most active lesion superonasally has irregular hyper- and hypofluorescence. D, Two years later, there is evidence of resolution of the most active lesion but multiple new lesions have appeared. A relapsing-remitting course is typical of this disorder, and ongoing surveillance for new CNV is critical. (Reproduced by permission from Singerman LJ, Novak MA. Subretinal neovascularization. In: Yannuzzi LA, ed. Laser photocoagulation of the macula. Philadelphia: JB Lippincott, 1989: 27–46.)

Subretinal neovascularization with disciform scar formation is an uncommon but reported complication of *rubella retinopathy* (100-104).

Several *hereditary dystrophies* may be associated with CNV. *Best's vitelliform dystrophy* is an autosomal dominant disease that usually has its onset in children 3 to 10 years of age. Uncommonly, affected patients develop CNV and macular detachment with subsequent disciform scarring and loss of vision to 20/100 or worse (57, p. 238; 105). *Fundus flavimaculatus* is characterized by yellowish flecks that resemble drusen but are more irregular and, on fluorescein angiography, either do not fluoresce or fluoresce irregularly (57, p. 256). Patients with this disease generally begin losing central vision in childhood or early adulthood. CNV and disciform macular detachment occur uncommonly (106,107).

Choroideremia is an X-linked recessive chorioretinal degenerative disease. It is characterized by progressive atrophy of the choroid and RPE. Until recently, it was believed that vision was unaffected until the macula became involved late in the course of the disease. However, CNV may rarely develop in association with choroideremia (108). Increased awareness by ophthalmologists of this complication may reveal more cases of neovascularization in choroideremia and other hereditary dystrophies, and some cases, if diagnosed early enough, may be treatable.

Probably any disease that affects the RPE may eventually be associated with CNV. The list of diseases that have been reported to be associated with CNV is constantly growing (57, p. 198). These include toxocara canis (57, p. 144), ocular toxoplasmosis (109), sarcoidosis (57, p. 144), Harada's disease (110,111), choroidal melanocytic nevus (112), demarcation lines caused by rhegmatogenous retinal detachment (57, p. 716), drainage sites for scleral buckling surgery, chorioretinal folds (113), photocoagulation (114), optic nerve drusen (115), focal

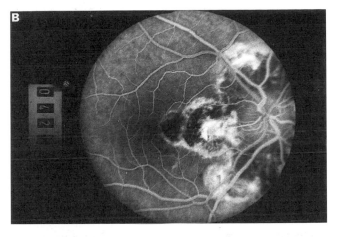

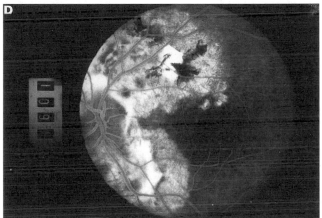

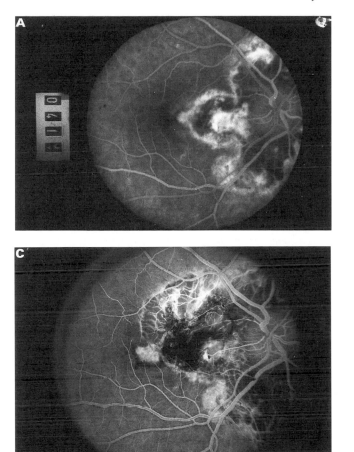

Fig. 6.18 Serpiginous choroidopathy and laser treatment of CNV. A, Angiogram in serpiginous choroidopathy reveals staining at the borders of the choroidopathy as well as late leakage from CNV at the foveal edge of the scar. B, Two months following krypton laser treatment of the extrafoveal CNV, there is no remaining activity. C, Five years later, there is juxtafoveal and subfoveal recurrence adjacent to the previously treated area. (Superiorly, there is atrophy corresponding to laser treatment of two other episodes of recurrent CNV.) D, The left eye of the same patient shows active neovascularization superior to the fovea. E, Complex angiogram of the same patient's left eye following laser treatment superior and temporal to the fovea. Acuity is 20/50. Superior to the disc is a crescent of fibrovascular tissue that stains. (Reproduced by permission from Singerman LJ, Novak MA. Subretinal neovascularization. In: Yannuzzi LA, ed. Laser photocoagulation of the macula. Philadelphia: JB Lippincott, 1989: 27–46.)

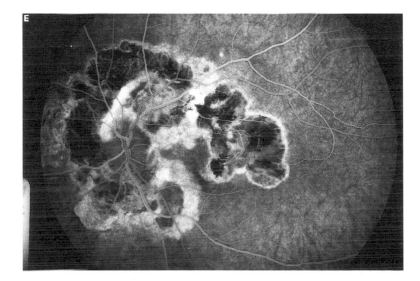

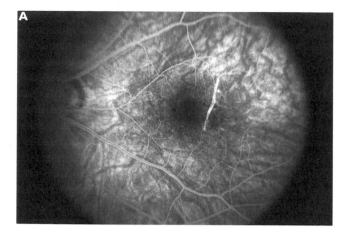

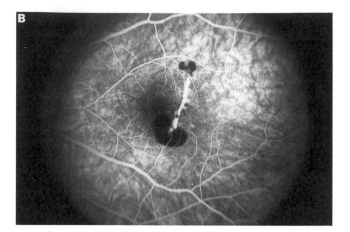

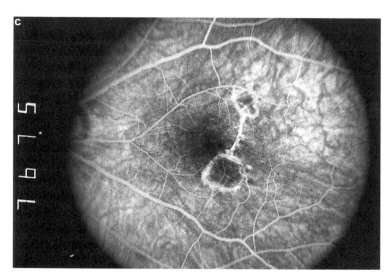

Fig. 6.19 Choroidal rupture and CNV. A, Angiogram of an asymptomatic 34-year-old man (acuity 20/20) reveals crescentic hyperfluorescence temporal to the fovea corresponding to staining of inactive fibrovascular tissue. B, Angiogram of the same patient after acute visual loss (acuity 20/80). Examination revealed serous/hemorrhage detachment of the temporal macula. Active CNV is obscured by hemorrhage at each end of the rupture. C, Two months after treatment, the macular detachment and hemorrhage has resolved, and there is no active leakage. Acuity has returned to 20/25. (Reproduced by permission from Singerman LJ, Novak MA. Subretinal neovascularization. In: Yannuzzi LA, ed. Laser photocoagulation of the macula. Philadelphia: JB Lippincott, 1989: 27–46.)

treatment of diabetic maculopathy (116), chronic papilledema (117), choroidal septic emboli (118), and many, many more.

In 1985, several investigators reported a newly recognized, unusual hemorrhagic disorder of the posterior pole, seen in middle-aged African American women (119). In 1990, three additional series describing similar cases were reported (120-122). Terms used to describe these cases vary but include "idiopathic polypoid choroidal vasculopathy" and "posterior uveal bleeding syndrome." The majority of affected patients are African American and women. Clinical findings include irregularly round serous and hemorrhagic detachments of the RPE apparently derived from large vascular channels. The lesions cluster around the optic nerve, and drusen and macular RPE changes are conspicuously absent (Fig. 6.22). Digital pressure on the globe will not collapse these lesions. Vitreous hemorrhage occurs commonly and is a significant cause of visual loss. In a minority of cases, fluorescein angiography discloses evidence of CNV. In the majority, however, the lesions appear smaller angiographically and do not leak. Spontaneous regression typically leaves subretinal scarring, however. The disorder follows a remitting-relapsing course. Laser photocoagulation to the polypoidal "feeding" vessels has led to resolution. In many cases, vitrectomy is required to clear the media and recover vision.

Laser Treatment Technique

Certain patterns of pretreatment, treatment, and posttreatment care are essential to the optimal management of all patients with CNV, regardless of etiology (123).

The ophthalmologist who does not treat CNV should promptly refer to an experienced laser surgeon any patient suspected of having CNV. This is preferable to ordering a fluorescein angiogram that may take days to weeks to be processed, interpreted, and returned. The delay can be disastrous because CNV can grow from an extrafoveal location to a subfoveal location in a very short time (124,125). The Moorfields study showed that patients

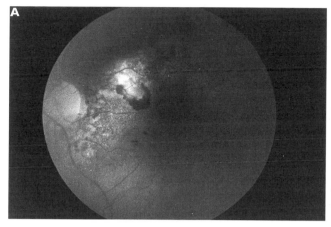

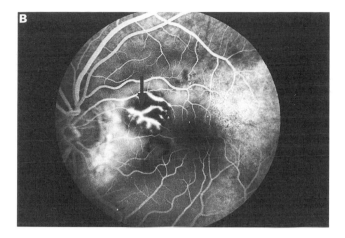

Fig. 6.20 Choroidal osteoma and CNV. A, Angiogram from a 24-year old woman with a choroidal osteoma. Superonasal to the fovea is a focus of intense hyperfluorescence surrounded by hemorrhage. Acuity is 20/30. B, Two days after treatment (with argon blue-green laser in 1975), all new vessels have been obliterated; however, there is hyperfluorescence from thermal retinal vasculitis (*arrow*). C, Eleven years later, a wide-angle angiogram shows further contraction and chorioretinal pucker at the treatment site (*arrow*), probably due to excessive absorption of blue wavelengths. (Reproduced by permission from Singerman LJ, Novak MA. Subretinal neovascularization. In: Yannuzzi LA, ed. Laser photocoagulation of the macula. Philadelphia: JB Lippincott, 1989: 27–46.)

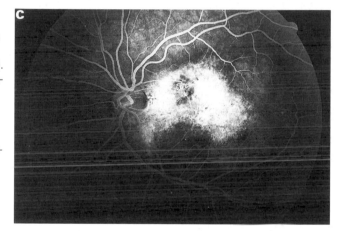

who were examined within a month of symptoms and who had good visual acuity had a high likelihood of showing treatable (which they essentially considered as extrafoveal) CNV, whereas patients who had symptoms for several months or presented with poor vision had a low likelihood of having such treatable vessels (126).

Once the ophthalmologist has decided to treat the CNV with laser, the patient should be informed that the aim of treatment is to prevent further visual loss, not to restore vision already lost. Because of the high incidence of recurrence of neovascularization, it is important to emphasize to the patient and family the importance of using the Amsler grid daily, and of calling the office promptly for an appointment if the patient notes any loss of vision or increased distortion. Furthermore, it is critical to instruct receptionists and technicians that any patient with potential CNV and new Amsler grid changes must be seen by the physician promptly.

If the patient has not had a fluorescein angiogram within 72 hours before treatment, an angiogram should be done. The angiogram serves as a guide for exact localization of the neovascularization to be photocoagulated and helps the laser surgeon to plan the treatment so that it can be accomplished as quickly and precisely as possible (127). Before the procedure, retrobulbar anesthesia often is administered, both for analgesia and to reduce eye movements that could lead to inadvertent laser damage to the fovea during treatment. This may not be necessary in cooperative patients with extrafoveal CNV.

Treatment should be performed only with a magnified image of the angiogram readily visible. Currently acceptable laser sources include argon green, krypton red, or dye yellow or red. Argon blue-green should be avoided due to greater absorption by foveal xanthophyll (Fig. 6.23). Red sources are particularly desirable in cases with significant cataract, turbid subretinal fluid, or considerable associated hemorrhage. Burn placement is more precise with red wavelengths, due to reduced lenticular scatter and less absorption by overlying hemoglobin. The complex of neovascularization and blocked fluorescence

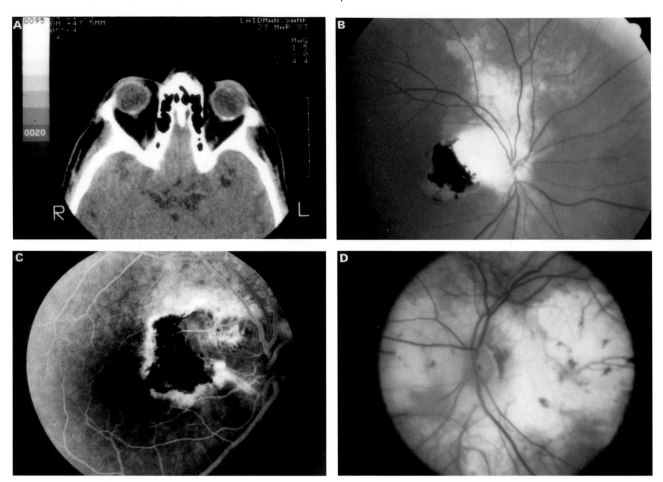

Fig. 6.21 Bilateral choroidal osteoma in a 34-year-old man. A, Computed tomography of the head reveals bilateral calcification of the posterior pole. B, Fundus photograph from the same patient 18 years after photocoagulation in the superior papillomacular bundle. The hyperpigmentation at the temporal end of the treated area is due to heavy blue-green absorption administered in 1974. The hypopigmentation superior to the superotemporal arcade is residual osteoma and overlying RPE change. C, Fluorescein angiogram of the treated area show staining of its borders with no active leakage. Visual acuity is 20/20. D, Left eye of the same patient. Note the severe macular changes from a larger tumor. Visual acuity is counting fingers.

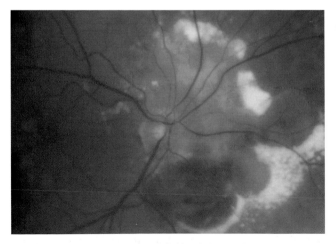

Fig. 6.22 Idiopathic polypoid choroidal vasculopathy. Note the several irregular and indistinct areas of serosanguineous RPE elevation with exudate at their margins. A polypoid vascular channel can be seen under the superior papillomacular bundle.

is first outlined with light 100 to 200-μm, 0.2-sec burns, placed noncontiguously 100 μm beyond its margins (Fig. 6.24A). The perimeter of the lesion closest to the fovea is treated initially, with 200-μm spots of 0.2- to 0.5-sec duration (Fig. 6.24B). The power is titrated to achieve a uniform white burn. Once the appropriate power is determined, the remainder of the perimeter is treated (Fig. 6.24C). The internal portion of the membrane is treated next, with overlapping 200-μm, 0.5- to 1.0-sec burns (Fig. 6.24D). The energy should be sufficient to cause dense whitening of the entire membrane, plus a surrounding rim 100 μm beyond angiographically evident lesion components (except blood). Treatment of recurrences should extend 300 μm into previously treated areas.

The goal of treatment is to obliterate the neovascularization without damage to the fovea. Argon and krypton laser photocoagulations are established, standard methods of treatment. The tunable dye laser offers theoretical

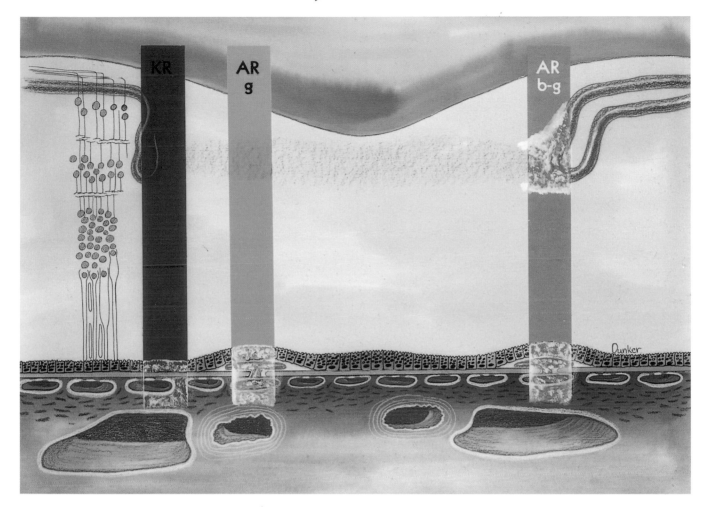

Fig. 6.23 Absorption characteristics for the various laser modalities commonly used in the treatment of CNV must be kept in mind. Argon blue-green was the laser used in the early MPS studies but is rarely used for macular treatment due to absorption by foveal xanthophyll. Argon green and dye yellow are minimally absorbed by xanthophyll and are most commonly used for these treatments. Krypton or dye red sources penetrate media opacities and blood far more effectively than argon green. Burn placement is probably most precise with red sources (burn intensity is enhanced, as well, with more laser-induced pain and a higher risk of complications). (Reproduced by permission from Singerman LJ [123].)

advantages in the management of CNV, and our clinical experience in thousands of cases suggests that it may allow improved results (128). We now prefer to treat the majority of cases of CNV with sequential red-yellow laser photocoagulation (Fig. 6.25). The CNV first is outlined with the red wavelength (630 to 647 nm). Red deeply penetrates the choroid and whitens the background, against which the CNV can be seen. The dye laser then can be tuned to the yellow wavelength (577 nm), which is absorbed directly into the hemoglobin in the new blood vessels, presumably enhancing the likelihood of their closure. Although the precise mechanism, or, more likely, combination of mechanisms, of the effect of laser treatment for CNV remains poorly understood, it does seem reasonable that enhancing uptake of laser energy in the choroidal new vessels should offer improved ability to close and obliterate them.

Areas where subretinal hemorrhage overlies the CNV are treated with the red wavelengths. Areas where the RPE is particularly atrophic are treated with the yellow wavelength, as are visibly red membranes and feeder vessels.

For those who do not have a dye laser, the argon-krypton laser may be used in a similar fashion, substituting krypton laser for red dye laser and green argon laser for the yellow dye laser (129,130).

Feeder vessels are treated directly, 100 μm beyond their lateral borders and 300 μm radially beyond their visible base. Retinal vessels should be scrupulously avoided. By MPS protocol, treatment of peripapillary lesions must spare 1.5 to 2 hours of the papillomacular bundle and not extend within 100 μm of the disc margin.

After treatment, fundus photographs are taken, both to document the treatment and to compare the

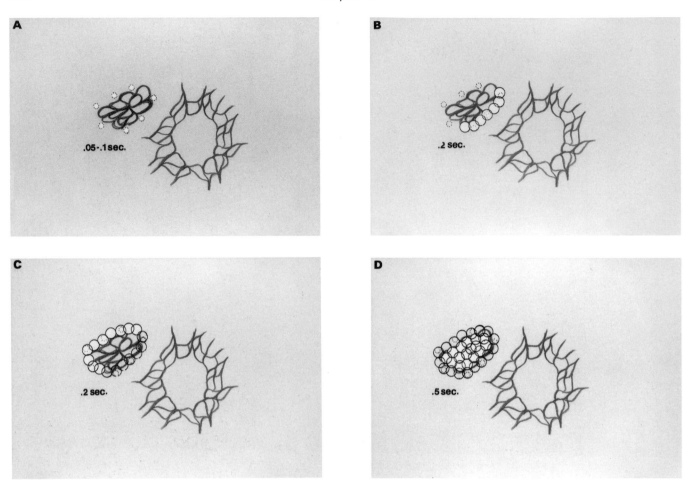

Fig. 6.24 Argon green laser treatment technique for extrafoveal and juxtafoveal CNV. A, The perimeter of the lesion is first lightly marked with noncontiguous 100 μm burns, 100 to 150 μm beyond its angiographically evident border. B, Next, the foveal side of the lesion's perimeter is covered with contiguous 200 μm burns. C, Next, the remainder of the lesion's perimeter is similarly treated. D, Finally, the center of the membrane is covered with 200- to 500-μm burns of longer duration (0.5 to 1.0 sec). (Reproduced by permission from Singerman LJ [123].)

immediate posttreatment appearance of the fundus with the pretreatment appearance and the appearance at follow-up visits. These photographs allow the laser surgeon to assess the accuracy and completeness of the treatment. If retrobulbar anesthesia was used, the eye is patched. The importance of using the Amsler grid and of prompt return to the office if any change in vision occurs is reiterated (Fig. 6.26).

Follow-up of laser treatment for CNV may be as important to its successful management as meticulous laser technique. Rigorous follow-up is essential to detect and treat persistent or recurrent neovascularization as promptly as possible. For the first several follow-up visits, fluorescein angiography is automatically repeated, and the laser surgeon performs slit-lamp fundus contact lens examination while studying the projected angiogram. An adequately treated membrane will develop an evenly hyperfluorescent rim, due to staining emanating from the adjacent untreated area. This should not be confused with

persistence, which will appear as focal hyperfluorescence. Leakage in the center of a treatment scar that has a broad rim of surrounding hypofluorescence need not be retreated. These areas usually resolve spontaneously, so treatment is avoided unless follow-up examination shows that the central hyperfluorescent area is enlarging.

The first follow-up examination often is scheduled 1 to 4 weeks after laser treatment. However, many experienced laser surgeons wait until 3 to 4 weeks after treatment. This is because, at 1 to 2 weeks after treatment, residual edema and retinal vasculitis may obscure the view of the fundus and prevent visualization of persistent neovascularization (see Fig. 6.20B). Therefore, only a positive fluorescein angiogram is helpful early, and this must be repeated by 1 month after treatment even if one was obtained at 1 to 2 weeks. An acceptable follow-up schedule might be as follows.

Length of time between laser treatment and follow-up visits:

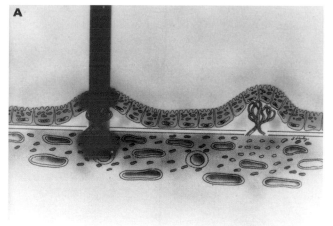

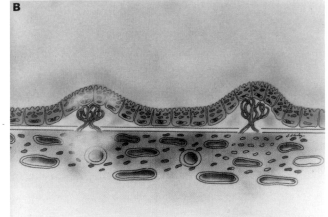

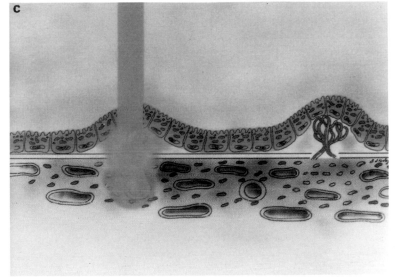

Fig. 6.25 Sequential red-yellow treatment of CNV. A, Red wavelengths (dye or krypton) are used to treat the membrane deeply, lightly whitening its background and highlighting its extent. B, Appearance at the conclusion of red treatment. The entire extent of the membrane has been lightly whitened due to choroidal and, possibly, outer retinal uptake. C, Intense yellow wavelength is then used to blanket the previously treated area. Enhanced uptake of yellow light by the new blood vessels is important for effective treatment. (Reproduced by permission from Singerman LJ, Kalski RS [128].)

Fig. 6.26 Critical points in the management of CNV include recent high-quality angiography magnified and projected in the treatment room, retrobulbar anesthesia for most juxtafoveal and subfoveal lesions, and close posttreatment surveillance for recurrence. (Reproduced by permission from Singerman LJ [123].)

1 to 2 weeks (optional)
3 to 4 weeks (mandatory)
2 months
4 months
6 to 7 months
9 to 12 months
Every 4 to 6 months in the second posttreatment year

Every 6 to 12 months indefinitely
Recurrence can occur years after treatment, so follow-up is carried on indefinitely.

Any sign of true recurrence should be promptly evaluated with angiography and treated, unless the extent of treatment exceeds MPS protocol (any case that does not meet MPS eligibility criteria must be considered for treatment on an individual basis). Visual acuity generally stabilizes within 6 months of successful treatment. Late loss of acuity should prompt careful evaluation for recurrence, but may result from late RPE atrophy due to "runoff" or spread of laser energy (14,16).

Complications of treatment are uncommon. Choroidal hemorrhage may be avoided by using spot sizes no smaller than 200 μm and durations of 0.2 sec or longer. Macular pucker, most commonly seen after blue-green treatment, is typically insignificant visually. The most serious complication in extrafoveal or juxtafoveal treatment is incidental foveal treatment. Projection of a recent, magnified, high-quality fluorescein angiogram in the treatment room is essential for avoiding this complication. Retrobulbar anesthesia is also helpful in this regard.

Conclusions

Until we learn to prevent CNV, the laser probably will be our best tool for treating selected cases. Randomized, controlled clinical trials are important in identifying appropriate cases in diseases in which such clinical trials are possible. For the less common diseases, such as angioid streaks, randomized trials would require many years and many centers to gain sufficient numbers to be meaningful. For even rarer diseases, such clinical trials are essentially impossible. We are therefore forced to extrapolate from the proven benefit of therapy in more common diseases in an effort to make an optimal judgment in more unusual diseases. Each disorder that is potentially associated with CNV has its own unique milieu, clinical setting, and natural history. Many factors must be kept in mind when considering photocoagulation, including the patient's age, visual needs, coexistent vision-limiting ocular conditions, and adverse effects of treatment. Each disorder has its own constellation of these factors, which must be weighed by the laser surgeon to assess properly the risk-benefit ratio of treatment.

References

1. Leibowitz HM, Krueger DE, Maunder LR, et al. The Framingham Eye Study Monograph: VI. Macular degeneration. Surv Ophthalmol 1988;24(suppl):428–457.
2. Sarks SH, Sarks JP. Age-related macular degeneration: atrophic form. In Ryan SJ, ed. Retina, vol 2. St. Louis: CV Mosby, 1990:149–173.
3. Haab O. Erkrankungen der Macula Lutea. Zentralbl Augenheilkd 1885;9:391–394. Cited by Duke-Elder S. System of Ophthalmology, vol 9. London: Kimpton, 1966:603.
4. Ghafour IM, Allan D, Foulds WS. Common causes of blindness and visual handicap in the west of Scotland. Br J Ophthalmol 1983;67:209–213.
5. Hyman LG, Lilienfeld AM, Ferris FL III, Fine SL. Senile macular degeneration: a case-control study. Am J Epidemiol 1983;118:213–227.
6. Tso MOM. Pathogenetic factors of aging macular degeneration. Ophthalmology 1985;92:628–635.
7. Blumenkranz MS, Russell SR, Robey MG, et al. Risk factors in age-related maculopathy complicated by choroidal neovascularization. Ophthalmology 1986;93:552–557.
8. West SK, Rosenthal FS, Bressler NM, et al. Exposure to sunlight and other risk factors for age-related macular degeneration. Arch Ophthalmol 1989;107:875–879.
9. Bressler NM, Bressler SB, Seddon JM, Gragoudas ES, Jacobson LP. Drusen characteristics in patients with exudative versus non-exudative age-related macular degeneration. Retina 1988;8:109–114.
10. Hogan MJ. Role of the retinal pigment epithelium in macular disease. Trans Am Acad Ophthalmol Otolaryngol 1972; 76:64–80.
11. Small ML, Green WR, Alpar JJ, et al. Senile macular degeneration: clinicopathologic correlation of two cases with neovascularization beneath the retinal pigment epithelium. Arch Ophthalmol 1976;94:601–607.
12. Bressler SB, Silva JC, Bressler NM, Alexander J, Green WR. Clinicopathologic correlation of occult choroidal neovascularization in age-related macular degeneration. Arch Ophthalmol 1992;110:827–832.
13. Bird AC. Pathogenesis of serous detachment of the retina and pigment epithelium. In: Ryan SJ, ed. Retina, vol 2. St. Louis: CV Mosby, 1989:99–105.
14. Elman MJ, Fine SL, Murphy RP, Patz A, Auer C. The natural history of serous retinal pigment epithelium detachment in patients with age-related macular degeneration. Ophthalmology 1986;93:224–230.
15. Gass JDM. Serous retinal pigment epithelial detachment with a notch. A sign of occult neovascularization. Retina 1984;4:215–220.
16. Rice TA, Murphy RP, Fine SL, Patz A. Stability of argon laser photocoagulation scars in ocular histoplasmosis. In: Fine SL, Owens SL, eds. Management of retinal vascular and macular disorders. Baltimore: Williams & Wilkins, 1983: 187–190.
17. Bressler NM, Bressler SB, Gragoudas ES. Clinical characteristics of choroidal neovascular membranes. Arch Ophthalmology 1987;105:209–213.
18. Macular Photocoagulation Study Group. Laser photocoagulation of subfoveal neovascular lesions in age-related macular degeneration. Results of a randomized clinical trial. Arch Ophthalmol 1991;109:1220–1231.
19. Macular Photocoagulation Study Group. Subfoveal neovascular lesions in age-related macular degeneration. Guidelines for evaluation and treatment in the Macular Photocoagulation Study. Arch Ophthalmol 1991;109:1242–1257.
20. Smiddy WE, Fine SL. Prognosis of patients with bilateral macular drusen. Ophthalmology 1984;91:271–277.
21. Elman MJ, Fine SL. Exudative age-related macular degeneration. In: Ryan SJ, ed. Retina, vol. 2. St. Louis: CV Mosby, 1990:175–199.
22. Macular Photocoagulation Study Group. Argon laser photocoagulation for neovascular maculopathy: three year results from randomized clinical trials. Arch Ophthalmol 1986; 104:694–701.
23. Berkow JW. Subretinal neovascularization in senile macular degeneration. Am J Ophthalmol 1984;97:143–147.
24. Bressler SB, Bressler NM, Fine SL, et al. Natural course of choroidal neovascular membranes within the foveal avascu-

lar zone in senile macular degeneration. Am J Ophthalmol 1982;93:157–163.

25. Guyer DR, Fine SL, Maguire MG, et al. Subfoveal choroidal neovascular membranes in age-related macular degeneration: visual prognosis in eyes with relatively good initial visual acuity. Arch Ophthalmol 1986;104:702–705.

26. Singerman LJ, Stockfish JH. Natural history of pigment epithelial detachment with associated choroidal neovascular membrane in age-related macular degeneration. Graef's Arch Clin Exp Ophthalmol 1989;227:507–510.

27. Macular Photocoagulation Study Group. Argon laser photocoagulation for senile macular degeneration: results of a randomized clinical trial. Arch Ophthalmol 1982;100:912–918.

28. Macular Photocoagulation Study Group. Recurrent choroidal neovascularization after argon laser photocoagulation for neovascular maculopathy. Arch Ophthalmol 1986;104:503–512.

29. Macular Photocoagulation Study Group. Krypton laser photocoagulation for neovascular lesions of age-related macular degeneration. Results of a randomized clinical trial. Arch Ophthalmol 1990;108:816–824.

30. Macular Photocoagulation Study Group. Persistent and recurrent neovascularization after krypton laser photocoagulation for neovascular lesions of age-related macular degeneration. Arch Ophthalmol 1990;108:825–831.

31. Macular Photocoagulation Study Group. Laser photocoagulation of subfoveal recurrent neovascular lesions in age-related macular degeneration. Results of a randomized clinical trial. Arch Ophthalmol 1991;109:1232–1241.

32. Moorfields Macular Study Group. Retinal pigment epithelial detachments in the elderly: a controlled trial of argon laser photocoagulation, Br J Ophthalmol 1982;66:1–16.

33. Pagliarini S, Barondes MJ, Chisholm IH, Hamilton AM, Bird AC. Detection of subpigment epithelial neovascularization in cases of retinal pigment epithelial detachments: a review of the Moorfields treatment trial. Br J Ophthalmol 1992;76:8–10.

34. Barondes MJ, Pagliarini S, Chisholm IH, Hamilton AM, Bird AC. Controlled trial of laser photocoagulation of pigment epithelial detachment in the elderly: a 4 year review. Br J Ophthalmol 1992;76:5–7.

35. Maguire JI, Benson WE, Brown GC. Treatment of foveal pigment epithelial detachments with contiguous extrafoveal choroidal neovascular membranes. Am J Ophthalmol 1990;109:523–529.

36. Singerman LJ. Laser photocoagulation for choroidal new vessel membrane complicating age-related macular degeneration associated with pigment epithelial detachment. Retina 1988;8:115–121.

37. Geeraets WJ, Berry ER. Ocular spectral characteristics as related to hazards from laser and other light sources. Am J Ophthalmol 1968;66:15–20.

38. Bischoff PM, Flower RW. Ten years' experience with choroidal angiography using indocyanine green dye: a new routine examination or an epilogue? Doc Ophthalmol 1985;60:235–291.

39. Kogure K, David NJ, Yamanouchi U, Choromoukos E. Infrared absorption angiography of the fundus circulation. Arch Ophthalmol 1970;83:209–214.

40. David NJ: Infra-red absorption fundus angiography. In: Amalric P, ed. Fluorescein angiography: Proceedings of the International Symposium, Albi, France 1969. Basel: Karger, 1969:189–192.

41. Flower RW. Infrared absorption angiography of the choroid and some observations on the effects of high intraocular pressures. Am J Ophthalmol 1972;4:600–614.

42. Flower RW, Hochheimer BF. A clinical technique and apparatus for simultaneous angiography of the separate retinal and choroidal circulations. Invest Ophthalmol Vis Sci 1971;12:248–261.

43. Patz A, Flower RW, Klein ML, et al. Clinical application of indocyanine green angiography. In: DeLaey JJ, ed. International Symposium on Fluorescein Angiography: Ghent, 28 March-1 April, 1976. The Hague: Dr. W. Junk, 1976:59–66. (Doc Ophthalmol Proc Ser; 9).

44. Hayashi K, DeLaey JJ. Indocyanine green angiography of choroidal neovascular membranes. Ophthalmologica 1985;190:30–39.

45. Destro M, Puliafito CA. Indocyanine green videoangiography of choroidal neovascularization. Ophthalmology 1989;96:846–853.

46. Guyer DR, Puliafito CA, Mones JM, et al. Digital indocyanine green angiography in chorioretinal disorders. Ophthalmology 1992;99:287–291.

47. Yannuzzi LA, Slakter JS, Sorenson JA, et al. Digital indocyanine green videoangiography and choroidal neovascularization. Retina 1992;12:191–223.

48. Puliafito CA, Destro M, To K, et al. Dye enhanced photocoagulation of choroidal neovascularization. Invest Ophthalmol Vis Sci 1988;29(suppl):414.

49. Balles MW, Puliafito CA, Kliman GH, et al. Indocyanine green dye enhanced diode laser photocoagulation of subretinal neovascular membranes. Invest Ophthalmol Vis Sci 1990;31(suppl):282.

50. Green WR. Retina. In: Spencer WH, ed. Ophthalmic pathology. An atlas and textbook. Philadelphia: WB Saunders, 1985.

51. Macular Photocoagulation Study Group. Argon laser for ocular histoplasmosis. Results of a randomized clinical trial. Arch Ophthalmol 1983;101:1347–1357.

52. Macular Photocoagulation Study Group. Argon laser for idiopathic neovascularization. Results of a randomized clinical trial. Arch Ophthalmol 1983;101:1358–1361.

53. Macular Photocoagulation Study Group. Krypton laser photocoagulation for neovascular lesions of ocular histoplasmosis. Results of a randomized clinical trial. Arch Ophthalmol 1987;105:1499–1507.

54. Fine SL, Wood WY, Isernhagen RD, et al. Laser photocoagulation of subfoveal neovascular lesions in ocular histoplasmosis: results of a pilot randomized clinical trial. Arch Ophthalmol 1993;111:19–20.

55. Schlaegel TF Jr. Letter. Ocular Histoplasmosis. New York: Grune & Stratton, 1977.

56. Woods AC, Whalen HE. The probable role of benign histoplasmosis in the etiology of granulomatous uveitis. Am J Ophthalmol 1960;49:205.

57. Gass JDM. Stereoscopic atlas of macular diseases. St. Louis: CV Mosby, 1987.

58. Schlaegel TF. Histoplasmic choroiditis. Ann Ophthalmol 1974;6:237–252.

59. Singerman LJ, Wong B, Ai E, Smith S. Spontaneous improvement in the first affected eye of patients with bilateral disciform scars. Retina 1985;5:135–143.

60. Orlando RG, Davidorf FH. Spontaneous recovery phenomenon in the presumed ocular histoplasmosis syndrome. Int Ophthalmol Clin 1983;23:137–149.

61. Jost BF, Alexander MF, Maguire MG, et al. Laser treatment for choroidal neovascularization outside randomized clinical trials. Arch Ophthalmol 1988;106:357–361.

62. Grossniklaus HE, Green WR. Pathologic findings in pathologic myopia. Retina 1992;12:127–133.

63. Hotchkiss ML, Fine SL. Myopia and choroidal neovascularization. Am J Ophthalmol 1981;91:177–193.

64. Avila MP, Weiter JJ, Jalkh AE, et al. Natural history of choroidal neovascularization in degenerative myopia. Ophthalmology 1984;91:1573–1581.

65. Fried M, Siebert A, Meyer-Schwickerath G, Wessig A. Natural history of Fuch's spot: a long-term follow-up study. Doc Ophthalmol Proc Ser 1981;28:215–221.

66. Soubrane G, Pisan J. Myopie degenerative: resultats de la photocoagulation des neovaisseaux sous-retiniens. In: Coscas G, Soubrane G, eds. Neovaisseaux Sous-retiniens Maculaires et Laser. Paris: Doin Editeurs, 1987: 180–184.

67. Brancato R, Pece A, Avanza P, Radrizzani E. Photocoagulation scar expansion after laser therapy for choroidal neovascularization in degenerative myopia. Retina 1990;10: 239–243.

68. Yannuzzi LA, Milch FA. Laser photocoagulation of subretinal neovascularization in pathological myopia. In: Brancato R, Coscas G, Lumbruso B, eds. Retinal diseases 2. Amsterdam-Berkeley: Kugler Publications/Milano, Ghedini Editore, 1987:53–68.

69. Gass JDM, Clarkson JG. Angioid streaks and disciform macular detachment in Paget's disease (osteitis deformans). Am J Ophthalmol 1983;75:576–586.

70. Green WR, Friedman-Kien A, Banfield WG. Angioid streaks in Ehlers-Danlos syndrome. Arch Ophthalmol 1976;76:197.

71. Singerman LJ: Angioid streaks in thalassemia major. Br J Ophthalmol 1983;67:558. Letter.

72. Singerman LJ, Hatem G. Laser treatment of choroidal neovascular membranes in angioid streaks. Retina 1981; 1:75–83.

73. Clarkson JG, Altman RD. Angioid streaks. Surv Ophthalmol 1982;26:235–246.

74. Lebwohl M, Phelps RG, Yannuzzi L, Chang S, Schwartz I, Fuchs W. Diagnosis of pseudoxanthoma elasticum by scar biopsy in patients without characteristic skin lesions. N Engl J Med 1987;317:347–350.

75. Singerman LJ, Rice TA, Novak MA, Passloff RW. Red krypton and/or green and/or blue-green argon laser photocoagulation in treatment of angioid streaks. Invest Ophthalmol Vis Sci 1984;25(suppl):89.

76. Singerman LJ. Stries angioides: traitement par le laser a argon et le laser a krypton. In: Coscas G, Soubrane G, eds. Neovaisseaux Sous-retiniens Maculaires et Laser. Paris: Doin Editeurs, 1987:221–223.

77. Gelisken O, Hendrikse F, Deutman AF. A long-term follow-up study of laser coagulation of neovascular membrane in angioid streaks. Am J Ophthalmol 1988;105:299–303.

78. Nozik RA, Dorsch W. A new chorioretinopathy associated with anterior uveitis. Am J Ophthalmol 1973;76:758–762.

79. Dreyer RF, Gass JDM. Multifocal choroiditis and panuveitis: a syndrome that mimics ocular histoplasmosis. Arch Ophthalmol 1984;102:1776–1784.

80. Watzke RC, Packer AJ, Folk JC, et al. Punctate inner choroidopathy. Am J Ophthalmol 1984;98:572–584.

81. Palestine AG, Nussenblatt RB, Parver LM, Knox DL. Progressive subretinal fibrosis and uveitis syndrome. Br J Ophthalmol 1984;68:667–673.

82. Palestine AG, Nussenblatt RB, Chan CC. Histopathology of the subretinal fibrosis and uveitis syndrome. Ophthalmology 1985;92:838–844.

83. Cantrill HL, Folk JC. Multifocal choroiditis associated with progressive subretinal fibrosis. Am J Ophthalmol 1986; 101:170–180.

84. Doran RML, Hamilton AM. Disciform macular degeneration in young adults. Trans Ophthalmol Soc UK 1982;102: 471–480.

85. Morgan CM, Schatz H. Recurrent multifocal choroiditis. Ophthalmology 1986;93:1138–1143.

86. Yannuzzi LA, Sorenson J, Shakin J, Milch F. Acute disseminated chorioretinal spots: the New York experience. Presented at the Eighth Annual Meeting of the Macular Society, 1985.

87. Singerman LJ. In discussion, Morgan CM, Schatz H. Recurrent multifocal choroiditis. Ophthalmology 1986;93: 1143–1147.

88. Coscas G, Soubrane G, Delayre T, Ramahefasolo C. Treatment of subretinal neovessels in idiopathic recurrent multifocal choroiditis. Bull Soc Ophthalmol Fr 1989; 89:1275–1279.

89. Mansour AM, Jampol LM, Packo KH, Hrisomalos NF. Macular serpiginous choroiditis. Retina 1988;8:125–131.

90. Jampol LM, Orth D, Daily MJ, Rabb MF. Subretinal neovascularization with geographic (serpiginous) choroiditis. Am J Ophthalmol 1979;88:683–689.

91. Schatz H, Maumenee AE, Patz A. Geographic helicoid peripapillary choroidopathy: clinical presentation and fluorescein angiographic findings. Trans Am Acad Ophthalmol Otolaryngol 1974;78:OP747–761.

92. Smith RE, Kelley JS. Late macular complications of choroidal ruptures. Am J Ophthalmol 1974;77:650–658.

93. Hart JCD, Natsikos VE, Riastrick ER, et al. Indirect choroidal tears at the posterior pole: a fluorescein angiographic and perimetric approach. Br J Ophthalmol 1980;64:59–67.

94. Fuller B, Gitter KA. Traumatic choroidal rupture with late serous detachment of the macula: report of successful argon laser treatment. Arch Ophthalmol 1973;89:354–355.

95. Gass JDM, Guerry RK, Jack RL, et al. Choroidal osteoma. Arch Ophthalmol 1978;96:428–435.

96. Burke JF, Brockhurst RJ. Argon laser photocoagulation of subretinal neovascular membrane associated with osteoma of the choroid. Retina 1983;3:304–307.

97. Avila MP, El-Markabi H, Azzolini C, et al. Bilateral choroidal osteoma with subretinal neovascularization. Ann Ophthalmol 1984;16:381–385.

98. Morrison DL, Magargal LE, Ehrlich DR, et al. Review of choroidal osteoma: successful krypton red laser photocoagulation of an associated subretinal neovascular membrane involving the fovea. Ophthalmic Surg 1987;18:299–303.

99. Rose SJ, Burke JF, Brockhurst RJ. Argon laser photoablation of a choroidal osteoma. Retina 1991;11:224–228.

100. Grand MG, Burgess DB, Singerman LJ, Ramsey J. Choroidal osteoma. Treatment of associated subretinal neovascular membranes. Retina 1984;4:84–89.

101. Deutman AF, Grizzard WS. Rubella retinopathy and subretinal neovascularization. Am J Ophthalmol 1987; 85:82–87.

102. Slusher MM, Tyler ME. Rubella retinopathy and subretinal neovascularization. Ann Ophthalmol 1982;14:292–294.

103. Orth DH, Fishman GA, Segall M, et al. Rubella maculopathy. Br J Ophthalmol 1980;64:201–205.

104. Frank KE, Purnell EW. Subretinal neovascularization following rubella retinopathy. Am J Ophthalmol 1978;86:462–466.

105. Miller SA, Bresnick GH, Chandra SR. Choroidal neovascular membrane in Best's vitelliform macular dystrophy. Am J Ophthalmol 1976;82:252.

106. Klein R, Lewis RA, Meyers SM, Myers FL. Subretinal neovascularization associated with fundus flavimaculatus. Arch Ophthalmol 1978;96:2054.

107. Leveille AS, Morse PH, Burch JV. Fundus flavimaculatus and subretinal neovascularization. Ann Ophthalmol 1982;14:331.

108. Robinson D, Tiedeman J. Choroideremia associated with a subretinal neovascular membrane: a case report. Retina 1987;7:70–74.

109. Gilbert HD: Unusual complications of ocular toxoplasmosis. In: Fine SL, Owens SL, eds. Management of retinal vascular and macular disorders. Baltimore: Williams & Wilkins, 1983:153–155.

110. Carlson MR, Kerman BM. Hemorrhagic macular detachment in Vogt-Koyanagi-Harada syndrome. Am J Ophthalmol 1977;84:632.

111. Snyder DA, Tessler HH. Vogt-Koyanagi-Harada syndrome. Am J Ophthalmol 1980;90:69–75.

112. Waltman DD, Gitter KA, Yannuzzi LA, Schatz H. Choroidal neovascularization associated with choroidal nevi. Am J Ophthalmol 1978;85:704–710.

113. Friberg TR, Grove AS Jr. Subretinal neovascularization and choroidal folds. Ann Ophthalmol 1980;12:245–250.

114. Benson WE, Townsend RE, Pheasant TR. Choriovitreal and subretinal proliferation: complications of photocoagulation. Ophthalmology 1979;86:283–289.

115. Harris MJ, Fine SL, Owens SL. Hemorrhagic complications of optic nerve drusen. Am J Ophthalmol 1981;92:70–76.

116. Varley MP, Frank E, Purnell EW. Subretinal neovascularization after focal argon laser for diabetic macular edema. Ophthalmology 1988;95:567–573.

117. Jamison RR. Subretinal neovascularization and papilledema associated with pseudotumor cerebri. Am J Ophthalmol 1978;85:78–81.

118. Munier F, Othenin-Girard P. Subretinal neovascularization secondary to choroidal septic metastasis from acute bacterial endocarditis. Retina 1992;12:108–112.

119. Stein RM, Zakov ZN, Zegarra HZ, Gutman FA. Multiple recurrent serosanguineous retinal pigment epithelial detachments in black women. Am J Ophthalmol 1985;100:560–569.

120. Yannuzzi LA, Sorenson J, Spaide RF, Lipson B. Idiopathic polypoidal choroidal vasculopathy (IPCV). Retina 1990;10:1–8.

121. Kleiner RC, Brucker AJ, Johnston RL. The posterior uveal bleeding syndrome. Retina 1990;10:9–17.

122. Perkovich BT, Zakov ZN, Berlin LA, Weidenthal D, Avins LR. An update on multiple recurrent serosanguineous retinal pigment epithelial detachments in black women. Retina 1990;10:18–26.

123. Singerman LJ. Important points in management of patients with choroidal neovascularization. Ophthalmology 1985;92:610–614.

124. Vander J, Morgan C, Schatz H. Growth rate of subretinal neovascularization in age-related macular degeneration. Ophthalmology 1989;96:1422–1426.

125. Singerman LJ, Hionis R. In discussion, Vander J, Morgan C, Schatz H. Growth rate of subretinal neovascularization in age-related macular degeneration. Ophthalmology 1989;96:1426–1469.

126. Moorfields Macular Study Group. Treatment of senile disciform macular degeneration: a single-blind randomised trial by argon laser photocoagulation. Br J Ophthalmol 1982;66:745–753.

127. Singerman LJ. Fluorescein angiography: practical role in the office management of macular diseases. Ophthalmology 1986;93:1209–1215.

128. Singerman LJ, Kalski RS. Tunable dye laser for choroidal neovascularization complicating age-related macular degeneration. Retina 1989;9:247–257.

129. Yannuzzi LA, Shakin JL. Krypton red laser photocoagulation of the ocular fundus. Retina 1982;2:1–14.

130. Singerman LJ. Red krypton laser therapy of macular and retinal vascular diseases. Retina 1982;2:15–28.

7

Laser Treatment of Retinal Vein Occlusions

Hernando Zegarra
Z. Nicholas Zakov
Lawrence J. Singerman
Jeffrey C. Lamkin

Retinal vein occlusion is one of the most common retinal vascular disorders after diabetic retinopathy. According to the retinal vessel involved, two distinct entities can develop: central retinal vein occlusion (CRVO) and branch retinal vein occlusion (BRVO). An intermediate form, referred to as hemispheric or hemicentral retinal vein occlusion (HRVO), has features common to both CRVO and BRVO and is discussed separately.

Central Retinal Vein Occlusion

Central retinal vein occlusion is a well-known entity that was accurately described by the late nineteenth century. Despite its early clinical recognition, the understanding of the etiology and pathogenesis of this condition is limited.

Pathogenesis

In 1878, Julius Von Michael recognized CRVO as a clinical entity produced by thrombus formation in the lumen of the central retina vein (1). Green and colleagues confirmed Von Michael's findings of thrombus formation in the central retinal vein near the lamina cribrosa producing variable degrees of obstruction accounting for the different presentations of CRVO (2). They also demonstrated secondary pathologic changes, such as thrombus recanalization, endothelial cell proliferation, inflammatory reaction, and fresh thrombus formation in an old recanalized occlusion. These changes are responsible for the variable clinical course and complications seen in this retinopathy.

A number of factors may induce thrombus formation near the lamina cribrosa, thereby causing CRVO. Focal compression by a sclerotic arterial wall on the adjacent central retinal vein may create increased turbulence and stagnation of flow in the area. In addition, systemic factors such as decreased perfusion, increased blood viscosity, and states of hypercoagulation may further induce the formation of a thrombus. Orbital and ocular disorders causing decreased venous outflow can also be significant factors in the pathogenesis of CRVO (3; Table 7.1). In approximately 15% to 20% of patients, no systemic abnormalities can be demonstrated (4).

Table 7.1 Associated Medical Conditions in Central Retinal Vein Occlusion

Small vessel disease
  Diabetes
  Hypertension
  Coronary artery disease
Hypoperfusion
  Carotid artery disease
  Carotid-cavernous fistula
  Vasculitis
    Takayasu's disease
    Syphilis
    Polyarteritis nodosa and other connective tissue disorders
    Sarcoidosis
    Wegener granulomatosis
    Temporal arteritis
  Hypotension
Hyperviscosity
  Waldenstrom macroglobulinemia
  Multiple myeloma
  Lymphoma
  Leukemia
  Polycythemia vera
  Chronic lung disease
  Cryoglobulinemia
  Sarcoidosis
  Hyperlipidemia, hypercholesterolemia
Hypercoagulation disorders
  Hemoglobinopathies
  Oral contraceptives
  Hyperfibrinogenemia
  Platelet, erythrocyte abnormalities

Table 7.1 Associated Medical Conditions in
Central Retinal Vein Occlusion (cont'd)

Orbital and ocular disorders causing decreased venous outflow

Orbital tumor, abscess, trauma (orbital fracture)

Mediastinal syndrome (tumor, inflammation)

Bilateral radical neck dissection

Thyroid ophthalmopathy

Sinusitis

Optic nerve glioma

Glaucoma

Optic nerve hemorrhage

Optic nerve drusen

Papilledema

Diagnosis and Clinical Course

The variable presentation and clinical course seen in
CRVO has led to a confusing classification and nomenclature, based on the severity of the retinopathy, the degree
of retinal hemorrhage, vascular damage, and loss of visual
function. Severe forms of CRVO have been termed complete or total CRVO or obstruction, hemorrhagic retinopathy (5), complete or total central retinal vein thrombosis,
and ischemic CRVO. Milder forms have been called partial or incomplete CRVO or obstruction, venous stasis
retinopathy (5) impending CRVO, central retinal vein
prethrombosis, and nonischemic CRVO.

The integrity of the capillary bed appears to be a distinctive feature differentiating the severe forms from the
milder forms of CRVO. Those with no evidence of significant capillary closure tend to follow a relatively benign
course (4-6), whereas those with the more severe forms
show extensive capillary closure, usually associated with
severe loss of visual function and complications such as
neovascular glaucoma. Currently, it is advisable to consider CRVO, at the time of its presentation or any time
during the course of the disease, as one of two types: the
nonischemic form or perfused CRVO and the ischemic or
nonperfused CRVO.

Nonischemic CRVO is characterized by congestion,
swelling of the optic nerve, venous engorgement, and
hemorrhages in all four quadrants (Fig. 7.1). This form of
vein occlusion can be asymptomatic or may cause decreased central vision if macular edema is present. The
most distinctive feature of this form of CRVO is the integrity of the capillary net throughout the retina as
demonstrated on fluorescein angiography (Fig. 7.2).

Patients with the nonischemic form of CRVO follow a
benign course, with complete resolution of the retinopathy in approximately 50% of the cases (6). Progression
from nonischemic to ischemic forms of CRVO was seen in
16 of 360 patients in a study by Minturn and Brown in
1986 (7). Approximately 30% of patients with CRVO will
have partial resolution of the retinopathy with segmental
clearing of the hemorrhage, simulating BRVO, and residual macular edema (6).

Ischemic CRVO has features similar to those of the nonischemic form but with increased severity and number of
retinal hemorrhage and the presence of microinfarcts (cotton wool spots) throughout the retina (Fig.
7.3). Visual acuity is usually decreased due to severe macular edema, macular hemorrhages, or capillary nonperfusion of the posterior pole (Fig. 7.4). An afferent pupillary
defect may be present (5,6), and severe visual field loss (8)
correlates with the degree of the peripheral ischemia.

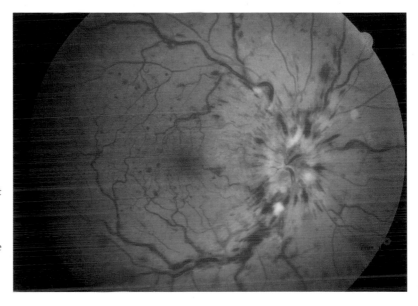

Fig. 7.1 Hypertensive man, aged 64,
with sudden loss of vision in his right
eye. There is moderately severe disc
edema with several nerve fiber layer
infarcts (cotton wool spots) and mild
to moderate retinal hemorrhages. The
nonischemic nature of this CRVO
cannot be determined without fluorescein angiography.

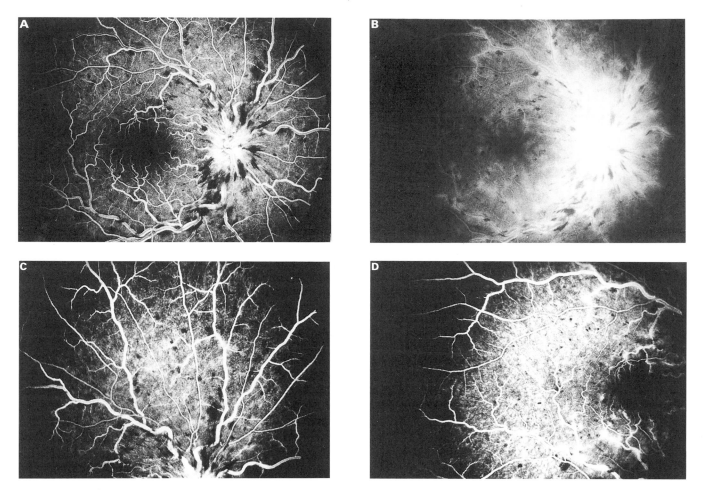

Fig. 7.2 Fluorescein angiography of the patient shown in Fig. 7.1. A, Early venous phase angiogram shows hyperfluorescence around the disc from leaking retinal capillaries. Patches of hypofluorescence correspond to retinal hemorrhages. Retinal capillary perfusion is relatively well preserved. B, Late views show persistent peripapillary leakage without significant macular edema. C, Midperipheral views show intact capillary perfusion. D, Further midperipheral views help classify this vein occlusion as nonischemic, or perfused.

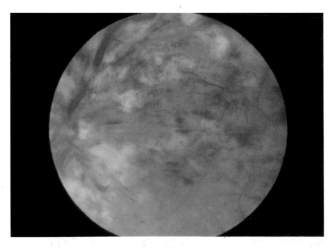

Fig. 7.3 Woman, aged 70, with sudden loss of vision in her left eye. Color fundus photography shows more extensive disc edema with more cotton wool spots than the case depicted in Fig. 7.1. Without fluorescein angiography, however, the degree of ischemia cannot be determined.

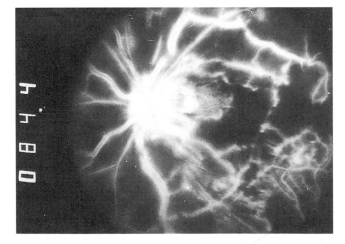

Fig. 7.4 Fluorescein angiography from the patient depicted in Fig. 7.3. There is extensive hypofluorescence not corresponding to retinal hemorrhage (capillary dropout). This is the defining feature of ischemic or nonperfused CRVO.

These cases have a poor visual prognosis with a significant number (20% to 50%) developing neovascular glaucoma, usually within the first 6 months after the occlusion (4,9,10).

Fluorescein Angiography

Fluorescein angiography is of critical importance in the management of cases of CRVO. This study should include photographs of the posterior pole and the midperipheral retina following the recommendations of the Diabetic Retinopathy Study (11; see Fig. 7.2).

In CRVO, the circulation time slows angiographically, with a marked delay in transit of dye. The choroidal circulation is angiographically normal. Confluent retinal hemorrhages and cotton wool spots, particularly in early cases, may block the underlying fluorescence. The disc may leak due to disc edema (see Fig. 7.2). The caliber of the arteries and veins may be variable with the veins often dilated and tortuous. Their walls may show sheathing and nonspecific leakage. The degree of ischemia can be evaluated in the macular region by evaluating the integrity of the perifoveal and macular capillary net. In the periphery, areas of capillary nonperfusion can also be measured (see Fig. 7.2). The late phases of the angiogram can also show the extent and severity of macular edema.

There is a group of patients in whom the status of retinal perfusion cannot be determined by fluorescein angiography because of extensive retinal hemorrhage (Fig. 7.5). Integrity of the capillary bed in these cases should be assessed by other clinical means, such as pupillary response, visual field defects, and electroretinographic findings. These patients must be considered to be at high risk for retinal ischemia (12).

Electroretinography

Recognition of the ischemic forms of CRVO by fluorescein angiography is of critical importance in identifying those cases prone to develop iris neovascularization and neovascular glaucoma (13). Unfortunately, in many patients adequate photography is not possible because of media opacity, small pupils, or the presence of confluent hemorrhage obscuring the underlying retinal capillaries (14).

Several authors have assessed the functional effects of retinal ischemia in the electroretinographic response, trying to identify those parameters that will predict the development of iris neovascularization (15-19).

Severe reductions of the B-wave amplitude producing a B:A ratio of less than 1.0 appeared to be a feature of some eyes that develop iris neovascularization (15; Fig. 7.6). Other predictors include reduction in oscillatory potential (20), delay on implicit time (21), and changes in the Log K (16,20). This last parameter determines the relative amount of light needed to produce half of the maximum amplitude of the B wave and has been shown to be more sensitive than fluorescein angiography in identifying eyes with CRVO that are prone to iris neovascularization. The Log K may represent a measurement of "retinal sensitivity" and may distinguish between hypoxic and anoxic or infarcted retina (14).

Hayreh and colleagues combined the electroretinographic response with relative afferent pupillary responses measured quantitatively and were able to differentiate ischemic from nonischemic CRVO in 97% to 100% of cases (8).

An ancillary study of the Central Vein Occlusion Study (CVOS) was designed to determine the value of electroretinography in predicting iris neovascularization and

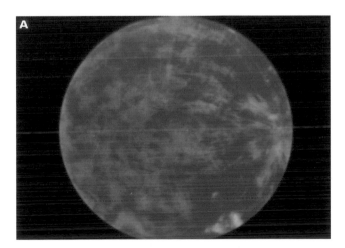

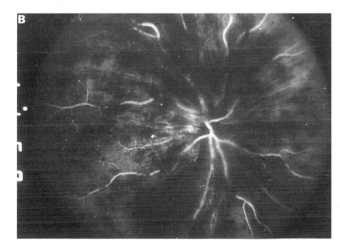

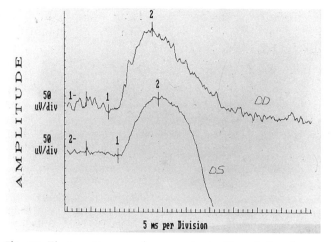

Fig. 7.6 Electroretinogram from a patient with an ischemic CRVO in the left eye. Note the diminution in A- and B-wave amplitudes, as well as the loss of oscillatory potential. These findings are associated with widespread nonperfusion.

neovascular glaucoma. Until the results of the ancillary study are available, clinicians should combine clinical and angiographic findings with functional parameters such as electroretinography and pupillary response to identify those eyes prone to iris neovascularization and neovascular glaucoma.

Treatment

Treatment in CRVO first should be directed to the underlying or associated systemic conditions, if identifiable, and then to the prevention or treatment of the ocular complications. The use of antiplatelet aggregation substances, such as aspirin or dipyridamole (Persantine), may be considered, although they have never been demonstrated to be effective. More potent anticoagulants carry a significant risk of central nervous system systemic bleeding and vitreous hemorrhage, with limited or no beneficial effect on the course and visual outcome of CRVO (22). Visual acuity may be improved by isovolemic hemodilution (23,24), but this is not commonly practiced clinically.

Laser Therapy

Laser therapy is indicated in the treatment or prevention of the complications of CRVO: neovascular glaucoma and macular edema.

Neovascular Glaucoma

Laser therapy in the form of panretinal laser photocoagulation (PRP) has been reported to be effective in the prevention of neovascular glaucoma in the ischemic forms of CRVO (10,25,26). Unfortunately, the extent of ischemia likely to lead to neovascular glaucoma was not established in these studies nor were adequate controls presented.

Furthermore, the angiographic evaluation of ischemia did not include the midperipheral retina. Hareh and coworkers studied 123 eyes with ischemic CRVO and found no difference in the incidence of neovascular glaucoma between laser-treated eyes and untreated eyes (27).

Although PRP appears to have a role in preventing neovascular glaucoma in ischemic CRVO, it is not clear when to treat. A national, randomized study, the CVOS, was undertaken to define the course of CRVO and to identify those patients in whom laser treatment will be beneficial, either for treating macular edema or for preventing neovascular glaucoma (12). Recruitment for the CVOS has ended, and the data is being analyzed.

Panretinal photocoagulation is indicated in all patients with CRVO and any degree of neovascularization of the iris, angle structures, or retina. Therefore, it is imperative that all patients with ischemic CRVO undergo frequent (every 4 to 6 weeks) gonioscopy and careful examination of the undilated iris to detect the earliest signs of iris or angle neovascularization. If follow-up evaluation is impractical or impossible, these patients should be considered for prophylactic PRP.

These treatments should be given following the guidelines of the Diabetic Retinopathy Study (11). Burns of 500 μm in size should be applied in all four quadrants. A total of 1000 to 2000 burns should be applied, spaced approximately 1/2 to one burn width apart. Treatment should not be applied over retinal hemorrhages/major retinal vessels, or to areas closer than 2 disc diameters temporal to the fovea or 500 μm nasal to the disc.

Argon green laser is the advisable modality in cases of ischemic CRVO or neovascular glaucoma. However, in cases with media opacity or confluent retinal hemorrhage, the use of krypton red laser or red wavelengths of the dye laser could be considered.

Treatment Parameters

Spot size: 500 μm
Intensity: sufficient to create a moderate gray or white burn
Duration: 0.1 to 0.2 sec
Anesthesia: topical or retrobulbar

In cases of neovascular glaucoma, the treatment should be more aggressive. We recommend two or three sessions of PRP, applying 1000 burns each at weekly intervals. Retrobulbar anesthesia may be necessary, and hyperosmotic agents may be needed in cases with corneal edema. In addition, medical treatment of neovascular glaucoma with acetazolamide (Diamox), cycloplegics, and topical steroids is advisable. These measures will decrease the discomfort produced by the increasing intraocular pressure and inflammatory reaction induced by neovascular glaucoma and aggressive laser therapy. Laser therapy is likely to be effective in early cases in which the anterior chamber angle is still open. In more severe cases, it will be necessary to use cyclocryotherapy or other cyclodestructive procedures in addition to PRP.

Macular Edema

Beneficial effects of macular grid photocoagulation in CRVO have been suggested in a pilot study by Klein and Finkelstein and reports by Gutman and Zegarra (28,29). Although angiographic improvement was noted, both studies found visual improvements to be variable.

CVOS may give us more specific indications on when to use photocoagulation for macula edema in CRVO (12). In the meantime, we advise that this therapy be considered in those patients with ischemic or nonischemic CRVO in which the macular edema produces a progressive decline in vision and persists for at least 6 months. It is extremely important to assess angiographically the status of the perifoveal capillaries whenever laser therapy of the macula is considered. Cases with significant posterior pole ischemia should not be considered for photocoagulation.

Argon green laser is currently recommended, using 100-μm burns of moderate intensity, with a duration of 0.1 or 0.2 sec, in a scatter fashion through areas of edema identified on the fluorescein angiogram. The burns should be spaced at least 100 μm apart and should not involve the foveal avascular zone (FAZ; Fig. 7.7). Treatment can be repeated in 3 to 4 months if the macular edema persists.

No significant complications have been reported with this form of therapy (28,29).

Branch Retinal Vein Occlusion

Obstruction of one of the tributaries of the central retinal vein constitutes a well-defined clinical entity different from CRVO. This vascular accident, BRVO, is more common than CRVO and carries a more benign visual prognosis.

Pathogenesis

The pathogenetic factors that induce thrombosis in BRVO are similar to those described for CRVO. Thrombus in BRVO forms in the lumen of the vein at the point of a retinal arteriovenous crossing where the artery and vein share a common adventitia (30). Systemic hypertension is the most commonly associated medical condition (31,32), although many other systemic vascular diseases have been associated with BRVO.

Diagnosis and Clinical Course

The clinical findings in BRVO are variable, depending on the location and size of the involved branch. If the affected vessel drains the macular area, visual acuity will be affected. Otherwise, the process may be asymptomatic, even with occlusions affecting large areas of the retina. The acute stage of BRVO is characterized by multiple hemorrhages that follow the distribution of a branch retinal vein. Microinfarcts are seen in some cases, and significant macular edema, with or without hemorrhage, occurs commonly in temporal vein occlusions (Fig. 7.8).

Studies of the natural history of BRVO have established the relatively good visual outcome in most untreated patients, 50% to 60% of whom spontaneously recover vision of 20/40 or better (31,32). Two distinct complications most commonly account for decreased visual function in BRVO: persistent macular edema and the late development of preretinal neovascularization with associated vitreous hemorrhage (31).

Fluorescein Angiography

Fluorescein angiography is of critical importance in evaluating patients with BRVO. The areas studied should always include the disc and macula, as well as the entire drainage bed of the occluded branch vein. The angiographic picture varies depending on the age of the BRVO (Fig. 7.9). In fresh cases, confluent hemorrhages and cotton wool spots may block underlying fluorescence. The obstructed vein shows slower filling times. The point of vein occlusion can be demonstrated in most cases. The affected vessel walls may stain and the affected branch vein is often engorged and tortuous. The extent of capillary nonperfusion can be evaluated in the macular region and in the periphery. Capillary leakage in the macular region and the extent and location of macular edema (often in a sector) can be demonstrated. Older BRVO may demonstrate large areas of vascular restructuring, varying degrees of capillary closure, telangiectaticvessels,collaterals, neovascularization of the disc, or neovascularization elsewhere (Fig. 7.10).

Treatment

As in CRVO, the management of BRVO should be directed first to the treatment of any associated medical condition, if identifiable, and then to the prevention or treatment of the ocular complications.

Systemic treatment with aspirin or anticoagulants has not had any clear benefit. Pilot studies have evaluated the possible benefit of hyperbaric oxygen in the treatment of chronic cystoid macular edema in BRVO (33). Surgical decompression of the occluded branch vein through vitrectomy techniques has been reported, but there are no series with suitable follow-up (34).

Through multicenter randomized, controlled clinical trials, the Branch Retinal Vein Occlusion Study Group established that laser photocoagulation is the preferred method of treating the complications of BRVO (35,36).

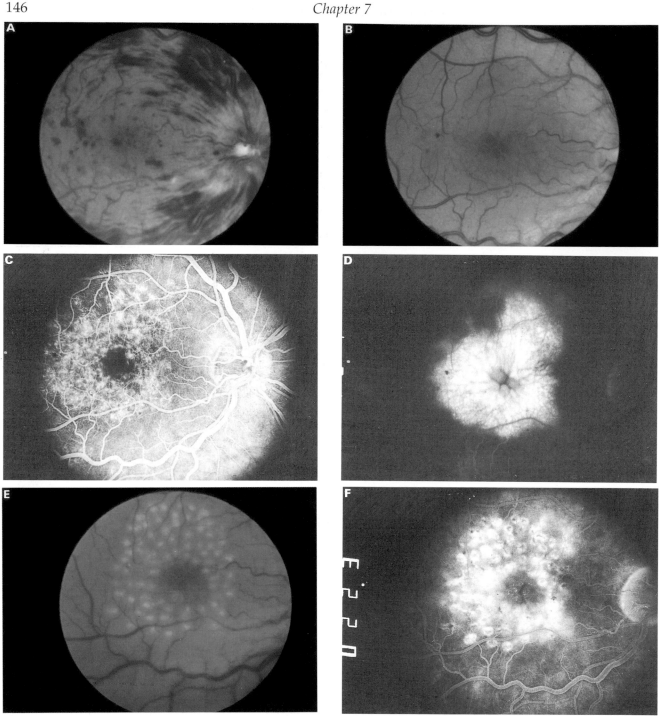

Fig. 7.7 CRVO complicated by macular edema. A, Acute central retinal vein occlusion. Visual acuity is 20/200. B, Six months after sudden visual loss, the acuity remains 20/200. Most of the hemorrhage has cleared, but there is significant cystoid macular edema. C, Midtransit fluorescein angiography reveals considerable leakage from the perifoveal retinal capillary net. D, Late transit views show striking cystoid macular edema. E, Immediate posttreatment photograph shows grid pattern of laser treatment. F, Fluorescein angiography later shows nearly complete resolution of cystoid macular edema 3 months following laser treatment. Visual acuity has improved to 20/40.

Macular Edema

The Branch Retinal Vein Occlusion Study Group demonstrated the beneficial effects of grid laser photocoagulation in BRVO associated with persistent macular edema and visual acuity of 20/40 or worse (35). Sixty-three percent of the treated patients gained two or more lines of vision, in contrast to 36% of the untreated patients. It is recommended to wait until clearing of the retinal hemorrhages allows angiographic evaluation of the integrity of the capillaries in the perifoveal area. The angiogram

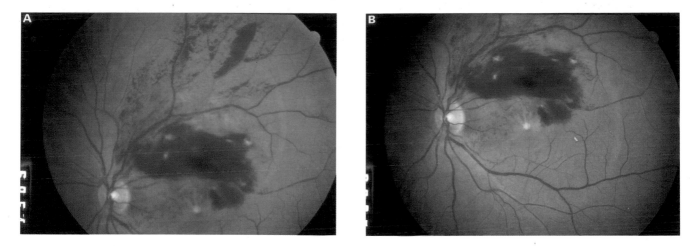

Fig. 7.8 Acute BRVO. A, Wide-angle photography documents the sectoral distribution of hemorrhages and nerve fiber layer infarction. B, Examination of the macula reveals cystoid macular edema and exudate deposition in the early stages of the occlusion.

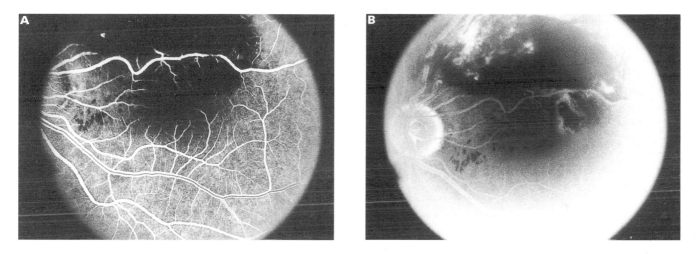

Fig. 7.9 Fluorescein angiography from an acute BRVO. A, On midtransit views, there is considerable blockage of underlying fluorescence by overlying retinal hemorrhage. B, Later views show leakage of fluorescein along the course of the obstructed venule.

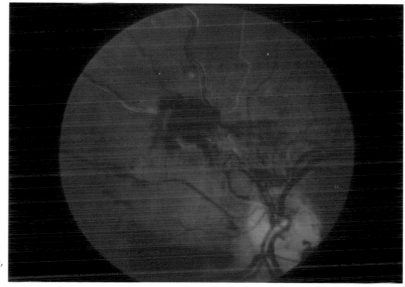

Fig. 7.10 Superonasal BRVO. There is severe neovascularization superior to the optic nerve with secondary preretinal hemorrhage inferonasally. Note the chronic changes in the occluded venule, including tortuosity and sheathing.

may then demonstrate the degree of macular ischemia and the capillary leakage producing macular edema. Cases with significant capillary closure in the foveal area should not be considered for laser therapy. Macular edema should be treated with argon green laser photocoagulation applied to the area of intraretinal leakage identified by angiography performed within the previous 4 weeks (Fig. 7.11). Mild intensity, 100-μm burns with a duration of at least 0.1 sec should be used. It is advisable to treat directly microaneurysms and vascular abnormalities outside of the FAZ. Collateral vessels should be avoided. Treatment over retinal hemorrhages is also not recommended because of the risk of excessive energy absorption.

Yellow wavelengths (577 nm) of the dye laser may be beneficial in the treatment of vascular abnormalities adjacent to the avascular zone. The use of red wavelengths (630 nm) of the krypton red laser (37) may be advantageous in the treatment of patients with confluent retinal hemorrhage that persists for more than 4 months, cataracts, or vitreous opacities.

Patients treated for macular edema should be reevaluated at 2-month intervals and considered for additional treatment if significant macular edema is recognized on angiography 4 months after the initial treatment.

Treatment complications are minimal. The Branch Vein Occlusion Study Group reported only one case of Bruch's membrane perforation, with no consequence on the visual outcome (35).

Preretinal Neovascularization

Retinal neovascularization develops in approximately 20% of BRVO (31). Retinal ischemia precedes retinal neovascularization; if the BRVO produces an area of ischemia of 5 disc diameters or larger, the chance of developing preretinal neovascularization increases to 40% within 6 to 12 months. Vitreous hemorrhage is likely to occur in 60% of these patients (36).

The Branch Vein Occlusion Study Group demonstrated that scatter laser therapy, when applied to the areas of nonperfusion, can prevent retinal neovascularization

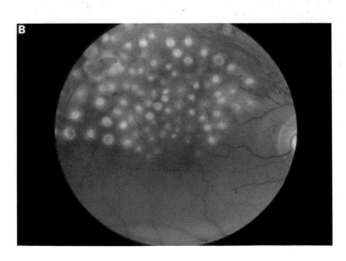

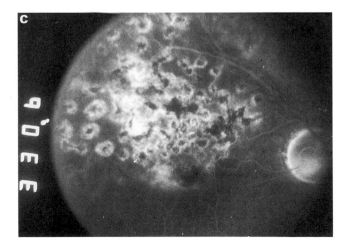

Fig. 7.11 Persistent visual loss 3 months after BRVO. A, Fluorescein angiogram, late transit view, shows significant retinal vascular leakage superotemporally with secondary macular edema. B, Fundus appearance following grid laser therapy for macular edema. C, Fluorescein angiography 3 months after laser therapy reveals significant improvement in macular edema.

and vitreous hemorrhage (36). However, over 60% of patients with nonperfused retina do not develop neovascularization. Therefore, the study recommends observing patients with BRVO and areas of ischemia and applying scatter treatment only if neovascularization is identified. We recommend treating all patients with any visible or angiographically demonstrated preretinal neovascularization, as well as those with areas of ischemia of 5 disc diameters or more in whom follow-up evaluation is impractical or impossible.

Scatter therapy should be applied using argon green laser with mild intensity, 200- to 500-μm burns, with 0.1 sec of duration and spaced one burn-width apart. Treatment should involve the areas of ischemia and should not be applied closer than 2 disc diameters from the FAZ (Fig. 7.12). Treatment should be repeated if the neovascularization persists at 4 to 6 weeks after the initial application of laser photocoagulation treatment.

Vitreous hemorrhage occurs in 60% of cases with neovascularization and in 29% of eyes already treated with scatter photocoagulation (36). Mild to moderate vitreous hemorrhage may preclude laser therapy. In some cases, the use of krypton red laser (37) or red wavelengths of the dye laser may penetrate the vitreous opacities better and make treatment possible. The use of the yellow wavelength (577 nm) may be beneficial for focal treatment of areas of persistent neovascularization.

No serious complications occur in scatter laser therapy in BRVO. One case of preretinal fibrosis has been reported in a patient in whom the treatment extended over in traretinal hemorrhage (36).

Hemispherical Retinal Vein Occlusion (HRVO)

This entity, also called hemiretinal vein occlusion or hemicentral retinal vein occlusion, has features of both CRVO and BRVO (Fig. 7.13). Even though the degree of venous occlusion in HRVO appears intermediate between the more extensive CRVO and the less extensive BRVO, Hayreh and Hayreh have stressed that this entity is much more closely related to CRVO probably as a variant of it; therefore, they prefer to call it hemi-CRVO (37). Recent reports support this view (38,39).

We have, however, seen and reported on atypical venous occlusive patterns affecting one third, two thirds, or three quarters of the venous tree. These unusual cases are probably related to anomalous branching patterns of venous tributaries to the central retinal vein at the disc and in the optic nerve (Fig. 7.14). The most common pattern of HRVO involves either the superior or the inferior branch of the central retinal vein. We have also reported an HRVO progressing to CRVO, possibly due to extension of the occluding thrombus.

Hemispherical retinal vein occlusion has been reported more commonly in older individuals and in men (37). As-

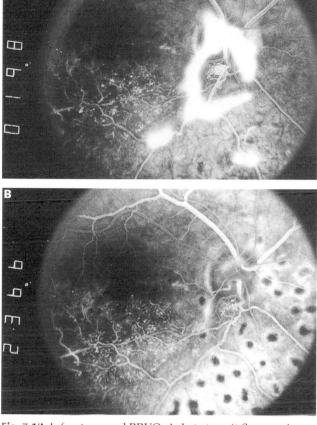

Fig. 7.12 Inferotemporal BRVO. A, Late transit fluorescein angiogram confirms the presence of severe neovascularization of the disc and elsewhere. B, Three months after quadrantic scatter photocoagulation, the neovascularization has completely regressed.

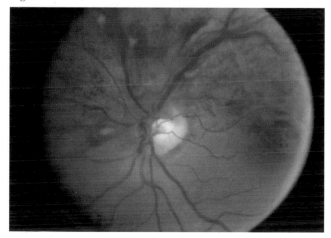

Fig. 7.13 Superior HRVO.

sociated conditions include hypertension (63%), diabetes mellitus (20%), and open angle glaucoma (25%). CRVO, BRVO, and HRVO in the fellow eye have also been reported. Two thirds of HRVOs are nonischemic (37), with

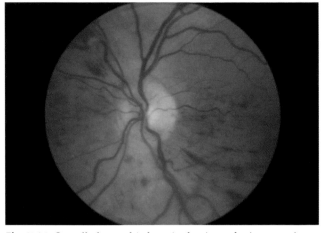

Fig. 7.14 So-called two-thirds retinal vein occlusion, sparing the superotemporal circulation.

better visual prognosis; the remaining third are more severe, with a poorer prognosis.

The complications of HRVO leading to visual loss are similar to those seen in CRVO and BRVO and include macular edema, macular ischemia, and neovascularization. Neovascularization of the disc and elsewhere may lead to vitreous hemorrhage, and the peripheral ischemic changes may produce iris and angle neovascularization in 9% of patients and neovascular glaucoma in 3% (37).

Even though series and controlled trials on the use of lasers in the treatment of these complications are lacking due to the lower incidence of HRVO relative to CRVO and BRVO, the treatment guidelines for macular edema in other vein occlusions can be successfully applied in the treatment of macular edema associated with HRVO. If areas of neovascularization of the disc or elsewhere develop, hemispheric scatter photocoagulation treatment is recommended to decrease the risk of blinding vitreous hemorrhages. Similarly, if iris and angle neovascularization develops, a similar treatment pattern should be considered to reduce the risk of neovascular glaucoma.

References

1. Von Michael J. Die spontane Thrombose der Vena Centralis des Opticus. Albrecht von Graefe's Arch Ophthalmol 1878;24:37–70.
2. Green WR, Chan CC, Hutchins GM, et al. Central retinal vein occlusion: a prospective histopathologic study of 29 eyes in 28 cases. Retina 1981;1:27–55.
3. Elman MJ. Systemic associations of retinal vein occlusion. Int Ophthalmol Clin 1991;31:15–22.
4. Zegarra H, Gutman FA, Conforto J. The natural course of central retinal vein occlusion. Ophthalmology 1979;86:1931–1939.
5. Hayreh SS. Classification of central vein occlusion. Ophthalmology 1983;90:458–474.
6. Zegarra H, Gutman FA, Zakov ZN, et al. Partial occlusion of the central retinal vein. Am J Ophthalmol 1983;96:330–337.
7. Minturn J, Brown GC. Progression of nonischemic central retinal vein occlusion. Ophthalmology 1986;93:1158–1162.
8. Hayreh SS, Klugman MR, Podhajsky P, Kolder HE. Electroretinography in central retinal vein occlusion. Correlation of electroretinographic changes with pupillary abnormalities. Graefs Arch Clin Exp Ophthalmol 1989;227:549–561.
9. Hayreh SS. So-called "central retinal vein occlusion." I. Pathogenesis, terminology, clinical features. Ophthalmologica (Basel) 1976;172:1–13.
10. Magargal LE, Brown GC, Augsburger JJ, Donoso LA. Efficacy of panretinal photocoagulation in preventing neovascular glaucoma following ischemic central retinal vein obstruction. Ophthalmology 1982;89:780–784.
11. Diabetic Retinopathy Study Research Group. Report 7. A modification of the Airlie House classification of diabetic retinopathy. Invest Ophthalmol Vis Sci 1981;21:210–226.
12. Clarkson JG. Photocoagulation for central retinal vein occlusion. Central Vein Occlusion Study. Arch Ophthalmol 1991;109:1218–1219.
13. Magargal LE, Donoso LA, Sanborn GE. Retinal ischemia and risk of neovascularization following central retinal vein occlusion. Ophthalmology 1982;89:1241–1245.
14. Bresnick GH. Following up patients with central retinal vein occlusion. Arch Ophthalmol 1988;106:324–326.
15. Sabates R, Hirose T, McMeel W. Electroretinography in the prognosis and classification of central retinal vein occlusion. Arch Ophthalmol 1983;101:232–235.
16. Johnson MA, Marcus S, Elman MJ, McPhee TJ. Neovascularization in central retinal vein occlusion: electroretinographic findings. Arch Ophthalmol 1988;106:348–352.
17. Kaye SB, Harding SP. Early electroretinography in unilateral central retinal vein occlusion as a predictor of rubeosis iridis. Arch Ophthalmol 1988;106:353–356.
18. Johnson MA. Use of electroretinographic ratios in assessment of vascular occlusion and ischemia. In: Heckenlively JR, Arden GB, eds. Principles and practice of clinical electrophysiology of vision. St. Louis: Mosby-Year Book, 1991:613–618.
19. Servais GE, Thompson HS, Hayreh SS. Relative afferent pupillary defect in central retinal vein occlusion. Ophthalmology 1986;93:301–303.
20. Johnson MA, Procope J, Quinlan PM. Electroretinographic oscillatory potentials and their role in predicting treatable complications in patients with central retinal vein occlusion. Opt Soc Am Techn Dig 1990;3:62–65.
21. Breton ME, Quinn GE, Keene SS, Dahman JC, Brucker AJ. Electroretinogram parameters at presentation as predictors of rubeosis in central retinal vein occlusion patients. Ophthalmology 1989;96:1343–1352.
22. Kohner EM, Retitt JE, Hamilton AM, Bulpitt CJ, Dollery CT. Streptokinase in central retinal vein occlusion. A controlled clinical trial. Br Med J 1976;1:550–553.
23. Hansen LL, Wiek J, Schade M, Muller-Stolzenburg N, Wiederholt M. Effect and compatibility of isovolaemic haemodilution in the treatment of ischemic and nonischemic central retinal vein occlusion. Ophthalmologica 1989;199:90–99.
24. Hansen LL, Wiek J, Weiderholt M. A randomized prospective study of treatment of nonischemic central retinal vein occlusion by isovolaemic haemodilution. Br J Ophthalmol 1989;73:895–899.

25. May DR, Klein ML, Peyman GA, Raichand M. Xenon arc panretinal photocoagulation for central retinal vein occlusion: a randomized controlled clinical study. Br J. Ophthalmol 1979;63:725–734.

26. Laatikainen L, Kohner EM, Khoury D, Blach RK. Panretinal photocoagulation in central retinal vein occlusion: a randomized controlled clinical study. Br J Ophthalmol 1977; 61:741–753.

27. Hayreh SS, Klugman MR, Podhajsky P, Servais GE, Perkins ES. Argon laser panretinal photocoagulation in ischemic central retinal vein occlusion. A 10-year prospective study. Graefs Arch Clin Exp Ophthalmol 1990;228:281–296.

28. Klein ML, Finkelstein D. Macular grid photocoagulation for macular edema in central retinal vein occlusion. Arch Ophthalmol 1989;107:1297–1302.

29. Gutman FA, Zegarra H, Nothnagel A. Laser treatment of macular edema secondary to central retinal vein occlusion. Int Ophthalmol 1987;10:100.

30. Frangieh GT, Green WR, Barraquer-Somers E, Finkelstein D. Histopathologic study of nine branch retinal vein occlusions. Arch Ophthalmol 1982;100:1132–1140.

31. Gutman FA, Zegarra H. The natural course of temporal retinal branch vein occlusion. Trans Am Acad Ophthalmol Otolaryngol 1974;78:OP178–192.

32. Michels RG, Gass JDM. The natural course of retinal branch vein occlusion. Trans Am Acad Ophthalmol Otolarnyngol 1974;78:OP166–177.

33. Ogura Y, Takehoshi M, Ueno S, Honde Y. Hyperbaric oxygen treatment for chronic cystoid macular edema after branch retinal vein occlusion. Am J Ophthalmol 1987; 104:301–302.

34. Osterloh MD, Charles S. Surgical decompression of branch retinal vein occlusions. Arch Ophthalmol 1988;106:1469–1471.

35. Branch Vein Occlusion Study Group. Argon laser photocoagulation for macular edema in branch vein occlusion. Am J Ophthalmol 1984;98:271–282.

36. Branch Vein Occlusion Study Group. Argon laser scatter photocoagulation for prevention of neovascularization and vitreous hemorrhage in branch vein occlusion. Arch Ophthalmol 1986;104:34–41.

37. Hayreh SS, Hayreh MS. Hemi-central retinal vein occlusion. Arch Ophthalmol 1980;98:1600–1609.

38. Appiah AP, Trempe CL. Differences in contributing factors among hemicentral, central and branch retinal vein occlusions. Ophthalmology 1989;96:364–366.

39. Gomez-Ulla de Izazazabal FJ, Cadorso Sugrez L, Orduna DE. Hemispheric central retinal vein occlusions. Ophthalmologica 1986;(1–2):14–22.

8

Laser Treatment of Less Common Macular Diseases

Lawrence J. Singerman
Rafael Addiego
Jeffrey C. Lamkin
Hernando Zegarra

Choroidal neovascularization (CNV) and diabetic maculopathy are the most common macular diseases, but a number of other, less common diseases, taken together, constitute a significant proportion of the diseases encountered by a laser surgeon.

Idiopathic Central Serous Choroidopathy

Overview

Central serous choroidopathy (CSC) is a condition of uncertain etiology (1-14). This disease is much more common in men (in some reports, by a ratio of over 10:1). It usually presents in the third, fourth, or fifth decades, although some patients older than 60 years have developed classic findings. It has also been reported (rarely) in children (15,16). In patients over 55 years old with findings consistent with CSC, exudative age-related macular degeneration (AMD) should be ruled out (1,17). Affected patients are generally healthy, although psychologic stress and certain personality profiles ("type A") are thought to be predisposing factors (1,2,18-21). CSC has also been associated with pregnancy (22,23). Systemic corticosteroid treatment may be another precipitant, although this association may be coincidental (9). There is no clear relationship with other ocular diseases, although there are isolated reports of CSC coexisting with retinitis pigmentosa and Hallermann-Streiff syndrome (16,24).

Pathology and Pathogenesis

Central serous choroidopathy is probably not a vascular problem but rather a primary disturbance of the retinal pigment epithelium (RPE; 8,12,21,25-29). There may be an as yet ill-defined precipitating insult to the RPE leading to poor adherence to Bruch's membrane or to impairment of ionic flow at the level of the RPE. In any case, this disturbance results in loss of the barrier function of the RPE with subsequent pigment epithelial detachment (PED) or sensory macular detachment or both.

Clinical Features

The condition typically presents with unilateral symptoms, although examination may reveal bilateral signs (1,4,6,7,9,11,12,14,18,30-32). One variant, which features multifocal RPE abnormalities, bullous exudative retinal detachment, and multiple sites of RPE disturbance, is more often bilateral (8). Vision is usually mildly reduced but may be improved with low-power plus lenses (1,4,5,6,11,12,18,29,31-33). Certain patients seem more likely to suffer severe visual loss: older patients (over 60 years old), patients with multiple recurrences or delayed resolution, patients with bullous exudative retinal detachments, and patients with RPE atrophy or tracks in the macula (8,14,26,28,34). Besides decreased vision, common complaints include metamorphopsia, micropsia, and eccentric scotoma (1,4-6,17,18,31). Special tests that may be abnormal during acute attacks include color vision, contrast sensitivity, dark adaptation, central threshold sensitivity, visual evoked potentials, and foveal densitometry (31,32,35-39).

The classic finding in CSC is a focal disturbance in the RPE with overlying serous retinal detachment (3,4,12,21, 31,33). The RPE disturbances are usually pinpoint areas of leakage, but the area of disturbance may be larger than $1/2$ disc diameter. These areas are usually central (within one disc diameter of the fovea; 10,13,40). There may be multiple foci of RPE leakage and disruption (6,8,26,33). PEDs develop at the source of leakage in a minority of cases; these are also usually central, small, and associated with overlying serous retinal detachment (1,12,41). Larger PEDs (occasionally greater than a disc diameter) may also be seen, more frequently in bilateral cases (2,6,18). PEDs may arise outside of or in the absence of associated serous retinal detachment (1,14,41). Multiple PEDs may be more common in bilateral cases and in older patients (14,18). A variant of CSC featuring bullous exudative retinal detachment (usually inferior and bilateral) has been reported and often features multiple or large PEDs underlying the detachment (2,8,28).

Another variant of CSC is characterized by atrophic RPE tracks descending from the macula and connecting a macular RPE leak to a dependent exudative detachment (26). The atrophic tracks may themselves leak. Serous detachment of the macula may coexist, and PEDs have been reported.

Other RPE changes noted with CSC include RPE mottling, hyperplasia, atrophy, clumping, and bone spicule or perivascular intraretinal migration (1,3,26). These changes often follow resolution of a serous retinal detachment or PED but may be found outside an obviously affected area of the retina or in the fellow eye. This is highly suggestive of previous attacks of CSC (1,6). RPE alterations are particularly noticeable in chronic or recurring cases (11,33).

In CSC, the serous retinal detachment almost always involves the macula and usually the fovea (1,12-14, 30-32,41,42). It is generally a well-defined, round or oval area overlying a focal leak or PED. Its size can vary widely, from approximately ½ disc diameter to over 10 disc diameters (33,41). Classic serous detachments outside the macula have also been reported (1,19). As described above, the inferior periphery is another region frequently involved with serous detachment. The subretinal fluid of an inferior detachment is often more turbid than in the classic form, obscuring the underlying RPE changes as well as the diagnosis (2,8,28). Subretinal precipitates are seen in a minority of cases. Fine intraretinal lipid deposition has been reported, but hemorrhage is distinctly uncommon (4,11,17,26). The presence of hemorrhage should prompt a thorough search for CNV (43,44). In the variant of CSC described above (tracks to inferior detachment), other retinal changes such as cystoid macular edema (CME), cystic degeneration, parafoveal telangiectasis with leakage, choroidal folds, and atrophy of the choriocapillaris have also been reported (26).

Progressive, often bilateral RPE decompensation has been reported as a distinct, chronic form of CSC (although not all such cases have clearly followed earlier attacks of classic CSC; 12,34,42,45). Sites previously affected by typical CSC seem to be predisposed to this chronic, progressive manifestation. Significant and progressive visual decline is associated with this variant despite the fact that involved areas may appear normal or only mildly affected. Fluorescein angiography reveals multiple patches of RPE window defects, often with focal areas of leakage or late staining. CNV has developed in eyes with this variant, both with and without treatment.

Fluorescein Angiography

Several patterns of fluorescein leakage have been noted in typical CSC. The vast majority of angiograms reveal isolated leaks, but multifocal leakage is not uncommon (5,10,41). Most leaks arise in the macula (10,13,21,40,41). The most common pattern is a pinpoint leak that slowly enlarges ("ink blot"; 3,5,10,12,13,26,31). The classic "smokestack" pattern (Fig. 8.1A—a stream of hyperfluorescence rising from a pinpoint leak) is seen in a minority of patients. There may be a PED under a pinpoint leak, with an overlying serous retinal detachment (12,14). Leakage from the RPE disturbance manifests as early hyperfluorescence, with later diffusion of dye into the serous retinal detachment. Window defects due to focal or diffuse RPE atrophy are another frequent cause of early hyperfluorescence. This may be seen within tracks connecting macular leaks to inferior detachments.

Prognosis

The course of CSC is variable, but the visual prognosis in typical forms is usually good (1,17,21,30,35,45). Most cases spontaneously resolve within 3 to 6 months, with

A

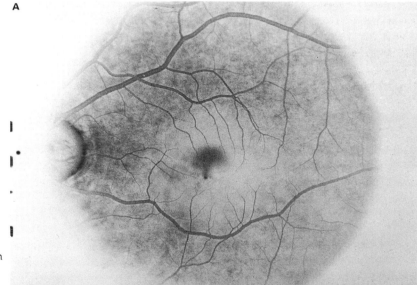

Fig. 8.1A CSC. A, Fluorescein angiogram from a 38-year-old man with sudden onset of metamorphopsia in his left eye. Examination of the retinal periphery was normal. Classic, but uncommon, smokestack pattern of fluorescein leakage through the RPE into an overlying sensory retinal detachment is seen.

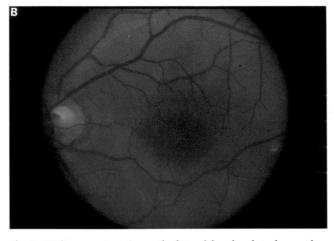

Fig. 8.1B Same patient 3 months later. Macular detachment has entirely resolved without treatment. RPE disturbances are evident.

retention of normal or near-normal visual acuity (Fig. 8.1B). However, many patients who recover good central acuity note subtle visual disturbances after resolution, and even more have abnormalities of visual function tests (32,37,38,41). A small percentage of patients may suffer significant, permanent reduction in vision following a severe attack.

A minority of patients develop chronic disease, or more severe or atypical forms, with large exudative detachments, multifocal leakage, or extensive RPE atrophy (8,9, 17,18,21,33). In these cases, the visual prognosis is not as favorable. CSC in older patients (over 60 years old) may have a poorer prognosis as well (14). In all cases, recurrences are common and may be more so at or near a previously affected site. Like initial attacks, recurrences tend to resolve spontaneously. Multiple recurrences, reflective of widespread RPE changes, are another poor prognostic indicator.

Treatment

No treatment other than laser (e.g., antibiotics, corticosteroids, tranquilizers) has been found to be effective (1,2,4,8,18). Photocoagulation using argon, krypton, xenon, or ruby sources has been studied. It is now widely accepted that laser treatment decreases the duration of the attack but does not alter the final visual acuity (4,6,21,31, 35,43,45). Whether the recurrence rate is affected by laser treatment is controversial (6,31,33,41,42,45). There is probably no relationship of final vision to presenting vision or worst vision to help determine if and when to treat (7).

Because of the disorder's (generally) benign course and favorable prognosis, as well as its predilection to involve the fovea, photocoagulation is reserved for only certain cases of CSC. Generally, observation for at least 4 months is advisable because typical attacks often resolve spontaneously (14,17,29,31,37,41). Treatment may be considered

after multiple recurrences, if the attack has significant visual impact, or for more severe cases (multiple leaks or severe visual loss). Lesions close to the fovea should be observed for as long as possible.

Argon green and krypton red lasers have been used, generally at settings of 200 μm and 0.1 to 0.2 sec, creating light burns (6,10,7,21,28,29,31,33,41). Treatment should be directed at the site of the leakage because indirect treatment has not been found to be effective (31,43). Treatment close to the fovea or within the papillomacular bundle should be avoided if possible. If either is necessary, the lightest possible treatment should be applied using a krypton red source. The red wavelengths may be more selectively absorbed at the level of the RPE, and one study suggested that recurrence rates may be lower following treatment with a krypton source (41). In most cases, one treatment session is sufficient to induce resolution of the serous retinal detachment within several weeks. For PED with associated exudative bullous retinal detachment, treatment of the entire PED is recommended unless it is large or central. For CSC associated with atrophic RPE tracks and inferior retinal detachments, treatment may be directed to the focal areas of leakage usually seen in or near the macula. (Argon green laser treatments of 50 to 100 μm, 0.2 to 0.3 sec, and 50 to 150 mW have been used (46). This treatment produced a gray burn at the level of the RPE without whitening of the overlying retina and succeeded in stabilizing or slowly improving vision in the majority of patients.)

Juxtafoveal Telangiectasis

Overview

Telangiectasis of the juxtafoveal capillary bed can arise secondary to numerous other conditions, including diabetes mellitus, venous occlusive disease, radiation retinopathy, sickle cell vasculopathy, Coats' disease, and ocular ischemia. However, certain cases of juxtafoveal capillary telangiectasis are idiopathic.

Several subgroups of idiopathic juxtafoveal telangiectasis (IJT) have been described (47-52). In each, the juxtafoveal capillary bed develops irregular dilation and beading. Typically, findings are more prominent temporally, but the nasal juxtafoveal vasculature may also be affected. Cases with circumfoveal involvement are also seen. The irregular, dilated capillaries are often incompetent, and resultant edema, exudate, and RPE changes account for mild to moderate visual loss. CNV is an uncommon but well-recognized cause of visual loss.

Pathology and Pathogenesis

The pathogenesis of this condition is unknown, and only one familial case has been reported (48). Most investigators consider the unilateral form to be a distinct developmental process similar to Coats' disease, strictly affecting the macula. It has been hypothesized that the bilateral forms are due to chronic, low-grade congestion related to the pattern of venules draining the affected areas. The disease is distinctly unlike venous occlusion, however—it gradually progresses above *and* below the raphe and is frequently bilateral. Another theory holds that juxtafoveal telangiectasis results from low perfusion pressure, with resultant stagnation and chronic hypoxia leading to microangiopathy. Others have suggested that the retinal vascular changes in the bilateral forms are secondary to a primary disorder of the RPE. Finally, there is a bidirectional relationship between IJT and diabetes mellitus. Patients with bilateral IJT have an apparently higher incidence of abnormal glucose tolerance tests, and classic juxtafoveal telangiectasis, with *no* other retinal vascular changes, has been seen in some patients with diabetes mellitus. The significance of this relationship is unclear (51).

A report of histopathologic findings is available from one patient with typical bilateral disease (53). Ironically, there was no dilation or telangiectasia of the affected vessels. Rather, capillary walls were markedly thickened, with luminal narrowing secondary to multilayered basement membrane proliferation. Trapped within this aberrant basement membrane layer was debris from desquamated endothelial cells and pericytes along with lamellar lipid. Pericyte and endothelial degeneration were also seen. These changes were detectable (to a lesser degree) throughout the entire retinal vascular bed. The findings were thought to represent primary endothelial cell degeneration and regeneration, with successive waves of basement membrane production, secondary degeneration of pericytes, and associated retinal edema, especially inner retinal edema. Some of the findings appeared strikingly similar to changes found in diabetic retinopathy. The apparent telangiectasis noted on fluorescein angiography was thought to result from rapid diffusion of dye into thickened vessel walls.

Clinical Features

The first of the four subtypes (1A) of IJT is unilateral. Middle-aged men are most frequently affected. The temporal half of the macula is usually more severely involved, and the extent of involvement is typically greater than one disc diameter, with equal involvement above and below the raphe. Funduscopic manifestations include dilated, telangiectatic vessels and microaneurysms. Macular edema and exudate (sometimes circinate) may cause significant visual loss or distortion. There are also reports of associated peripheral telangiectasia. Subretinal abnormalities and right angle venules (described below) are seen in a minority of patients of this subtype. The second

subtype (1B) is unilateral as well but is seen in older men with less dramatic leakage and mild visual loss.

The other two subtypes (2 and 3) of IJT are bilateral. Like type 1B, the bilateral types are disorders of middle age; unlike the unilateral subtypes, they are more likely to affect women. Bilateral disease tends to be symmetric, again affecting primarily the temporal macula above and below the raphe. Bilateral disease tends to affect smaller areas of the macula (less than one disc diameter) than does type 1A, with less edema and exudate and greater outer retinal and subretinal disruption than in unilateral disease. These deep changes may include right angle venules draining telangiectatic capillaries in the deep capillary plexus. These vessels may form retinochoroidal anastomoses and become dilated and tortuous; they also have been associated with stellate subretinal RPE hyperplasia or pigmentary plaques, fibrous metaplasia of the RPE, subretinal fibrosis, subretinal exudate, hemorrhage, and CNV. Cystic degeneration and RPE atrophy may complicate cases with significant macular edema. Peripheral retinal vascular changes have been reported but to a lesser degree than in the unilateral group.

One form of bilateral disease (type 2) features gray haloes of discoloration with retinal thickening along with multiple, punctate yellow refractile opacities near the inner retinal surface (Fig. 8.2; 49,54). The refractile bodies are often seen in association with typical capillary changes, and, in a study by one of us (IJS, unpublished data), they were found in 60% of eyes with this subtype. High-magnification biomicroscopy may be required for the examiner to see these refractile bodies. Although perhaps not pathognomonic for parafoveal telangiectasis, they are distinctly less common and less numerous in other diseases. Yellow, oval, subfoveal deposits, generally less than $1/4$ disc diameter, may also be seen in this subgroup. Type 3 features foveal capillary nonperfusion and cystic atrophy.

Fluorescein Angiography

Clinical findings in IJT may be very subtle, and mild edema may be the only visible change on examination. Fluorescein angiography may be required to define the vascular abnormalities in one or both eyes. Angiography in juxtafoveal telangiectasis shows fine, fusiform, tortuous, variably sized capillaries and vessel tortuosity affecting the superficial and deep capillary plexus (see Fig. 8.2). The deeper plexus may also show dilated, club-shaped, angulated, or branched capillaries. Microaneurysms are common in the unilateral subtype. The affected vessels fill completely and promptly, and leakage of dye is seen in late phases (see Fig. 8.2). Typical CME may develop. Hypofluorescence results from RPE hyperplasia or hemorrhage (in the setting of CNV). Besides capillary leakage,

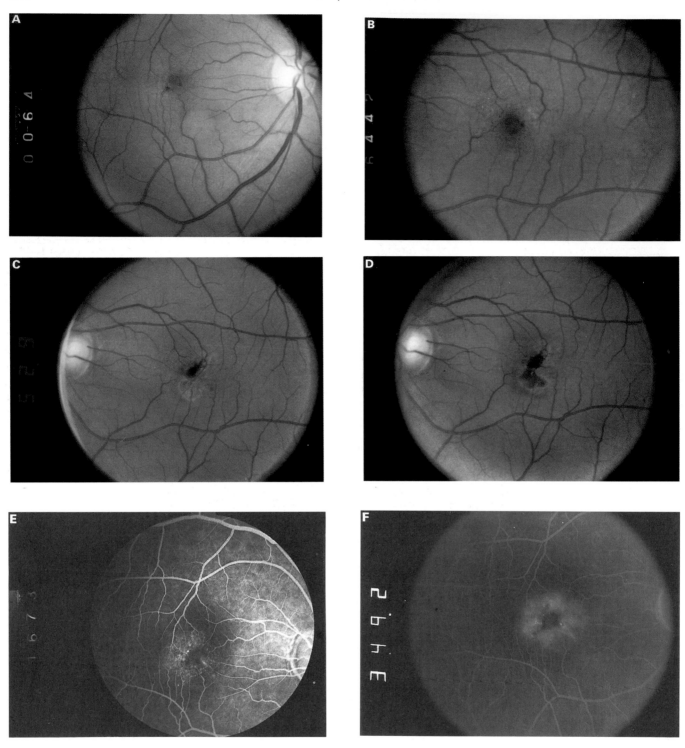

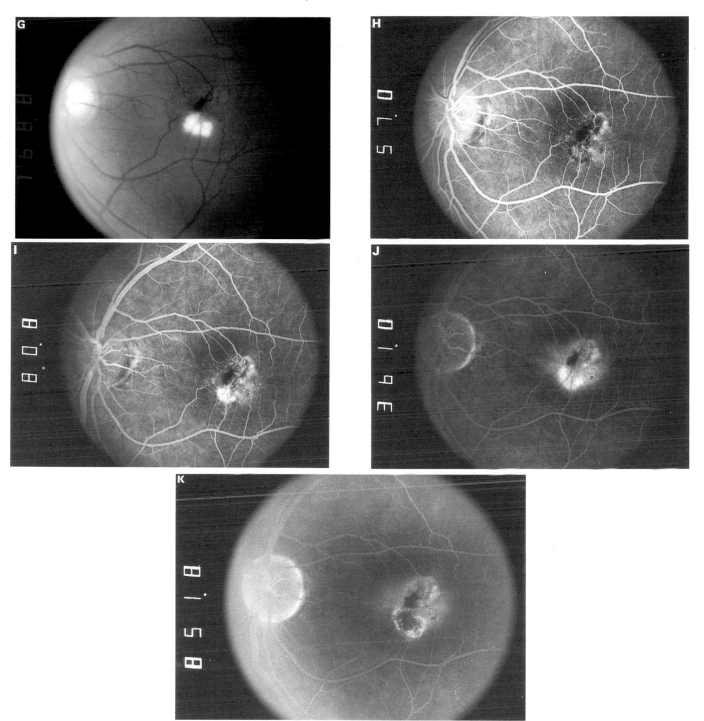

Fig. 8.2 Fifty-three-year-old man with gradually progressive visual blurring in both eyes. Visual acuity is 20/50 OU. A, Right eye. Note the retinal vascular irregularity along with mild intraretinal edema and discoloration temporal to the fovea. There is a stellate RPE figure temporal to the fovea. B, Monochromatic green light highlights the retinal vascular abnormalities, as well as the crystalline deposits nasal to the fovea. C, Left eye. A smaller pigment figure is present temporally, along with crystalline deposits nasally. These findings are consistent with the diagnosis of juxtafoveal telangiectasis, type 2. D, Left eye viewed with green light. E, Fluorescein angiogram of the right eye of the same patient. There is already mild leakage on midtransit views. F, Late transit views reveal significant leakage in a petaloid pattern. G, Two years later, the visual acuity has decreased to 20/100 in the left eye. There is a subretinal hemorrhage inferotemporal to the fovea, as well as a dirty gray area of retinal elevation inferior to the fovea. H, Fluorescein angiogram reveals an area of lacy early hyperfluorescence inferior to the fovea. Early hyperfluorescence superiorly corresponded to areas of RPE atrophy. I, The area of hyperfluorescence inferiorly has increased in intensity as dye transit continues. The window defects have not changed appreciably. J, Late views reveal considerable leakage inferior to the fovea, consistent with CNV complicating juxtafoveal telangiectasis. The window defects superiorly have faded. K, Fluorescein of left macula immediately after sequential red-yellow photocoagulation for CNV.

RPE window defects also account for hyperfluorescence, especially in bilateral disease.

Prognosis

The course and visual prognosis of juxtafoveal telangiectasis is somewhat variable. The major forms, both unilateral and bilateral, usually cause mildly decreased vision and metamorphopsia. There may be a slow progression with time, but patients generally maintain good vision in at least one eye for many years. Visual decline in unilateral juxtafoveal telangiectasis is caused by intraretinal edema and exudate and is usually minimal. With bilateral disease, retinal edema and exudate are less prominent. Unfortunately, right angle venules and subretinal findings are more common. Subretinal hemorrhage and exudate and CNV may occur, as well as RPE hyperplasia, metaplasia, and atrophy. Subsequent visual loss is generally more severe than with unilateral disease. Cystic retinal changes and lamellar macular holes have also been reported as causes of visual decline in both unilateral and bilateral juxtafoveal telangiectasis (49,52).

Treatment

Photocoagulation in this condition has had variable success. Treatment of unilateral disease frequently induces resolution of edema and exudate. However, because the natural history of this form is often self-limited, observation is probably warranted. If there is persistent or progressive visual loss, particularly with increasing macular edema and exudate, judicious treatment with argon green or dye yellow laser should be considered. Laser applications of 100 to 500 µm and a duration of 0.05 to 0.1 sec should create burns of light to moderate intensity. Treatment should be applied in a grid pattern to areas of leakage outside the foveal avascular zone (Fig. 8.3). Multiple treatment sessions are preferable to a heavier single treatment, and not all abnormal vessels need to be destroyed or treated directly. Treatment should be performed sparingly, with the visual effects of extensive macular photocoagulation kept in mind. Choroidal neovascular membranes complicating IJT should also be considered for laser treatment (see Fig. 8.2E through K).

Retinal Arterial Macroaneurysms

Overview

Retinal arterial macroaneurysms are acquired dilatations of the retinal arterial systems (55-65). The exact incidence is unknown, but these macroaneurysms are uncommon. The incidence clearly increases with age, peaking in the seventh and eighth decades. Women are more commonly affected than men by a ratio of approximately 4:1.

There is a strong association with hypertension, which is present in approximately 75% of patients with retinal macroaneurysms (56,57,59,60,62,66-69). Atherosclerotic heart disease, dyslipidemias, and polycythemia are also associated with macroaneurysms, although less strongly than is hypertension (58,59,61-63,68). Affected patients also seem to be at a higher risk for stroke (59,61,64,70). Because of these associations with systemic disease, patients with retinal arterial macroaneurysms should be considered for thorough medical evaluation.

Arterial macroaneurysms may not be the only retinal vascular anomaly in an affected eye. Coexistent findings may include generalized arteriolar narrowing, vascular tortuosity, and caliber irregularity and sheathing as well

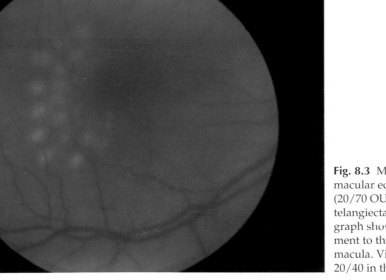

Fig. 8.3 Man, aged 58, with a history of macular edema and reduced vision (20/70 OU) secondary to juxtafoveal telangiectasis. Posttreatment photograph shows the grid pattern of treatment to the temporal half of the macula. Visual acuity improved to 20/40 in the treated eye.

as intra-arterial plaques and emboli. Central and branch vein occlusions (in the same or fellow eye) may also be seen, as well as occlusion of the affected artery distal to the macroaneurysm. Arterial changes similar to macroaneurysms have also been seen with congenital arteriovenous malformations of the retina (71).

Pathology and Pathogenesis

Histopathologically, the affected arterial wall is thickened by hyalin, fibrin, lipid, and foamy macrophages (69). Aneurysms vary in severity from simple cuff-like lesions to hemorrhagic "blow-outs." There may be fresh or organized thrombus partially occluding the vessel lumen, as well as atheromas in adjacent arterial branches. Dilated capillaries and accumulations of collagen, hemosiderin, and lipid surround the aneurysm itself, a focal outpouching of the retinal arterial wall (64). Paramacular lipid and protein exudates are located primarily in the outer retinal layers but may also be subretinal. The adjacent retina may become disorganized, with loss of photoreceptors, glial proliferation, and scar formation.

These histopathologic changes, along with the associated systemic and ocular findings, have led to the hypothesis that arterial macroaneurysms result from focal vascular decompensation following injury by systemic hypertension or local vaso-occlusion (thromboembolic disease; 56,57,65,69,70). In support of this theory, Giuffre and colleagues observed focal arterial hyalinization preceding macroaneurysm formation (66). Similarly, Lewis reported macroaneurysmal changes following branch retinal artery occlusion (70).

Clinical Features

Retinal arterial macroaneurysms are more often unilateral than bilateral; they may arise multiply, even along the same vessel, although most lesions are solitary (56-59,61,65,68-70). Right and left eyes are equally affected. Macroaneurysms are most commonly located along a temporal arcade, typically before the third-order arteriole (Fig. 8.4). The nasal arcades and cilioretinal arteries are less commonly involved. Peripapillary macroaneurysms have also been reported.

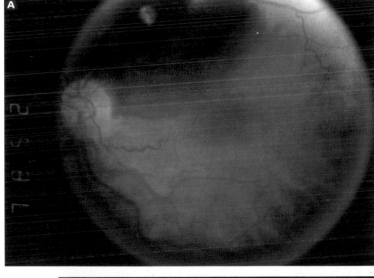

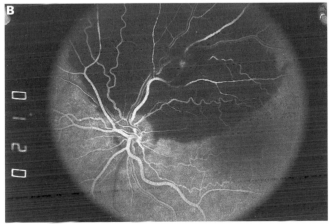

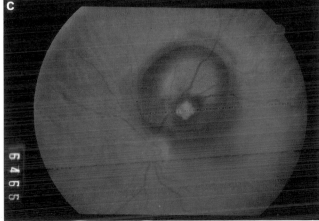

Fig. 8.4 Woman, aged 64, presenting with a "shadow" in her left eye. A, Sub-RPE and subretinal hemorrhage predominate, with limited intraretinal hemorrhage surrounding a white sclerotic lesion along the superotemporal arcade. B, Fluorescein angiogram from the same patient. Early transit views reveal rapid filling of a round lesion along the course of a second order arteriole. Surrounding hypofluorescence is secondary to intraretinal and subretinal hemorrhage. C, One week following direct treatment with argon green photocoagulation. Note the confluent treatment over the lesion.

Although they may be silent, many retinal arterial macroaneurysms present with visual loss, either acute (secondary to hemorrhage or rupture) or chronic (secondary to macular edema, exudate, and detachment).

The aneurysm itself appears as a focal, red, saccular, or fusiform dilation of the arterial wall. The saccular type may be more prone to hemorrhage (58). The size of a macroaneurysm tends to vary directly with the size of the affected artery and may grow to several times its diameter. A ring of vascular hyalinization and thickening, along with glial proliferation, is frequently found surrounding the aneurysm. Adjacent edema and exudate are common and result from the aneurysm's altered vascular permeability. The exudate often surrounds the macroaneurysm in a circinate pattern but may migrate into the macula, regardless of aneurysm location. Macular edema is common; serous macular detachment may also occur. Hemorrhage from macroaneurysm is initially intraretinal but may settle into the subretinal space (more common) or break through the internal limiting membrane into the vitreous (less common). A combination of these two produce the so-called "dumbbell" hemorrhage. Macroaneurysms located closer to the optic nerve seem more likely to bleed or rupture (see Fig. 8.4A). Distal macroaneurysms are usually exudative and less prone to hemorrhage, as are macroaneurysms associated with vein occlusions. Some retinal arterial macroaneurysms pulsate. Whether this finding is associated with an increased risk of rupture is uncertain. Macroaneurysms are sometimes obscured by the associated exudate, hemorrhage, and scarring, making diagnosis difficult (Fig. 8.5). Involuted macroaneurysms appear as translucent, vascular outpouchings or shrunken, round, gray-white lesions along an artery. Arterial irregularity, kinking, and sheathing can also be seen with involution.

The perianeurysmal vasculature often shows characteristic changes including microaneurysms, telangiectasis, capillary nonperfusion, widening of the capillary-free zone, intraretinal microvascular abnormalities (IRMA), and collateral vessel formation. These changes may be adjacent to the macroaneurysm as well as in areas with significant exudate (e.g., the macula). Any of these abnormalities may leak. It has been hypothesized that a macroaneurysm disrupts blood flow through the involved artery; the resultant hypoperfusion and hypoxia of the adjacent capillary bed is thought to cause these capillary irregularities and leakage (64). Other secondary changes include vein and artery occlusions, arterial thromboemboli, and vascular sheathing.

Fluorescein Angiography

Fluorescein angiography typically demonstrates rapid filling of a macroaneurysm in the early arterial phase (56,57,66,70,72). If there are multiple lesions, filling of distal lesions may be delayed. The rate of filling seems to be determined by the size of the macroaneurysm neck. The fusiform variety may fill more rapidly than the saccular type. Filling may be delayed, incomplete, or irregular due to intraluminal thrombus, endothelial cell proliferation, or involution. Hemorrhage, exudate, or arterial hyalinization may block the typical hyperfluorescence (see Fig. 8.4B). Late staining and leakage are common at the wall of the macroaneurysm, as well as along the proximal arterial segment. Surrounding capillary changes (e.g., capillary nonperfusion, telangiectasis, microaneurysm, IRMA, and collateralization) will be highlighted by angiography and typically leak. Macular capillary leakage and edema may also be demonstrated.

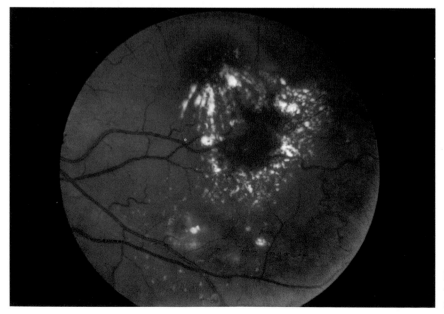

Fig. 8.5 A more distal macroaneurysm with perianeurysmal hemorrhage and marked exudative maculopathy.

Prognosis

Retinal arterial macroaneurysms may remain stable for long periods, and many patients are asymptomatic as long as the aneurysm does not affect the macula (56-59,62,65,70). Many macroaneurysms close spontaneously, without causing visual loss. With spontaneous resolution, the lumen of the involved artery may be fully or partially restored, or it may become entirely occluded. Arterial sheathing may be another sequela, along with residual edema. Rupture or hemorrhage of a macroaneurysm is typically followed directly by involution. Uncommonly, recurrent hemorrhage or reactivation of a quiescent or "involuted" macroaneurysm occurs (57).

The visual prognosis for symptomatic macroaneurysms is guarded. A permanent, significant decrease of vision may be seen in the setting of long-standing and severe macular edema, exudate, and hemorrhage, particularly subfoveal (59,61,63,70). Secondary changes, including subretinal fibrosis, epiretinal membrane formation, RPE atrophy, and macular cysts or holes, also limit recovery (56,58,61). The prognosis with macroaneurysms associated with acute preretinal or vitreous hemorrhage seems better than that with macroaneurysms associated with exudate affecting the macula. Simple intraretinal hemorrhage often clears without sequelae (57).

Treatment

Laser photocoagulation of macroaneurysms significantly shortens the duration of patency and may expedite visual recovery (56,57,70). Treatment should be considered for cases in which the macroaneurysm shows significant or increasing leakage affecting or threatening the fovea, especially if there has been a persistent loss of vision after one to 3 months of observation. In patients with good vision, exudative lesions that do not affect the macula may be observed, although a rapid increase in exudation (within one month) from these lesions may occur. Unless persistent, dense vitreous hemorrhage prompts vitrectomy, a hemorrhagic or ruptured macroaneurysm without active leakage usually does not require treatment because spontaneous involution usually follows. Treatment should be considered if there is recurrent hemorrhage or leakage from the macroaneurysm after hemorrhage. Pulsatile lesions may be observed because rupture is not necessarily imminent.

The goal of laser treatment is the elimination of leakage without occlusion or perforation of the artery (73). Extra care should be taken in the setting of vitreous hemorrhage, and overtreatment avoided, because this increases the likelihood of distal arteriolar occlusion (55,74,75). Due to their absorption by hemoglobin, argon green or dye yellow wavelengths are recommended for laser treatment of retinal macroaneurysms (55-57,73). Photocoagulation treatment strategies can be direct, indirect, or a combination of the two. Both techniques use low to moderate energy 200- to 500-μm burns with a duration of 0.2 to 0.5 sec. With the direct method, the laser is applied to the macroaneurysm itself. Treatment generally begins near the edge, overlapping onto adjacent retina. The center of the macroaneurysm is then partially or fully treated with larger, lighter burns, proceeding proximally to distally and avoiding feeder vessels (see Fig. 8.4C). The larger and lighter burns may decrease the risk of hemorrhage and artery occlusions. With the indirect strategy, laser is applied in a pattern of one to three rows of nearly confluent laser burns around and adjacent to the macroaneurysm, again beginning proximally.

Response to laser treatment is not immediate, but closure of the macroaneurysm is usually accelerated by the reaction that is stimulated (57,63). Retreatment may occasionally be necessary (58,73). Involution of the lesion after treatment occurs over several months, and resolution of exudate and hemorrhage may require even longer. Serous retinal detachment usually resolves promptly, but exudate may transiently increase as this occurs (59). Fluorescein angiographic evidence of persistent leakage may indicate that repeat treatment is necessary. With resolution of a macroaneurysm, visual acuity often improves, except in the setting of significant foveal exudate, edema, or hemorrhage (55-57). Complications of laser treatment include branch retinal artery occlusion (which may be more likely with the direct treatment technique and with the dye yellow source), hemorrhage, choroidal rupture, and subretinal neovascularization (56,57,67,72,76).

Coats' Disease

Overview

Coats' disease is a primary disorder of the retinal vasculature featuring prominent irregular, incompetent, telangiectasis of large and small retinal vessels. The disorder is most likely developmental, with no evident genetic basis (77,78).

Coats' disease primarily affects men (approximately 80% of cases) and is usually unilateral (at least 90% of cases). When bilateral, it is usually asymmetric (79-82). Findings indistinguishable from Coats' disease are seen in 3% to 5% of patients with retinitis pigmentosa and have been reported in association with several other inherited disorders (facioscapulohumeral muscular dystrophy, Senior-Loken syndrome, Turner's syndrome) and with various chromosomal defects (83-87). However, there is usually no specific etiology, systemic correlate, or inheritance pattern (77,81).

Pathology and Pathogenesis

Pathophysiologically, the disease process causes structural or functional breakdown of retinal vessels (88-90).

The findings are consistent with a noninflammatory, exudative vasculopathy. Apparent loss of the blood-retina barrier leads to telangiectasis and leakage, with secondary changes in the retina, especially the inner retina. Vessels are thickened and hyalinized. Plasmoid and fibrinoid infiltration of vessel walls leads to aneurysmal dilation or obliteration. Endothelial cells and pericytes are lost; glial cells proliferate. The vascular leakage leads to inner retinal cysts, exudates, hemorrhage, diffuse glial proliferation, and RPE hyperplasia. There is a mild leukocytic response to the exudate, with destruction of the retinal architecture, including the photoreceptors and subretinal space. The exudate, derived from plasma, is associated with fibrin, subretinal macrophages, and cholesterol clefts. Metaplastic or secondary calcification of detached, disorganized retina has been reported. Optic atrophy may ensue.

Clinical Features

The peak incidence of the disorder is at the end of the first decade, with the vast majority of affected patients presenting by age 30 (77,79-82). It has been diagnosed in infants. Young children, especially those less than four years old, often present with poor or no fixation, decreased vision, strabismus, and leukocoria, and are often referred for evaluation to rule out retinoblastoma. Older children may complain of blurred vision, although many are asymptomatic with normal or mildly decreased visual acuity initially detected by screening examinations. Some adults also present with minimal visual loss. Other presentations include neovascular glaucoma and severe exudative retinal detachment with profound visual loss.

Coats' disease features a wide variety of clinical findings. It is painless unless secondary glaucoma is present. The vascular changes are most commonly seen in the temporal fundus, particularly the superotemporal quadrant. The only sign of mild disease may be capillary telangiectasis, the most common sign (82,91,92). This may be subtle and associated with minimal leakage. With more severe disease, tortuosity, kinking, and telangiectasis increase, with involvement of venules and arterioles as well as capillaries (77). The major vessels develop "grape cluster" or "light bulb" configurations, beading, aneurysmal changes, and other irregularities (77,79,80,88-90,93,94). Associated changes include vascular obstruction, sheathed and sclerotic vessels, microaneurysms, small vessel and capillary dropout, and abnormal arteriovenous shunting.

Secondary effects of these abnormal vessels stem from inherent vascular incompetence. Retinal thickening, edema, and hemorrhage (subretinal, intraretinal, and preretinal), along with intraretinal and subretinal exudate, are often seen. Serous or cloudy yellow exudate may be marked. As with other exudative disorders, lipoprotein deposits often migrate into the macula regardless of their origin. Exudative deposits may be circinate or form a yellow, elevated mass (Fig. 8.6). Particularly with diffuse disease, serous detachment of the sensory retina, sometimes total, may develop. Subretinal refractile crystals and pigmentary changes frequently follow exudative detachment. Retinal and iris neovascularization, with neovascular glaucoma, iridocyclitis, cataracts, and disc edema, is a manifestation of severe posterior disease. Vitreous condensations, veils, and bands can form and progress to traction retinal detachment, with or without neovascularization.

Various combinations of primary and secondary manifestations threaten vision, most often as a result of leakage and exudation. CME, circinate maculopathy, and exudative macular detachment can develop with either macular or peripheral retinal vasculopathy (see Figs. 8.6 and 8.7).

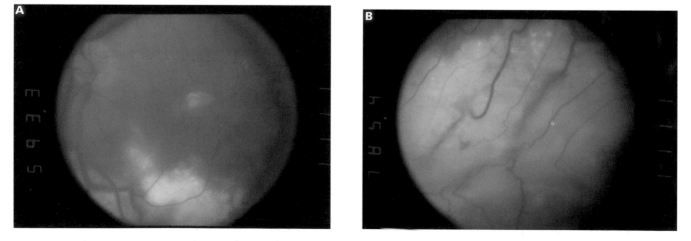

Fig. 8.6 An 8-year-old boy had recently failed a school eye examination. A, Exudative maculopathy, including subfoveal exudate. B, Inferonasal quadrant of the same eye. Extensive subretinal exudate with overlying retinal vascular abnormalities consistent with Coats' disease.

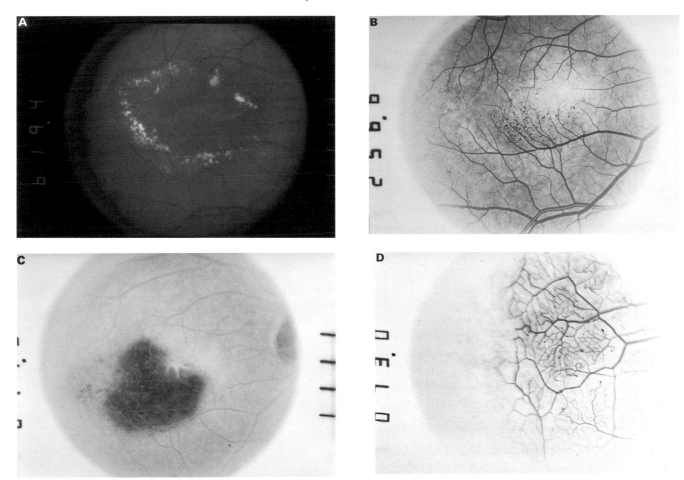

Fig. 8.7 A 15-year-old boy complained of worsening vision in his right eye. A, A circinate figure surrounds a diffusely thickened macula. B, Fluorescein angiogram from the same patient. Note microaneurysmal and telangiectatic changes, more severe inferiorly. C, Late transit views from the same angiogram. There is marked leakage and CME, worse inferiorly. D, Peripheral views of the same eye. Note the capillary dropout, microaneurysms, telangiectasis, and anomalous vascular communications.

In severe cases, a disciform mass may form centrally. Capillary nonperfusion of the macula may further contribute to visual loss.

Fluorescein Angiography

Fluorescein angiography plays an important role in demonstrating the typical vascular changes, as well as in determining their extent. Angiography may demonstrate changes not readily seen on examination and highlight the irregular telangiectasis of capillary beds (see Fig. 8.7B and D) and associated venules and arterioles (77,80,81). Capillary nonperfusion, microaneurysms, vascular beading, and abnormal vascular communications ("shunting" through dilated capillaries) are common (see Fig. 8.7D). Occasionally, there may also be broad intraretinal neovascular channels originating from the abnormal arteriovenous communications. With prominent arteriovenous channels or aneurysms, fluorescein transit may be delayed through the affected area. Intraretinal and subreti-

nal leakage of fluorescein begins early in the venous phase and persists (see Fig. 8.7B and C; 78,95). Characteristic CME may develop (see Fig. 8.7C), and subretinal pooling may be seen locally or in dependent areas remote from the abnormal vessels. The solid yellow intraretinal or subretinal exudates usually do not fluoresce, unless serous exudate is also present. In fact, they may obscure vascular changes if sufficiently large. Slight disc leakage may occasionally be seen. Usually, fluorescein does not "spill over" into the vitreous.

Prognosis

The natural history of Coats' disease is variable, and rare remissions have been reported (77,79,82,94). Limited disease may fluctuate, with little or no progression. Some patients, such as those with limited paramacular telangiectasis and mild edema and exudate, may be observed without treatment. Regardless of its initial severity, the condition may progress to involve all quadrants, causing total exudative retinal detachment, secondary glaucoma, or other complications. Progression may be gradual or rapid, progressing from limited disease to total exudative retinal detachment within a year. Significant progression is more likely with more extensive vascular involvement. The prognosis seems to be worse if three or more quadrants of the retina are involved. Coats' disease tends to be more severe in young children (less than 4 years old); patients who are younger at presentation are more likely to have widespread disease and extensive sequelae. The end stages of advanced disease may include severe visual loss, subtotal or total exudative retinal detachment, organized exudate simulating a neoplasm, subretinal or vitreous hemorrhage, traction retinal detachment, massive gliosis, rubeosis with neovascular glaucoma, and phthisis (77,79-82,96).

Treatment

Treatment is recommended in Coats' disease to preserve vision and prevent eye-threatening sequelae (77,79-81,89-91,97). Treatment is effective in stabilizing (and occasionally improving) vision in the majority of patients, as well as in preserving the eye. Early treatment seems to be more effective, particularly when there is a flat, attached retina. Close observation may be considered in older, reliable patients with good visual acuity and limited disease sparing the macula. Extramacular lesions with subretinal exudate should be treated before frank retinal detachment or macular exudate develops. Among patients with macular disease, those with recent loss of vision and exudate from focal paramacular telangiectasis may be among the best candidates for treatment. Extra care should be used in treating disease near the fovea, especially in the papillomacular bundle.

Treatment outcomes are less favorable for children (especially those less than 4 years old), who may also require more treatment sessions. Treatment of children should be prompt and aggressive. The prognosis is also guarded in eyes presenting with three or more quadrants of involvement, extensive exudative retinal detachment, heavy foveal lipid deposition, or subfoveal fibrous plaque formation. Disease associated with retinitis pigmentosa also seems more refractory to treatment. In severe cases, all peripheral lesions should be treated, even when the prognosis for central vision is guarded, to prevent large exudative retinal detachments. Even blind eyes can be considered for treatment, with the goals of comfort, cosmesis, and retention of the globe. Therapeutic modes have included, alone or in combination, photocoagulation, cryotherapy, diathermy, scleral buckling, external drainage of subretinal fluid, and even pars plana vitrectomy for significant traction detachment. The choice of modality depends on the extent, duration, and location of the vascular abnormalities and exudate.

Photocoagulation should be guided by clinical examination, as well as fluorescein angiography, to ensure that all affected areas are treated. Currently, laser photocoagulation is performed with the argon green or dye yellow laser, using a spot size of 100 to 500 µm for a duration of 0.2 to 0.5 sec. Burns are applied directly to the anomalous vessels to cause spasm or whitening. The therapeutic end point is obliteration of the telangiectatic vessels. Therapy can also be directed to adjacent retina and abnormal capillary beds. Extra care is necessary when treating the macula. Photocoagulation may need to be combined with other modalities. Cryotherapy is needed in lesions that are peripheral or accompanied by large exudative retinal detachments; such cases may require prior drainage of subretinal fluid. Diathermy and scleral buckling, along with drainage of subretinal fluid, have also been used.

Despite treatment, progression still occurs in a significant percentage of patients, and multiple sessions are often needed, especially in young patients. Resolution of the disease is gradual, usually beginning 4 to 6 weeks after therapy. Complete resolution of exudate may take over a year. Subfoveal nodules of organized exudate may persist indefinitely. A temporary increase of exudate and subretinal fluid may occur after cryotherapy, potentially leading to total exudative retinal detachment and proliferative vitreoretinopathy (PVR). Epiretinal membrane formation, pigmentary changes, hemorrhage, inflammation, and scotoma have also developed after laser treatment or cryotherapy (78,82,95,98).

Even with successful treatment, the disease can recur in areas of previously normal vessels, even many years after initial therapy. Long-term follow-up, at least biannually, is recommended.

Capillary Hemangiomas

Overview

Capillary hemangiomas are benign vascular hamartomas of the retina and, occasionally, the optic nerve (99,100). These lesions may be isolated or part of a familial syndrome (von Hippel-Lindau disease; 100–110). There are no clinical findings unique to either the sporadic and familial presentations, although patients with multiple or bilateral lesions are probably more likely to have von Hippel-Lindau disease (104,107). Capillary hemangioma like lesions have also been reported rarely in association with retinitis pigmentosa and neurofibromatosis (111-113).

Capillary hemangiomas of the retina are uncommon, with a similar incidence in men and women (102,104,108, 109,114,115). New lesions have been discovered at all ages but most often present in the second and third decades and rarely after the fourth. Younger patients often have a positive family history.

Von Hippel-Lindau disease is inherited as an autosomal dominant trait with high penetrance and variable expressivity (102,104,106). It is unusual for an affected patient to have all the manifestations of the syndrome. Family history is not always positive, however, due to the late and silent manifestations of von Hippel-Lindau disease. It is not clear what percentage of retinal angiomas are truly familial, but it may be more than the accepted 20% (100,104,107,116). Two thirds (or more) of patients with von Hippel-Lindau disease develop retinal capillary hemangiomas, making this its most common manifestation (102,108). It also causes the presenting symptoms in most patients. Cerebellar hemangioblastoma and renal cell carcinoma are also seen frequently in von Hippel-Lindau disease and are the most common cause of death (102,106,108,115). Other associated abnormalities include pheochromocytoma and, less frequently, polycythemia, medullary and spinal hemangioblastomas, angiomas of the skin, and cysts of the liver, kidney, pancreas, epididymis, adrenal glands, ovaries, lung, bone, omentum, and thyroid (102,104,106-108,115,117). Bladder hemangiomas and islet cell tumors of the pancreas have also been reported (102,106).

Pathology and Pathogenesis

Histopathologically, capillary hemangiomas are benign vascular hamartomas composed of multiple large, irregular, tortuous, branching, interconnected capillary proliferations of variable caliber (103,117,118). They may arise in various layers of the retina, causing architectural disruption and full-thickness displacement in some cases. Smaller hemangiomas may contain fairly normal capillaries and arterioles, with normal-appearing endothelium, basement membrane, and pericytes. Larger lesions are obviously disturbed, including endothelial cells with irregular thickness and fenestrations, decreased numbers of pericytes, and basement membrane duplication. The interstitium of the tumor contains foamy, vacuolated cells along with scattered erythrocytes. Other findings include lipid exudates, gliosis, dilated feeder vessels, RPE proliferation, congestion of the adjacent choroid, and retinal and choroidal vascular communications. Breaches of the internal limiting membrane are common with large tumors and lead to preretinal neovascularization and overlying vitreous condensations. Regressed lesions develop a hyperplastic RPE response, fibroglial scarring, and retinal thinning. The remainder of the retinal vasculature appears normal.

Clinical Features

Capillary hemangiomas of the retina can represent singly or multiply (101,102,106,107,117-119). The reported incidence of bilaterality is variable but may be as high as 50% (100,107). Capillary hemangiomas most frequently affect the midperiphery and periphery.

Growth patterns are variable. Typical endophytic capillary hemangiomas appear to arise from the inner retina and initially appear similar to microaneurysms—small, red, single or multiple enlarged capillary nodules without evident afferent or efferent vessels. Larger lesions form fleshy, well-defined, elevated, oval to round, solitary orange-red nodules (Fig. 8.8A; 100,102,104–106,119,120). These are found in all locations, including at the optic nerve, and may enlarge to many disc diameters in size. Except for those near the optic nerve, larger tumors develop afferent and efferent vessels. Initially, these feeder vessels may not be markedly abnormal, particularly if the lesion is smaller than a disc diameter; however, in larger lesions, they develop tortuosity and dilatation, along with arterialization of the draining vein. The afferent and efferent vessels assume a similar color due to admixture of the arterial and venous circulations.

Sessile and exophytic lesions involve the deeper or outer retina and can extend into the subretinal space. They seem to arise more frequently around the optic nerve. These lesions often do not develop obvious feeder vessels. They are usually indistinct, flatter areas of red-orange discoloration with thickening and whitening of the overlying retina. Examination may show only a whitening of the overlying retina and a few dilated retinal capillaries extending posteriorly into the tumor. Surface hemorrhage may be another sign.

Regardless of type or growth pattern, hemangiomas may cause macular edema (sometimes cystoid), retinal exudate (intraretinal or subretinal), retinal hemorrhage (preretinal, intraretinal, or subretinal), and exudative retinal detachment (99,103-105,107,121-123). Exudate often migrates into the macula, regardless of tumor location. Vitreous reaction and preretinal fibrosis, macular pucker, and preretinal neovascularization are not uncommon and can lead to traction retinal detachment (100,104, 107,115,124-127). This may be further complicated by rhegmatogenous retinal detachment following breaks caused by surface traction, especially at the posterior base of the lesion between the afferent and efferent vessels.

Many lesions, perhaps up to 50%, are clinically silent (102). In symptomatic patients, the spectrum of presentation includes painless blurred vision, floaters, visual field loss, scotoma, metamorphopsia, micropsia, or even a blind, painful eye (99,102-105,115). Decreased vision is the most common symptom, usually due to chronic macular edema. Leukocoria may be the presenting sign in young patients if exudate is extensive.

Patients presenting with retinal capillary hemangiomas should be evaluated for von Hippel-Lindau disease (102,107,115). Work-up should include a careful family history (which may be falsely negative) and neurologic and physical examinations, including standing and

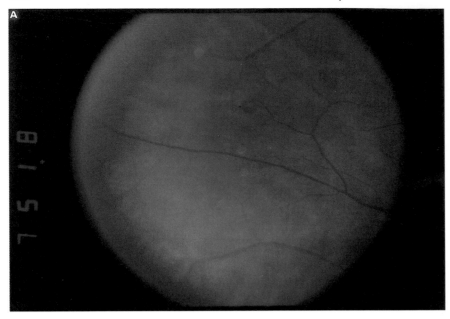

Fig. 8.8 A, An asymptomatic 19-year-old myope. A moderately small peripheral, endophytic capillary hemangioma. A careful medical and neurologic review of systems was normal.

supine blood pressures. Tests to be performed at presentation and annually thereafter include complete blood counts, urine catecholamines and metanephrines, and renal ultrasound. Tests to be performed at presentation and biannually thereafter include head and abdominal computed tomography (CT) scans. Examination of family members, particularly children and young adults, should be considered. Retinal examinations, including fluorescein angiography, should be performed at least annually in patients with suspected von Hippel-Lindau disease. In patients with previous capillary hemangioma, lifetime surveillance for new or recurrent lesions, with examinations at least every 6 months, is recommended.

Fluorescein Angiography

Fluorescein angiography typically demonstrates early perfusion of the tumor, which appears to be made up of small-caliber vessels (99,103-105,123). Perfusion of the angioma is retinal in origin. The transit of dye is rapid. Afferent and efferent vessels often are dilated and tortuous, particularly with larger tumors. Fluorescein leakage and staining may be confined to within the tumor or extend intraretinally, intravitreally, or into the subretinal space. Very small or encapsulated lesions may not leak (107,121). In fact, they may be difficult to demonstrate. There usually is no macular leakage found, even with significant exudate. Fluorescein angiography of deeper tumors, particularly juxtapapillary and optic nerve tumors, demonstrates fine vascular networks, also filling early (99,105). This vascular network appears to fill earlier than the surrounding retinal capillary bed, suggesting additional blood supply from a deeper optic nerve plexus. Afferent and efferent vessels are rarely evident with these exophytic tumors. Other secondary changes in the an-

giography are due to heavy exudate, macular edema, preretinal neovascularization, and RPE disruption.

Prognosis

The clinical course of retinal capillary hemangiomas is generally one of slow progression (104,107,116,117). Some lesions, particularly smaller ones, are static or progress very slowly. Other lesions may grow rapidly, with worsening exudate leading to exudative or tractional retinal detachment, neovascular glaucoma, blindness, and phthisis. Progression to severe visual loss or other end-stage complications occurs in at least 50% of patients, even with treatment. Progression can be rapid and aggressive, but spontaneous regression has also been reported (106,117). Maximal growth occurs before puberty, but the size of capillary hemangiomas can increase into the third and fourth decades and sometimes later. New lesions can arise anywhere, including near areas of previous treatment. The development of new lesions may occur more often in eyes with multiple lesions.

Treatment

Retinal capillary hemangiomas should be treated promptly because they often cause visual loss and because treatment is significantly easier and more effective for smaller lesions with less exudate (107,109,114,115). The exception to this rule is an optic nerve tumor (99,105). Here, the approach should be more conservative because treatment itself can significantly diminish vision. It is probably better to follow these, at least until there is significant associated exudate. Photocoagulation, cryotherapy, diathermy, scleral buckling, drainage of subretinal fluid, and pars plana vitrectomy have all been used, often in combination, to treat capillary hemangiomas and their sequelae (100,101,104-107,109,114,115,119,120,121,124,125). The choice of the therapeutic mode depends on factors including lesion size, location, and media clarity.

Laser photocoagulation has been used, with good results, in the treatment of smaller lesions. Although complete histologic ablation of these tumors may be less likely with lesions larger than 0.8 to 1 disc diameter, reasonable clinical responses have occurred in lesions smaller than 2.5 disc diameters. Argon green or dye yellow laser has been used to treat retinal capillary hemangiomas directly with confluent burns of 100 to 1000 μm (depending on lesion size) and long duration (0.2 to 0.5 sec). The end point is a significant whitening or blanching over the entire angioma (Fig. 8.8B). Small spot size and high intensity are avoided to minimize the risk of hemorrhage. The goal of treatment should be complete obliteration of the tumor with visible shrinkage and whitening, decreased afferent and efferent vessel caliber, decreased exudate, and nonperfusion on fluorescein angiogram. Response to treatment can be delayed, especially with larger lesions, and multiple sessions are often necessary (and may also be safer). Treatment sessions should be separated by approximately one to 2 weeks. Because of the possibility of recurrence, regular follow-up, including fluorescein angiography, should be performed every 6 months, with retreatment if reperfusion occurs. New lesions should be sought and treated. Laser photocoagulation of feeder vessels has also been performed in addition to or preceding direct treatment. This is not a widely accepted practice, however, due to higher risk of significant scotoma from vascular occlusion or full thickness retinal damage. Feeder vessel treatment may also require more sessions than direct photocoagulation. Its most beneficial role

may be in conjunction with direct treatment to obliterate larger lesions.

As described above, optic nerve and juxtapapillary lesions must be managed carefully because treatment may significantly reduce vision. "Partial success" (decreased exudate and partial regression without significant loss of vision) has been obtained using low to moderate surface photocoagulation repeated over several months. Treatment of "selected portions" of the tumors may also be beneficial, but the overall prognosis is still poor. High-intensity treatment to larger areas contributes to visual loss, scotoma, and epiretinal membrane formation. Consideration might also be given to "barrier laser treatment," attempting to protect the macula from encroaching exudate.

Although the response to treatment of smaller retinal capillary hemangiomas is often good, recurrences and treatment failures do occur, with progression to rubeosis, neovascular glaucoma, exudative retinal detachment, and phthisis. Complications of photocoagulation include epiretinal membrane, scotoma, and hemorrhage. Worsened subretinal fluid or exudate is common but usually mild and transient and may be worse following cryotherapy. The exact incidence of these complications is uncertain and is difficult to distinguish from the natural history of the disorder itself.

Larger lesions have been treated with photocoagulation but may respond better to cryotherapy. Cryotherapy is also preferred for anterior lesions or in eyes with hazy media. The double-freeze thaw technique is recommended, with no more than 12 cycles per session to avoid an increased risk of PVR. Multiple sessions may be necessary, repeated at intervals of approximately 6 to 8 weeks. Complications of cryotherapy are similar to those of laser

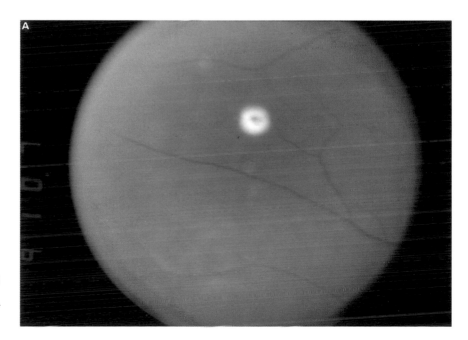

Fig. 8.8 B The same patient following laser photocoagulation of the hemangioma. Treatment was undertaken before the lesion began to leak or grow.

treatment or untreated capillary hemangiomas. Excessively vigorous cryotherapy may be associated with higher rates of PVR.

Other treatments have been used in very large or unresponsive capillary hemangiomas or those complicated by traction, exudative, or rhegmatogenous retinal detachment. Combinations of pars plana vitrectomy, scleral buckling, drainage of subretinal fluid, and cryotherapy may be needed for these cases. Transscleral diathermy has also been used, as has surgical eyewall resection. Epiretinal membranes should be managed by treating the associated tumor and waiting at least 6 months because successful treatment of the hemangioma may induce spontaneous regression of the epiretinal membrane. When necessary, pars plana vitrectomy with epiretinal membrane dissection has been used with good results.

Visual outcome following treatment is better when the lesion is smaller than 2.5 disc diameters. Furthermore, the chance of successful destruction of the tumor seems to be greater than the chances for improved vision, and good tumor response is not always accompanied by a good visual result. Even with successful treatment of the tumor, permanent visual deficit, caused by sequelae including subfoveal hemorrhage, subfoveal lipid epiretinal membrane, and traction retinal detachment, is not uncommon.

Cavernous Hemangiomas of the Retina

Overview

Cavernous hemangiomas are benign vascular hamartomas affecting the retina and, occasionally, the optic nerve (100,128-133). Their clinical appearance and behavior, as well as characteristic histopathology, distinguish them from capillary hemangiomas. The demographics of these hemangiomas are similar to those of the capillary variety—they are equally rare in men and women and typically present in early adulthood. Although they are frequently isolated congenital malformations, they have also been seen in association with similar neurologic and cutaneous lesions, suggestive of a phakomatosis (113,130-132,134-139). Individuals affected by such a syndrome may develop angiomas anywhere in the central nervous system (CNS), heralded by seizure, cranial nerve palsy, paresthesia, or focal neurologic deficits. Cutaneous angiomas have also been reported but are an inconsistent manifestation of this syndrome, which is transmitted in an autosomal dominant pattern.

Pathology and Pathogenesis

Histopathologically, cavernous hemangiomas arise within the inner half of the retina, but large lesions may involve outer retina as well (130,139,140). These tumors consist of numerous dilated, thin-walled vessels that interconnect. The luminal caliber is greater than that seen in the capillary variety. Normal endothelial cells and pericytes account for the characteristic absence of leakage, exudate, and edema.

Clinical Features

Most patients do not have visual symptoms. The lesions are almost always monocular and solitary (130,131,135, 136). They are frequently posterior to the equator but outside the temporal arcades and appear as sessile, thin-walled, grapelike clusters of saccular aneurysms. Macular hemangiomas have been reported and can cause visual loss due to direct macular involvement or secondary traction. They are usually elevated. The individual saccules can vary in size from small microaneurysms up to as large as one disc diameter, and the overall lesion size can be several disc diameters, projecting into the vitreous. These tumors may be seen along the course of a major vein. The saccules themselves are usually filled with dark venous blood and may appear only partially filled—sluggish flow leads to separation of clear plasma above from erythrocytes below. Additionally, portions of the tumor may be white or fibrous or even cystic.

Small clumps or satellites of isolated aneurysms are frequently seen around the main body of the mass. The remaining retina and major vessels, however, generally appear uninvolved, although twin vessels have been associated. Abnormal feeder vessels and arteriovenous shunts are not seen, and exudation is rare. A gray-white fibrous epiretinal membrane often partially covers its surface and may become more prominent with time or following partial obliteration. Occasionally, adjacent pigmentary clumping or hypopigmentation develops.

Cavernous hemangiomas occasionally have small superficial hemorrhages. Vitreous hemorrhage complicates up to 10% of cases and is the most common cause of visual loss. Subretinal and intraretinal hemorrhage also occur but are usually mild (100,129-131).

Patients with newly developed cavernous hemangioma of the retina should undergo a careful family history, a thorough physical evaluation with attention to the skin and neurologic systems, and CT or magnetic resonance imaging scan of the brain. Family members should also be examined, particularly in the setting of a positive family history or systemic findings consistent with a hereditary syndrome.

Fluorescein Angiography

Fluorescein angiography of cavernous hemangiomas demonstrates delayed perfusion, suggesting that the lesions are relatively isolated from the retinal circulation (128-131). There is hypofluorescence in the arterial phase with slow-filling occurring in the mid to late venous phase. Filling may occur from the periphery of the lesion toward the center, with obvious draining venules, or it may be incomplete. Some darker lesions show minimal or no filling. Venous drainage is often extremely delayed, and fluorescence of the mass can persist into the recirculation phases. Plasma-erythrocyte layering is particularly prominent on fluorescein angiography, with hyperfluorescent caps in the saccules, particularly in the late phases. Satellite clusters are often seen surrounding the main body of the cavernous hemangioma. Usually there is no leakage of dye, although there may be mild late diffusion into the overlying vitreous. The tumor itself may stain. The blood-retinal barrier is intact in most cases. There are also no arteriovenous shunts, significant feeder vessels, or involvement of the remainder of the retinal circulation.

Prognosis

The course of cavernous hemangiomas is usually nonprogressive, although growth has rarely been seen (129-131, 134). Some lesions show progressive thickening and hyalinization, possibly due to thrombosis and organization. Exudation does not usually occur, but surface fibroglial tissue may increase over time. Visual prognosis is excellent in most cavernous hemangiomas, and the lesions usually may be followed without treatment.

Treatment

Ablation with photocoagulation or cryotherapy may be considered in cases of significant recurrent hemorrhage (100,129,131,135). Laser photocoagulation, if required, should be applied confluently to the surface of the tumor and possibly the adjacent retina, avoiding major vessels. Ablation may prove to be incomplete, and retreatment may be necessary. Optic nerve lesions should rarely, if ever, be treated, due to the potential for optic nerve injury with visual field loss or decreased vision. Other potential complications of laser treatment include growth of the lesion, vitreous hemorrhage, and epiretinal membrane formation, with subsequent macular distortion.

Arteriovenous Communications of the Retina

Overview

Arteriovenous communications of the retina are rare, congenital, direct communications between the arterial and venous circulations without an intervening normal capillary bed (100,141-147). These shunts may appear as sporadic, isolated findings or as part of the systemic Wyburn-Mason syndrome. They affect men and women equally and are most often diagnosed in young adults (typically younger than 30 years old).

Arteriovenous communications generally do not demonstrate a well-defined inheritance pattern, even when part of the Wyburn-Mason syndrome (100,141-143). This rare phakomatosis is characterized by monocular retinal shunts associated with similar arteriovenous malformations of the ipsilateral CNS, including the midbrain, cerebral hemispheres, and, often, the visual pathways (142, 146-148). The incidence of CNS lesions in patients with retinal shunts is hard to identify precisely, and estimates range from 17% to 81% (146). Other sites for potential arteriovenous malformations include the orbit, ipsilateral face and paranasal structures, eyelids, skin, lung, and spine (100,142,149). Accompanying neurologic symptoms are variable, depending on the size and location of the lesion (146,147,150). Visual field loss (particularly hemianopia), cranial nerve palsies, seizures, headaches, bruits, pupillary abnormalities, speech dysfunction, and hemiplegia have all been reported secondary to these lesions. Cutaneous findings are infrequent and include nevus flammeus and ipsilateral facial vessel dilation (142,145, 151). Due to its prominent systemic findings and relatively larger ocular lesions, the Wyburn-Mason syndrome is usually diagnosed earlier in life than are isolated arteriovenous malformations.

Pathology and Pathogenesis

Histopathologically, large arteriovenous communications occupy the full thickness of the retina (147,148). Involved arteries and veins are difficult to distinguish from each other. Each vessel has a fibromuscular medial coat of variable thickness and a wide, almost acellular fibrohyaline adventitial coat. Adjacent retinal changes include loss of ganglion cells and nerve fibers, as well as attenuation and cystic degeneration. Thrombi may be seen in some of the vessels. Outside the lesion, the retina and its vasculature appear normal. An arteriovenous malformation of the optic nerve can replace much of the nerve's normal structure.

Clinical Features

Arteriovenous communications of the retina usually present unilaterally. They can be single or multiple in an affected eye. They can involve any part of the retina but seem to arise more frequently in the temporal quadrants and the papillomacular bundle. The arteriovenous communications vary in appearance from obscure, barely visible arteriovenous anastomoses to a "bag of worms" or mass of dilated vessels with indistinct arterial and venous components. In larger lesions, there is arterialization of the veins, thickening of all vessel walls, and dilatation of the vascular channels to over 500 μm (146). Retinal vessels in the area of the arteriovenous malformation are often increased in number, size, and tortuosity. Other potential findings in the vessels of larger lesions include sheathing, beading, kinking, and increased filling pressure. There is no pulsation. There may be small foci of retinal degeneration and pigmentation. Usually, no optic atrophy is seen.

Arteriovenous malformations have been divided into three grades (141,142). Grade 1 lesions are communications between a small arteriole and a small venule; grade 2 lesions are communications between a branch artery and a branch vein (Fig. 8.9); and grade 3 ("diffuse type") arteriovenous communications of the retina demonstrate widespread, marked dilation of most of or all of the vascular system (Fig. 8.10). The Wyburn-Mason syndrome usually associated with grade 2 and 3 lesions.

Visual acuity typically correlates inversely with the clinical grade (141,142). Patients with grade 3 lesions often have visual acuity no greater than finger counting. This severe visual loss often leads to earlier diagnosis. Location is also important because vascular malformations directly involving the macula or disc produce more visual compromise. At the other end of the spectrum are smaller peripheral lesions that are clinically silent.

Complications of arteriovenous communications of the retina are infrequent but include intraretinal hemorrhage, vitreous or preretinal hemorrhage, vascular occlusion, optic atrophy, choroidal and retinal ischemia, and neovascular glaucoma (141,142,152). These lesions have been associated with other vascular anomalies such as retinal macrovessels (with grade 1 lesions), leaking macroaneurysms, and twin vessels, but they are usually seen without other retinal vascular anomalies (153).

Fluorescein Angiography

Typically, angiography shows rapid filling of these malformations in the arterial phase, with a greatly reduced transit time and venous filling immediately after arterial filling (see Fig. 8.10B; 141,142). As a result, there may be axial rather than peripheral filling of the involved veins ("arterial laminar flow"), especially in larger lesions. Late staining of affected veins is possible, and slight leakage may be present in some larger, decompensating malformations. Accompanying capillary changes include capillary leakage inside the area affected by the malformation, adjacent capillary dropout, microaneurysms, and microvascular dilations. Choroidal and retinal ischemia may also be seen.

Prognosis

Many arteriovenous communications of the retina are asymptomatic and stationary (especially grade 1 lesions), although some increased tortuosity, sclerosis, and remodeling may occur (141,142,149,152). Spontaneous regression of these lesions has been reported (154). Although vein occlusion, hemorrhage, and neovascular glaucoma are possible, significant edema or exudate is rare and usually is seen only in grade 3 lesions (141,143,144). Visual loss may occur due to macular edema, macular hemorrhage, direct macular involvement, visual field loss secondary to optic pathway lesions, and optic atrophy of the fellow eye if there has been chiasmal involvement. Amblyopia may significantly limit the response to treatment (142,143,149,151).

Treatment

Treatment is usually not indicated unless the lesions are complicated by vein occlusion or neovascular glaucoma (144,149,152). Panretinal photocoagulation or peripheral cryotherapy are better options than is direct photocoagulation, which may be complicated by bleeding,

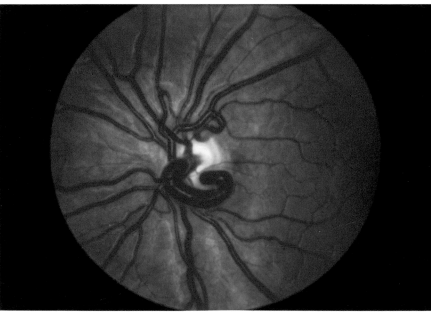

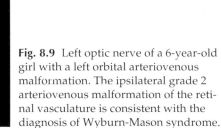

Fig. 8.9 Left optic nerve of a 6-year-old girl with a left orbital arteriovenous malformation. The ipsilateral grade 2 arteriovenous malformation of the retinal vasculature is consistent with the diagnosis of Wyburn-Mason syndrome.

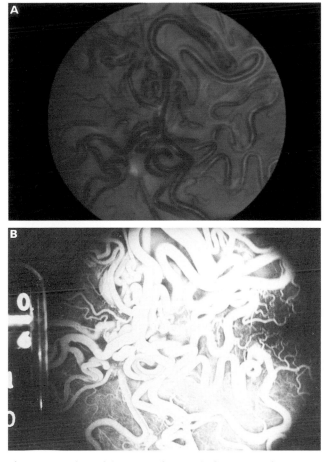

Fig. 8.10 Wyburn-Mason syndrome. A, Severe, grade 3 arteriovenous malformation from a patient with an ipsilateral cerebellar vascular malformation. B, Fluorescein angiogram of patient. Direct treatment of such lesions is obviously ill-advised.

secondary ischemia, and failure to close the malformation. Patients with grade 3 lesions should be referred for systemic evaluation and possible neuroimaging to rule out intracranial lesions. Grades 1 and 2 arteriovenous communications of the retina, however, are usually isolated anomalies, and patients with such lesions generally require systemic evaluation only if there are associated signs and symptoms of systemic arteriovenous communications, such as visual field loss, neurologic changes, or cutaneous hemangiomas.

Radiation Retinopathy

Overview

Radiation retinopathy is an occlusive microangiopathy that has been reported following local or external radiation therapies for many conditions, including Graves' disease, uveal melanoma, retinoblastoma, choroidal metastasis, and tumors of the CNS, sinus, nasopharynx, and orbit (155-174). External beam doses of less than 3000 rads, in daily fractions of no more than 200 rads, are be-

lieved to be significantly less likely to lead to radiation retinopathy, but the condition has been reported following dosages of 1500 to 2000 rads (157,159,161,171,172). Significantly higher doses of local radiation modalities (plaques, implants) may be needed to produce equivalent disease (161).

Radiation retinopathy usually presents 6 months to 3 years after treatment but may occur several weeks to decades later (156,157,160,161,165,170,171,173,175,176). There may be a slightly shorter latency period with plaque treatment (161). The retinopathy is usually slowly progressive. The condition is often more severe in patients receiving chemotherapy and those with diabetes (155,161, 167,170,173,176,177). Other diseases that compromise retinal circulation, such as hypertension and collagen vascular disease, have also been postulated as risk factors for the development or exacerbation of radiation retinopathy (168,170). Some patients with hereditary retinoblastoma may have a defect in the repair of x-ray-induced DNA damage and show an unusually severe response to radiation therapy (165).

Pathology and Pathogenesis

The damage to the retina, choroid, and optic nerve in radiation retinopathy is probably a result of primary vascular insult, with occlusion and decompensation (157,160, 161,163,167,177). Studies in monkeys have shown involvement of both the retinal vasculature and the choriocapillaris, with a focal decrease in pericytes and capillary endothelial cells as the earliest change. Capillary nonperfusion is the next abnormality detected. These areas become confluent and correspond to cotton wool spots seen clinically. Smaller vessels are occluded before larger vessels. Studies in human beings have shown similar findings—early endothelial cell loss, limited recanalization, vessel fenestration, and thickening of some vascular walls with secondary lumens (161,163,165,172,177). These changes may be among the most consistent lesions in radiation retinopathy. Other retinal vascular changes include degenerative changes of the media and adventitia, loss of endothelial cells and pericytes, multifocal inner retinal ischemic atrophy, RPE changes, and cystic intraretinal changes and exudates (165,172,177). Ganglion cell death and subsequent nerve fiber layer atrophy may be a primary effect or secondary to the glaucoma also seen in certain patients. Photoreceptors are more resistant than the inner retina to radiation changes and thus show less damage. Narrowing of the posterior ciliary arteries secondary to myointimal proliferation has also been noted. Ischemic optic nerve changes also occur (radiation neuropathy).

Clinical Features

Patients often present with symptoms of blurred vision, either mild or severe, or floaters (155,157,160,161,169,172,

173). The most common signs on examination include intraretinal hard exudates and hemorrhage, telangiectasis of retinal capillaries, microaneurysms, and cotton wool spots (155,157-162,166-171,173,174). Other changes include intraretinal and macular edema, RPE hyperplasia or atrophy, vascular sheathing, arterial attenuation and occlusion, and segmental vascular dilatation (Fig. 8.11A and B). Proliferative retinopathy (of the disc or elsewhere) with sequelae including vitreous hemorrhage and traction retinal detachment may be seen. CNV has been reported (165,172,174). Radiation retinopathy is generally most severe in the posterior pole; as reflected in animal studies, the smallest vessels are affected first, and the largest last (160,161). The retinopathy following external beam modalities is usually more severe than that following local modalities. Numerous extraretinal findings such as papillitis and optic atrophy, cataract, corneal changes, and rubeosis iridis are common. Local infarcts of the choroid following cobalt 60 plaques for retinoblastoma have also been reported (164).

Fluorescein Angiography

Fluorescein angiography readily demonstrates the angiopathic nature of this disease (155,157,159-161,166,167, 169,174,175). Capillary nonperfusion can be extensive (Fig. 8.11C), and, if severe, occlusion of larger arterioles may be seen. Irregular, telangiectatic capillaries and microaneurysms often leak, and further leakage may be noted at the disc or from areas of neovascularization. Hyperfluorescence or hypofluorescence due to pigmentary alterations and defects are common in chronic and severe cases.

Prognosis and Treatment

Laser photocoagulation has been reported to be useful in the treatment of macular edema associated with radiation retinopathy (157,166,168,169,174). Indications and techniques similar to those developed for diabetic macular edema can be used to direct treatment. In one report,

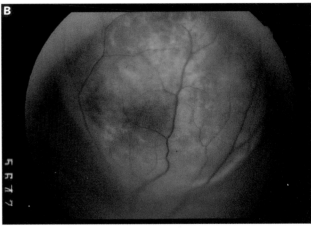

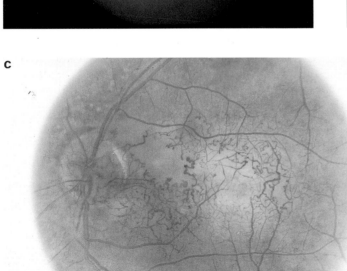

Fig. 8.11 Man, aged 48, with gradually progressive visual distortion 8 months after external beam irradiation (proton beam) for choroidal melanoma. A, Note the macular edema with exudates, cotton wool spots, and vascular sheathing, consistent with the diagnosis of radiation retinopathy. B, Large choroidal melanoma superior to the optic nerve, stable without growth following proton beam irradiation. C, Fluorescein angiogram from the same patient. Note the prominent capillary dropout, microaneurysms, and telangiectasis. Late views showed diffuse leakage.

argon green laser applications at settings of 50 to 100 μm and 0.05 to 0.1 sec were applied to focal microaneurysms and other sites of leakage (157). Alternatively, a grid pattern with spacing of approximately one burn-width was used for areas of diffuse leakage and capillary nonperfusion associated with macular edema. Other investigators have reported effectively stopping leakage from telangiectatic parafoveal vessels and microaneurysms using the krypton laser (50 to 100 μm, 0.05 sec in a grid pattern to the RPE in the area of the vascular changes; 166). Additional light treatments may be necessary. For proliferative retinopathy, panretinal photocoagulation has been effective in inducing regression (157,175). Early treatment of radiation retinopathy has been suggested for macular edema or neovascularization because the prognosis is generally poor without treatment (166,174). Cases most likely to benefit from treatment include those with mild to moderate edema without cystoid changes, severe nonperfusion, or severe visual loss. Significant macular ischemia is a contraindication to laser treatment. Because there is some variability in the amount of radiation exposure necessary to produce radiation retinopathy, repeated evaluation of patients receiving as little as 2000 rads should be performed for at least 3 years after radiation treatment (159,174,176).

Nonarterial Macroaneurysms

Macroaneurysms may develop from retinal veins, capillaries, or collateral vessels following venous occlusion (178-181). These macroaneurysms tend to be saccular and may arise multiply in a given eye. They are similar in size to arterial macroaneurysms and have been graded as small (100 to 149 μm), medium (150 to 249 μm), and large (250 μm or larger; 180). Most are of medium size. These nonarterial macroaneurysms are found in the areas of distribution of the occluded vein and are associated with retinal ischemia and capillary nonperfusion. This ischemia, combined with elevated hydrostatic pressure, has been postulated to play a role in the development of these macroaneurysms.

On fluorescein angiography, venous macroaneurysms are usually associated with major branch veins or venules and are well circumscribed, saccular lesions that hyperfluoresce in the mid to late phases of the angiogram. Capillary macroaneurysms appear to be on the venous side and fill from adjacent capillary beds. Filling is delayed, and there may be late staining of the walls as well as adjacent capillary bed irregularity. Macroaneurysms of collateral vessels are usually obvious.

Nonarterial macroaneurysms have been associated with surrounding retinal edema, serous macular detachment, intraretinal hemorrhage, and exudates. These lesions usually do not affect visual acuity, but if these complications affect the macula, photocoagulation may be indicated. Argon laser treatment has been used to obliterate capillary macroaneurysms and to treat venous aneurysms indirectly, with some visual benefit. Before treatment, the visual impact of the macroaneurysm must be carefully weighed against other potential coincident causes of visual loss (CME, ischemia, neovascularization, vitreous hemorrhage, etc).

Cystoid Macular Edema

In aphakic or pseudophakic CME associated with vitreous strand incarceration in the surgical wound, several investigators have used yttrium-aluminum-garnet (YAG) vitreolysis, with variable success in improving vision (182-186). Most clinical studies done to date, however, have been small, nonrandomized, and poorly controlled. Therefore, the efficacy of this technique is not well established (182,183,184,187,188). There is no clear correlation between CME and anterior anatomic derangement, and some investigators believe that response to YAG vitreolysis is the exception rather than the rule (183). However, in certain clinical situations, this technique may be useful, and significant complications are rare (182,184). Prophylactic vitreolysis is probably not warranted, and chronic CME is probably less likely to respond (182).

Vitreolysis is generally performed with a contact lens to enhance magnification, focus, and energy delivery (182,184). Treatment near the corneal scleral wound, where the vitreous strands are narrower and more easily visualized, is probably more effective. Disruption of the thinnest accessible distal portion of the strand is recommended (182). Single pulses of low energy (1.0 to 1.5 mJ) are usually sufficient. Several attempts over multiple sessions are often necessary to lyse the vitreous adhesions completely. Transient corneal stromal white opacities or small iris hemorrhages may occur, but these resolve spontaneously. Rare complications, including retinal detachment and elevated intraocular pressure, have also been reported (185). Prophylactic topical anti-inflammatory and antiglaucoma agents are commonly used.

Direct retinal photocoagulation of aphakic CME has been performed with various modes but has not been widely adopted (183,189,190).

Photocoagulation of CME associated with retinitis pigmentosa has also been attempted, with encouraging results (191). Argon green is used to place 100 μm, 0.1-sec applications in two to three rows around the macula, no closer than 500 μm from the center of the fovea. The energy level is titrated to produce a barely visible reaction. Additional clinical trials of this approach are required to define its efficacy fully. The available information is insufficient to warrant widespread recommendations, and it is probably premature to use laser photocoagulation to treat CME in retinitis pigmentosa (192).

References

1. Gass JDM. Pathogenesis of disciform detachment of the neuroepithelium. II. Idiopathic central serous retinopathy. Am J Ophthalmol 1967;63(suppl):1–139.

2. Gass JDM. Bullous retinal detachment. An unusual manifestation of idiopathic central serous choroidopathy. Am J Ophthalmol 1973;75:810–821.

3. Wessig A. Changing concept of central serous retinopathy and its treatment. Trans Am Acad Ophthalmol Otolaryngol 1973;77:275–280.

4. Klein ML, Van Buskirk M, Freidman E, Gragoudas E, Chandra S. Experience with nontreatment of central serous choroidopathy. Arch Ophthalmol 1974;91:247–250.

5. Schatz H. Central serous chorioretinopathy and serous detachment of the retinal pigment epithelium. Int Ophthalmol Clin 1975;15:159–169.

6. Gass JDM. Photocoagulation treatment of idiopathic central serous choroidopathy. Trans Am Acad Ophthalmol Otolarnyngol 1977;83:456–467.

7. Lyons DE. Conservative management of central serous retinopathy. Trans Ophthalmol Soc UK 1977;97:214–216.

8. Kayazawa F. Central serous choroidopathy with exudative retinal detachment. Ann Ophthalmol 1982;114:1035–1042.

9. Harada T, Harada K. Six cases of central serous choroidopathy induced by systemic corticosteroid therapy. Doc Ophthalmologica 1985;60:37–44.

10. Spitznas M, Huke J. Number, shape, and topography of leakage points in acute type 1 central serous retinopathy. Graefes Arch Clin Exp Ophthalmol 1987;225:437–440.

11. Roseman RL, Olk RJ. Grid laser photocoagulation for atypical central serous chorioretinopathy. Ophthalmic Surg 1988;19:786–791.

12. Levine R, Brucker AJ, Robinson F. Long-term follow-up of idiopathic central serous chorioretinopathy by fluorescein angiography. Ophthalmology 1989;96:854–859.

13. Mutlak JA, Dutton GN. Fluorescein angiographic features of acute central serous retinopathy. Acta Ophthalmologica 1989;67:467–469.

14. Schatz H, Madeira D, Johnson RN, McDonald HR. Central serous chorioretinopathy occurring in patients 60 years of age and older. Ophthalmology 1992;99:63–67.

15. Fine SL, Owens SL. Central serous retinopathy in a 7-year-old girl. Am J Ophthalmol 1980;90:871–873.

16. Blair NP, Brockhurst RJ, Lee W. Central serous choroidopathy in Hallermann-Streiff syndrome. Ann Ophthalmol 1981;13:987–990.

17. Robertson DM. Argon laser photocoagulation treatment in central serous chorioretinopathy. Ophthalmology 1986;93:972–974.

18. O'Connor PR. Multifocal serous choroidopathy. Ann Ophthalmol 1975;7:237–245.

19. Mandelcorn M, Mednick E. Eccentric serous choroidopathy: a case report. Can J Ophthalmol 1979;14:102–105.

20. Yannuzzi LA. Type-A behavior and central serous chorioretinopathy. Retina 1987;7:111–130.

21. Weinberger D, Kremer I, Sira IB. The treatment of foveal central serous choroidopathy by krypton red laser. Ann Ophthalmol 1990;22:35–38.

22. Cruysberg JRM, Deutman AF. Visual disturbances during pregnancy caused by central serous choroidopathy. Br J Ophthalmol 1982;66:240–241.

23. Fastenberg DM, Ober RR. Central serous choroidopathy in pregnancy. Arch Ophthalmol 1983;101:1055–1058.

24. Lewis ML. Coexisting central serous choroidopathy and retinitis pigmentosa. South Med J 1980;73:77–80.

25. Piccolino FC. Central serous chorioretinopathy: some considerations on the pathogenesis. Ophthalmologica 1981;182:204–210.

26. Yannuzzi LA, Shakin JL, Fisher YL, Altomonte MA. Peripheral retinal detachments and retinal pigment epithelial atrophic tracts secondary to central serous pigment epitheliopathy. Ophthalmology 1984;91:1554–1572.

27. Spitznas M. Pathogenesis of central serous retinopathy: a new working hypothesis. Graefes Arch Clin Exp Ophthalmol 1986;224:321–324.

28. Mazzuca DE, Benson WE. Central serous retinopathy: variants. Surv Ophthalmol 1986;31:170–174.

29. Slusher MM. Krypton red laser photocoagulation in selected cases of central serous chorioretinopathy. Retina 1986;6:81–84.

30. Urrets-Zavalia A. Recurrence of central serous choroidopathy after photocoagulation. Can J Ophthalmol 1973;8:404–407.

31. Robertson DM, Ilstrup D. Direct, indirect, and sham laser photocoagulation in the management of central serous chorioretinopathy. Am J Ophthalmol 1983;95:457–466.

32. Mutlak JA, Dutton GN, Zeini M, Allan D, Wail A. Central visual function in patients with resolved central serous retinopathy. Acta Ophthalmologica 1989;67:532–536.

33. Annesley WH, Augsburger JJ, Shakin JL. Ten year follow-up of photocoagulated central serous choroidopathy. Trans Am Ophthalmol Soc 1981;79:335–346.

34. Gilbert M, Owens SL, Smith PD, Fine SL. Long-term follow-up of central serous chorioretinopathy. Br J Ophthalmol 1984;68:815–820.

35. Leaver P, Williams C. Argon laser photocoagulation in the treatment of central serous retinopathy. Br J Ophthalmol 1979;63:674–677.

36. Kayazawa F, Yamamoto T, Itoi M. Temporal contrast sensitivity in central serous choroidopathy. Ann Ophthalmol 1982;14:272–275.

37. van Meel GJ, Smith VC, Pokorny J, van Norren D. Foveal densitometry in central serous choroidopathy. Am J Ophthalmol 1984;98:359–368.

38. Folk JC, Thompson S, Han DP, Brown CK. Visual function abnormalities in central serous retinopathy. Arch Ophthalmol 1984;102:1299–1302.

39. Chuang EL, Sharp DM, Fitzke FW, Kemp CM, Holden L, Bird AC. Retinal dysfunction in central serous retinopathy. Eye 1987;1:120–125.

40. Landers MB, Shaw HE, Anderson WB, Sinyai AJ. Argon laser treatment of central serous chorioretinopathy. Ann Ophthalmol 1977;9:1567–1572.

41. Novak MA, Singerman LJ, Rice TA. Krypton and argon laser photocoagulation for central serous chorioretinopathy. Retina 1987;7:162–169.

42. Ficker L, Vafidis G, While A, Leaver P. Longterm results of treatment of central serous retinopathy—a preliminary report. Trans Ophthalmol Soc UK 1986;105:473–475.

43. Watzke RC, Burton TC, Woolson RF. Direct and indirect laser photocoagulation of central serous choroidopathy. Am J Ophthalmol 1979;88:914–918.

44. Gomolin JES. Choroidal neovascularization and central serous chorioretinopathy. Can J Ophthalmol 1989;24:20–23.

45. Ficker L, Vafidis G, While A, Leaver P. Long-term follow-up of a prospective trial of argon laser photocoagulation in the treatment of central serous retinopathy. Br J Ophthalmol 1988;72:829–834.

46. Jalkh AE, Jabbour N, Avila MP, Trempe CL, Schepens CL. Retinal pigment epithelium decompensation. II. Laser treatment. Ophthalmology 1984;91:1549–1553.

47. Chopdar S. Retinal telangiectasis in adults: fluorescein angiographic findings and treatment by argon laser. Br J Ophthalmol 1978;62:243–250.

48. Hutton WL, Snyder WB, Fuller D, Vaiser A. Focal parafoveal retinal telangiectasis. Arch Ophthalmol 1978;96:1362–1367.

49. Gass JDM. Idiopathic juxtafoveal retinal telangiectasia. Arch Ophthalmol 1982;100:769–780.

50. Millay RH, Klein ML, Handelman IL, Watzke RC. Abnormal glucose metabolism and parafoveal telangiectasia. Am J Ophthalmol 1986;102.363–370.

51. Chew EY, Murphy RP, Newsome DA, Fine SL. Parafoveal telangiectasis and diabetic retinopathy. Arch Ophthalmol 1986;104:71–75.

52. Casswell AG, Chaine G, Rush P, Bird AC. Paramacular telangiectasis. Trans Ophthalmol Soc UK 1986;105:683–692.

53. Green WR, Quigley HA, de la Cruz Z, Cohen B. Parafoveal retinal telangiectasis. Light and electron microscopy studies. Trans Ophthalmol Soc UK 1980;100:162–170.

54. Moisseiev J, Lewis H, Bartov E, Fine SL, Murphy RP. Superficial retinal refractile deposits in juxtafoveal telangiectasis. Am J Ophthalmol 1990;109:604–605.

55. Joondeph BC, Joondeph HC, Blair NP. Retinal macroaneurysms treated with the yellow dye laser. Retina 1989;9: 187–192.

56. Rabb MF, Gagliano DA, Teske MP. Retinal arterial macroaneurysm. Surv Ophthalmol 1988;33:73–96.

57. Lavin ML, Marsh RJ, Peart S, Rehman A. Retinal arterial macroaneurysms: a retrospective study of 40 patients. Br J Ophthalmol 1987;71:817–825.

58. Abdel-Khalek MN, Richardson J. Retinal macroaneurysm: natural history and guidelines for treatment. Br J Ophthalmol 1986;70:2–11.

59. Palestine AG, Robertson DM, Goldstein BG. Macroaneurysms of the retinal arteries. Am J Ophthalmol 1982;93: 164–171.

60. Asdourian GK, Goldberg MF, Jampol L, Rabb M. Retinal macroaneurysms. Arch Ophthalmol 1977;95:624–628.

61. Cleary PE, Kohner EM, Hamilton AM, Bird AC. Retinal macroaneurysms. Br J Ophthalmol 1975;59:355–361.

62. Robertson DM. Macroaneurysms of the retinal arteries. Trans Am Acad Ophthalmol Otolarnyngol 1973;77:55–67.

63. Hudomel J, Imre G. Photocoagulation treatment of the solitary aneurysm near the macula lutea. Acta Ophthalmologica 1973;51:633–638.

64. Gold DH, La Piana F, Zimmerman LE. Isolated retinal arterial aneurysms. Am J Ophthalmol 1976;82:848–857.

65. Khalil M, Lorenzette DWC. Acquired retinal macroaneurysms. Can J Ophthalmol 1979;14:163–168.

66. Giuffre G, Montalto FP, Amodei G. Development of an isolated retinal macroaneurysm of the cilioretinal artery. Br J Ophthalmol 1987;71:445–448.

67. Panton RW, Goldberg MF, Farber MD. Retinal arterial macroaneurysms: risk factors and natural history. Br J Ophthalmol 1990;74:595–600.

68. Nadel AJ, Gupta KK. Macroaneurysms of the retinal arteries. Arch Ophthalmol 1976;94:1092–1096.

69. Fichte C, Streeten BW, Friedman AH. A histopathologic study of retinal artery aneurysms. Am J Ophthalmol 1978;85; 509–518.

70. Lewis RA, Norton EW, Gass JDM. Acquired arterial macroaneurysms of the retina. Br J Ophthalmol 1987;60:21–30.

71. Tilanus MD, Hoyng C, Deutman AF, Cruysberg, Aandekerk A. Congenital arteriovenous communications and the development of two types of leaking retinal macroaneurysms. Am J Ophthalmol 1991;112:31–33.

72. Shults WT, Swan KC. Pulsatile aneurysms of the retinal arterial tree. Am J Ophthalmol 1974;77:304–309.

73. Mainster MA, Whitacre MM. Dye yellow photocoagulation of retinal arterial macroaneurysms. Am J Ophthalmol 1988; 105:97–98.

74. Russell SP. Retina 1990;10:229. Letter.

75. Joondeph HC, Joondeph BC. Retina 1990;10:321. Letter.

76. Russell SR, Folk JC. Branch retinal artery occlusion after dye yellow photocoagulation of an arterial macroaneurysm. Am J Ophthalmol 1987;104:186–187.

77. Gass JDM. A fluorescein angiographic study of macular dysfunction secondary to retinal vascular disease. V. Retinal telangiectasis. Arch Ophthalmol 1968;80:592–605.

78. McGrand JC. Photocoagulation in Coats' disease. Trans Ophthalmol Soc UK 1970; 90:47–56.

79. Ridley ME, Shields JA, Brown GC, Tasman W. Coats' disease. Evaluation of management. Ophthalmology 1982;89:1381–1387.

80. Egerer I, Tasman W, Tomer TL. Coats disease. Arch Ophthalmol 1974;92:109–112.

81. Harris GS. Coats' disease, diagnosis and treatment. Can J Ophthalmol 1970;5:311–320.

82. Gomez-Morales A. Coats' disease. Natural history and results of treatment. Am J Ophthalmol 1965;60:855–865.

83. Skuta GL, France TD, Stevens TS, Laxova R. Apparent Coats' disease and pericentric inversion of chromosome 3. Am J Ophthalmol 1987;104:84–86.

84. Tolmie JL, Brown BH, McGettrick PM, Stephenson JBP. A familial syndrome with Coats' reaction retinal angiomas, hair and nail defects and intracranial calcification. Eye 1988;2:297–303.

85. Kondra L, Cangemi FE, Pitta CG. Alport's syndrome and retinal telangiectasis. Ann Ophthalmol 1983;15:550–551.

86. Gurwin EB, Fitzsimons RB, Sehmi KS, Bird AC. Retinal telangiectasis in facioscapulohumeral muscular dystrophy. Arch Ophthalmol 1985;103:1695–1700.

87. Schuman JS, Lieberman KV, Freidman AH, Berger M, Schoeneman MJ. Senior-Loken syndrome (familial renal-retinal dystrophy) and Coats' disease. Am J Ophthalmol 1985;100:822–827.

88. Tripathi K, Ashton N. Electron microscopical study of Coats' disease. Br J Ophthalmol 1971;55:289–301.

89. Green WR. Bilateral Coats' disease. Massive gliosis of the retina. Arch Ophthalmol 1967;77:378–383.

90. McGettrick PM, Loeffler KU. Bilateral Coats' disease in an infant (a clinical, angiographic, light and electron microscopic study). Eye 1987;1:136–145.

91. DeSai UR, Sabates FN. Long-term follow-up of facioscapulohumeral muscular dystrophy and Coats' disease. Am J Ophthalmol 1990;110:568–569.

92. Pe'er J. Calcification on Coats' disease. Am J Ophthalmol 1988;106:742–743.

93. Farkas TG, Potts AM, Boone C. Some pathological and biochemical aspects of Coats' disease. Am J Ophthalmol 1973;75:289–301.

94. Deutsch TA, Rabb MF, Jampol LM. Spontaneous regression of retinal lesions in Coats' disease. Can J Ophthalmol 1982;17.169–172.

95. Lee ST, Friedman SM, Rubin ML. Cystoid macular edema secondary to juxtafoveal telangiectasis in Coats' disease. Ophthalmic Surg 1991;22:218–221.

96. Tarkkanen A, Laatikainen L. Coats's disease: clinical, angiographic, histopathological findings and clinical management. Br J Ophthalmol 1983;67:766–776.

97. Sneed SR, Blodi CF, Pulido JS. Treatment of Coats' disease with the binocular indirect argon laser photocoagulator. Arch Ophthalmol 1989;107:789–790.

98. Arrig PG, Lahav M, Hutchins RK, Weiter JJ. Pigmentary retinal degeneration and Coats' disease: a case study. Ophthalmic Surg 1988;19:432–436.

99. Yimoyines DJ, Topilow HW, Abedin S, McMeel J. Bilateral peripapillary exophytic retinal hemangioblastoma. Ophthalmology 1982;89:1388–1392.

100. Gass JDM. Treatment of retinal vascular anomalies. Trans Am Acad Ophthalmol Otolarnyngol 1977;83:432–445.

101. Apple DJ, Goldberg MF, Wyhinny GJ. Argon laser treatment of von Hippel-Lindau retinal angiomas. II. Histopathology of treated lesions. Arch Ophthalmol 1974;92:126–130.

102. Hardwig P, Robertson DM. von Hippel-Lindau disease: a familial, often lethal, multisystem phakomatosis. Ophthalmology 1984;91:263–270.

103. Mottow-Lippa L, Tso MOM, Peyman GA, Chejfec G. von Hippel angiomatosis. A light, electron microscopic, and immunoperoxidase characterization. Ophthalmology 1983;90:848–855.

104. Schindler RF, Sarin LK, MacDonald PR. Hemangiomas of the optic disc. Can J Ophthalmol 1975;10:304–318.

105. Gass JDM, Braunstein R. Sessile and exophytic capillary angiomas of the juxtapapillary region and optic nerve head. Arch Ophthalmol 1980;98:1790–1797.

106. Welch RB. von Hippel-Lindau disease: the recognition and treatment of early angiomatosis retinae and the use of cryosurgery as an adjunct to therapy. Trans Am Ophthalmol Soc 1970;68:367–424.

107. Ridley M, Green J, Johnson G. Retinal angiomatosis: the ocular manifestations of von Hippel-Lindau disease. Can J Ophthalmol 1976;21:276–283.

108. Melmon KL, Rosen SW. Lindau's disease. Review of the literature and study of a large kindred. Am J Med 1964;36:595–617.

109. Blodi CF, Russell SR, Pulido JS, Folk JC. Direct and feeder vessel photocoagulation of retinal angiomas with dye yellow laser. Ophthalmology 1990;97:791–797.

110. DeJong PTVM, Verkaart RJF, van de Vooren MJ, Majoor-Krakauer DF, Wiegel AR. Twin vessels in von Hippel-Lindau disease. Am J Ophthalmol 1988;105:165–169.

111. Medlock RD, Shields JA, Shields CL, Yarian DL, Beyrer CR. Retinal hemangioma-like lesions in eyes with retinitis pigmentosa. Retina 1990;10:274–277.

112. Kollaritis CR, Mehelas TJ, Shealy TR, Zahn JR. Von Hippel tumors in siblings with retinitis pigmentosa. Ann Ophthalmol 1982;14:256–259.

113. Dobyns WB, Michels VV, Groover RV, et al. Familial cavernous malformation of the central nervous system and retina. Ann Neurol 1987;21:579–583.

114. Annesley WH, Leonard BC, Shields JA, Tasman WS. Fifteen year review of treated cases of retinal angiomatosis. Trans Am Acad Ophthalmol Otolarnyngol 1977;83:446–453.

115. Lane CM, Turner G, Gregor ZJ, Bird AC. Laser treatment of retinal angiomatosis. Eye 1989;3:33–38.

116. Usher CH. On a few hereditary eye affections. Trans Ophthalmol Soc UK 1935;55:164–193.

117. Whitson JT, Welch RB, Green WR. Von Hippel-Lindau disease: case report of a patient with spontaneous regression of a retinal angioma. Retina 1986;6:253–259.

118. Nicholson DH, Green WR, Kenyon KR. Light and electron microscopic study of early lesions in angiomatosis retinae. Am J Ophthalmol 1976;82:193–204.

119. Sellors PJ, Archer D. The management of retinal angiomatosis. Trans Ophthalmol Soc UK 1970;89:529–543.

120. Lowden BA, Harris GS. Pheochromocytoma and von Hippel-Lindau's disease. Can J Ophthalmol 1976;11: 282–288.

121. Goldberg MF, Koenig S. Argon laser treatment of von Hippel-Lindau retinal angiomas. Arch Ophthalmol 1974; 92:121–124.

122. Peyman GA, Rednam KRV, Mottow-Lippa L, Flood T. Treatment of large von Hippel tumors by eye wall resection. Ophthalmology 1983;90:840–847.

123. Kremer I, Gilad E, Ben-Sira I. Juxtapapillary exophytic retinal capillary hemangioma treated by yellow krypton (568 nm) laser photocoagulation. Ophthalmic Surg 1988;19:743–747.

124. Nicholson DH, Anderson LS, Blodi C. Rhegmatogenous retinal detachment in angiomatosis retinae. Am J Ophthalmol 1986;101:187–189.

125. Laatikainen L, Immonen I, Summanen P. Peripheral retinal angiomalike lesion and macular pucker. Am J Ophthalmol 1989;108:563–566.

126. Schwartz PL, Trubowitsi G, Fastenberg DM, Stein M. Macular pucker and retinal angioma. Ophthalmic Surg 1987;18:677–679.

127. Schwartz PL, Fastenberg DM, Shakin JL. Management of macular puckers associated with retinal angiomas. Ophthalmic Surg 1990;21:550–556.

128. Drummond JW, Hall D, Steen WH, Lusk JE. Cavernous hemangioma of the optic disc. Ann Ophthalmol 1980;12:1017–1018.

129. Klein M, Goldberg MF, Cotlier E. Cavernous hemangioma of the retina: report of four cases. Ann Ophthalmol 1975;7:1213–1221.

130. Gass JDM. Cavernous hemangioma of the retina. A neuro-oculo-cutaneous syndrome. Am J Ophthalmol 1971;71:799–814.

131. Lewis RA, Cohen MH, Wise GN. Cavernous hemangioma of the retina and optic disc. A report of three cases and a review of the literature. Br J Ophthalmol 1975;59:422–434.

132. Colvard DM, Robertson DM, Trautmann JC. Cavernous hemangioma of the retina. Arch Ophthalmol 1978;96: 2042–2044.

133. Moffat KP, Lee MS, Ghosh M. Retinal cavernous hemangioma. Can J Ophthalmol 1988;23:133–135.

134. Gautier-Smith PC, Sanders MD, Sanderson KV. Ocular and nervous system involvement in angioma serpiginosum. Br J Ophthalmol 1971;55:433–443.

135. Pancurak J, Goldberg MF, Frenkel M, Crowell RM. Cavernous hemangioma of the retina. Genetic and central nervous system involvement. Retina 1985;5:215–220.

136. Yamaguchi K, Yamaguchi K, Tamai M. Cavernous hemangioma of the retina in a pediatric patient. Ophthalmologica 1988;197:127–129.

137. Schwartz AC, Weaver RG, Bloomfield R, Tyler M. Cavernous hemangioma of the retina, cutaneous angiomas, and intracranial vascular lesion by computed tomography and nuclear magnetic resonance imaging. Am J Ophthalmol 1984;98:483–487.

138. Goldberg RE, Pheasant TR, Shields JA. Cavernous hemangiomas of the retina. A four-generation pedigree with neurocutaneous manifestations and an example of bilateral retinal involvement. Arch Ophthalmol 1979;97:2321–2324.

139. Bottoni F, Canevini MP, Canger R, Orzalesi N. Twin vessels in familial cavernous hemangioma. Am J Ophthalmol 1990;109:285–289.

140. Messmer E, Font RL, Laqua H, Hopping W, Naumann G. Cavernous hemangioma of the retina. Immunohistochemical and ultrastructural observations. Arch Ophthalmol 1984;102:413–418.

141. Archer DB, Deutman A, Ernests JT, Krill AE. Arteriovenous communications of the retina. Am J Ophthalmol 1973;75:225–241.

142. Mansour AM, Walsh JB, Henkind P. Arteriovenous anastomoses of the retina. Ophthalmology 1987;94:35–40.

143. Font RL, Ferry AP. The phakomatoses. Int Ophthalmol Clin 1972;12:1–50.

144. De Jong PTVM. Neovascular glaucoma and the occurrence of twin vessels in congenital arteriovenous communications of the retina. Doc Ophthalmol 1988;68:205–212.

145. Chakravarty A, Chatterjee S. Retino-cephalic vascular malformation. JAPI 1990;38:941–943.

146. Cameron ME. Congenital arterio-venous aneurysm of the retina. Br J Ophthalmol 1958;42:655.

147. Wyburn-Mason R. Arteriovenous aneurysm of midbrain and retina, facial naevi and mental changes. Brain 1943;66:164–203.

148. Cameron ME, Greer CH. Congenital arterio-venous aneurysm of the retina. A postmortem report. Br J Ophthalmol 1968;52:768–772.

149. Effron L, Zakov ZN, Tomsak RL. Neovascular glaucoma as a complication of the Wyburn-Mason syndrome. J Clin Neuro Ophthalmol 1985;5:95–98.

150. Iplikcioglu AC, Ozek MM, Ozean OE, Cizmeli O, Saglam S. Bilateral arteriovenous malformations of the choroid plexus and retina. Neurosurgery 1990;27:302–305.

151. Brodsky MC, Hoyt WF, Higashida RT, Hieshima GB, Halbach VV. Bonnet-Dechaume-Blanc Syndrome with large facial angioma. Arch Ophthalmol 1987;105:844–845.

152. Mansour AM, Wells CG, Jampol LM, Kalina RE. Ocular complications of arteriovenous communications of the retina. Arch Ophthalmol 1989;107:232–236.

153. Brown GC, Donoso LA, Magargal LE, Goldberg RE, Sarin LK. Congenital retinal macrovessels. Arch Ophthalmol 1982;100:1430–1436.

154. Varma R, Goldberg RE, Spaeth GL. Applications of digital image analysis: the topography of an optic disc coloboma and alterations in the retinal vessels in an arteriovenous malformation. Trans Pa Acad Ophthalmol Otolaryngol 1987;39:588–591.

155. Kinyoun JL, Kalina RE, Brower SA, Mills RP, Johnson RH. Radiation retinopathy after orbital irradication for Grave's ophthalmopathy. Arch Ophthalmol 1984;102:1473–1476.

156. Kinyoun JL, Orcutt JC. Radiation retinopathy. JAMA 1987;258:610–611. Letter.

157. Kinyoun JL, Chittum ME, Wells CG. Photocoagulation treatment of radiation retinopathy. Am J Ophthalmol 1988;105:470–478.

158. Nikoskelainen E, Joensuu H. Retinopathy after irradiation for Graves' ophthalmopathy. Lancet 1989;2:690–691. Letter.

159. Miller ML, Goldberg SH, Bullock JD. Radiation retinopathy after standard radiotherapy for thyroid-related ophthalmopathy. Am J Ophthalmol 1991; 112:600–601. Letter.

160. Hayreh SS. Post-radiation retinopathy. A fluorescence fundus angiographic study. Br J Ophthalmol 1970;54:705–714.

161. Brown GC, Shields JA, Sanborn G, Augsburger JJ, Savino PJ, Schatz NJ. Ophthalmology 1982;89:1494–1501.

162. Egbert PR, Donaldson SS, Moazed K, Rosenthal R. Visual results and ocular complications following radiotherapy for retinoblastoma. Arch Ophthalmol 1978;96:1826–1830.

163. Egbert PR, Fajardo LF, Donaldson SS, Moazed K. Posterior ocular abnormalities after irradiation for retinoblastoma: a histopathological study. Br J Ophthalmol 1980;64:660–665.

164. Ellmassri A. Radiation chorioretinopathy. Br J Ophthalmol 1986;70:326–329.

165. Albert DM, Walton DS, Weichselbaum RR, et al. Fibroblast radiosensitivity and intraocular fibrovascular proliferation following radiotherapy for bilateral retinoblastoma. Br J Ophthalmol 1986;70:336–342.

166. Axer-Siegel R, Kremer I, Ben-Sira I, Weiss J. Radiation retinopathy treated with red krypton laser. Ann Ophthalmol 1989;21:272–276.

167. Viebahn M, Barricks ME, Osterloh MD. Synergism between diabetic and radiation retinopathy: case report and review. Br J Ophthalmol 1991;75:629–632.

168. Chee PH. Radiation retinopathy. Am J Ophthalmol 1968;66:860–865.

169. Gass JDM. A fluorescein angiographic study of macular dysfunction secondary to retinal vascular disease. VI. X-ray irradiation, carotid artery occlusion, collagen vascular disease, and vitritis. Arch Ophthalmol 1968;80:606–617.

170. Wara WM, Irvine AR, Neger RE, Howes EL, Phillips TL. Radiation retinopathy. Int J Radiat Oncol Biol Phys 1979;5:81–83.

171. Bagan SM. Radiation retinopathy after irradiation of intracranial lesions. Am J Ophthalmol 1979;88:694–697.

172. Boozalis GT, Schachat AP, Green WR. Subretinal neovascularization from the retina in radiation retinopathy. Retina 1987;7:156–161.

173. Midena E, Segato T, Piermarrocchi S, Corti L, Zorat PL, Moro F. Retinopathy following radiation therapy of paranasal sinus and nasopharyngeal carcinoma. Retina 1987;7:142–147.

174. Amoaku WMK, Archer DB. Fluorescein angiographic features, natural course, and treatment of radiation retinopathy. Eye 1990;4:657–667.

175. Chaudhuri PR, Austin DJ, Rosenthal AR. Treatment of radiation retinopathy. Br J Ophthalmol 1981;65:623–625.

176. Amoaku WMK, Archer DB. Cephalic radiation and retinal vasculopathy. Eye 1990;4:195–203.

177. Archer DB, Amoaku WMK, Gardiner TA. Radiation retinopathy—clinical, histopathological, ultrastructural, and experimental correlation. Eye 1991;5:239–251.

178. Schulman J, Jampol LM, Goldberg MF. Large capillary aneurysms secondary to retinal venous obstruction. Br J Ophthalmol 1981;65:36–41.

179. Sanborn GE, Magargal LE. Venous macroaneurysm associated with branch retinal vein obstruction. Ann Ophthalmol 1984;16:464–468.

180. Cousins SW, Flynn HW, Clarkson JG. Macroaneurysms associated with retinal branch vein occlusion. Am J Ophthalmol 1990;109:567–570.

181. Magargal LE, Augsburger JJ, Hyman D, Townsend R. Venous macroaneurysm following branch retinal obstruction. Ann Ophthalmol 1980;12:685–689.

182. Katzen LE, Fleischman JA. YAG laser treatment of cystoid macular edema. Am J Ophthalmol 1983;95:589–592.

183. Yannuzzi LA. A perspective on the treatment of aphakic cystoid macular edema. Surv Ophthalmol 1984;28(suppl): 540–543.

184. Levy JH, Pisacano AM. Clinical experience with Nd:YAG laser vitreolysis in the anterior segment. J Cataract Refract Surg 1987;13:548–550.

185. Tchah H, Rosenberg M, Larson RS, Lindstrom RL. Neodymium: YAG laser vitreolysis for treatment and prophylaxis of cystoid macular edema. Aust N Z J Ophthalmol 1989;17:179–183.

186. Steinert RF, Wasson PJ. Neodymium: YAG laser anterior vitreolysis for Irvine-Gass cystoid macular edema. J Cataract Refract Surg 1989;15:304–307.

187. Reese LT. YAG laser treatment of cystoid macular edema. Am J Ophthalmol 1983;96:556. Letter.

188. Weingeist TA. YAG laser treatment of cystoid macular edema. Am J Ophthalmol 1983;96:407–409. Letter.

189. Saggau DD, Singerman LJ. Cystoid macular edema: causes, diagnosis, and treatment. In: Weinstock FJ, ed. Management and care of the cataract patient. Boston: Blackwell Scientific Publications, 1992.

190. Jampol LM, Sanders DR, Kraff MC. Prophylaxis and therapy of aphakic cystoid macular edema. Surv Ophthalmol 1984;28(suppl):535–539.

191. Newsome DA, Blacharski PA. Grid photocoagulation for macular edema in patients with retinitis pigmentosa. Am J Ophthalmol 1987;103:161–166.

192. Heckenlively JR. Grid photocoagulation for macular edema in patients with retinitis pigmentosa. Am J Ophthalmol 1987;104:94. Letter.

9

Laser Surgery for Retinal Tears, Retinal Detachment, Vitrectomy, and Posterior Segment Tumors

David B. Karlin

Retinal Tears

Historical Background

Before the noninvasive surgical development of lasers for retinal surgery, retinal tears were treated by intraoperative transcleral diathermy applications surrounding the break. This necessitated conjunctival dissection and resulted in scars in the sclera at places where the diathermy was applied. In the early 1960s, Lincoff and colleagues (1) introduced transconjunctival cryopexy as the treatment for retinal tears. In this procedure, a probe cooled by liquid nitrogen or carbon dioxide was applied to the intact conjunctival tissue overlying the retinal break to produce the chorioretinal adhesion. Conjunctiva and sclera were left relatively histopathologically intact, with most of the energy absorption taking place at the chorioretinal interface. However, with extensive treatment, a transient hyperemia, edema, iritis, and some discomfort were frequently produced.

The xenon arc photocoagulator (Fig. 9.1) developed by Meyer-Schwickerath (2) was the first instrument using white light to produce the necessary chorioretinal adhesion surrounding the retinal break. It was always used with the transpupillary approach. Its advantage was that it was noninvasive. Its disadvantage was that a retrobulbar anesthetic was required to reduce discomfort, photopsia, and ocular movement. The advent of retinal laser photocoagulation in the 1960s signalled the gradual demise of intraoperative diathermy and the cumbersome xenon arc photocoagulator as treatments of choice for retinal breaks.

The use of the laser for retinal tears has become the treatment of choice, especially when the tears are located at or posterior to the equator. It is also the preferred method in degenerative retinal disorders, especially in cases of lattice degeneration harboring retinal breaks. Rutnin and Schepens (3) and Byer (4) have shown that retinal tears may occur in as high as 7% of the population. Most of these eyes are asymptomatic. Only 1% to 2% of those eyes harboring retinal breaks will develop a retinal detachment according to Byer's study (4).

A retinal drawing of the fundus, using binocular indirect ophthalmoscopy, should be made before laser treatment. A Goldmann three-mirror lens examination is also advised. This permits greater magnification than that provided with the +20 diopter (D) condensing lens used with indirect ophthalmoscopy. Secondly, a Goldmann lens examination with slit-lamp biomicroscopy will determine if the ocular media are sufficiently clear to permit laser treatment through the slit-lamp delivery system.

Factors Contributing to Retinal Tear Formation

Many factors may lead to the formation of retinal tears. Myopia on the order of 2 to 10 D is a contributory factor because, as Karlin and Curtin (5) have shown, an increase in the axial length of the eye produces thinning and an increased incidence of tear formation in the retina. Many investigators believe the extremely myopic eye above 10 to 12 D is frequently immune from the development of retinal tears and retinal detachment. This is at least partially explainable on the basis of advanced chorioretinal degeneration in the periphery of such highly myopic eyes that produces a good chorioretinal adhesion between the pigment epithelium and the neurosensory retina. In addition, eyes above 10 to 15 D of myopia have almost a complete posterior vitreous detachment with complete syneresis of the vitreous body. This minimized the development of vitreoretinal adhesions, resulting in fewer retinal tears and detachments.

Aphakic and pseudophakic eyes are also at greater risk for the development of retinal tears and detachment than eyes still retaining the physiologic lens. Manipulations of the lens and zonules during cataract extraction produce forces that are transmitted to the peripheral retina, causing traction and the production of retinal tears. The study of Javitt and coworkers (6) demonstrated less risk of retinal tears and retinal detachment in patients undergoing planned extracapsular cataract extraction than in those eyes having intracapsular extraction. The main reason for this is that the posterior lens capsule is left intact. This prevents the vitreous from herniating forward anterior to the iris diaphragm, producing traction on the retina.

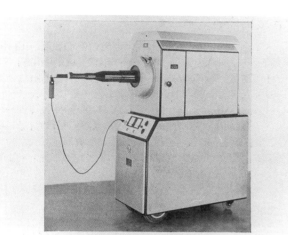

Fig. 9.1 The xenon arc light photocoagulator.

Phaco-emulsification, in which the posterior lens capsule is also left intact, has also lessened the incidence of retinal tears and retinal detachment. The recent study by Javitt and colleagues (7) has shown that once the posterior capsule has been violated through a yttrium-aluminum-garnet (YAG) laser capsulotomy, there is almost a fourfold increase in the incidence of retinal tears and retinal detachment. The latter study found that younger patients, male sex, and the Caucasian race were also associated with increased risk of retinal complications after extracapsular cataract extraction.

Today, proliferative diabetic retinopathy (PDR) has become a common predisposing factor leading to the development of traction retinal detachment (Fig. 9.2) with the formation of retinal breaks. Other blood dyscrasias, especially sickle cell retinopathy, predispose to retinal break formation. Trauma and retinopathy of prematurity are also causes of retinal tears. The rare hereditary disorders of Marfan's syndrome, juvenile retinoschisis, Goldmann-Favre syndrome, and Stickler's syndrome, may also contribute to the formation of retinal tears.

Lattice degeneration is one of the most common causes of retinal tears. This entity frequently accompanies progressive myopia and is discussed later in this chapter.

Technique of Laser Treatment of Retinal Tears

Topical anesthesia using proparacaine hydrochloride 0.5% is usually the only anesthetic required. Occasionally, when working in the macular area, akinesia and a retrobulbar anesthetic consisting of 4 ml Lidocaine 2% is given to prevent blepharospasm and extraocular muscle rotation, and to diminish photophobia.

Retinal tears should be completely surrounded by three concentric rows of laser application using 500- to 1000-μm size lesions (Fig. 9.3). The argon green or krypton laser wavelength is most commonly used. The duration of application is usually 0.2 sec. It is important to make the laser burns contiguous to ensure a good chorioretinal adhesion. It is also important to note that laser photocoagulation can frequently be given in those eyes in which a very flat elevation of the retina surrounds the retinal break. By increasing the power level or the duration time in such a case, one can frequently obtain an adequate 360° chorioretinal response.

The chorioretinal adhesion produced with argon and krypton laser photocoagulation results from the absorption of light energy by the retinal pigment epithelium (RPE). Light energy is converted into heat energy at the RPE level, causing an adhesion of the outer neurosensory retina, the RPE, and the inner layers of the choroid.

Anterior retinal tears located just posterior to the ora serrata are frequently difficult to treat with laser application in the older individual. Often, adequate laser reaction surrounding the anterior lip of the tear is

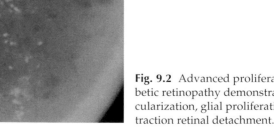

Fig. 9.2 Advanced proliferative diabetic retinopathy demonstrates neovascularization, glial proliferation, and a traction retinal detachment.

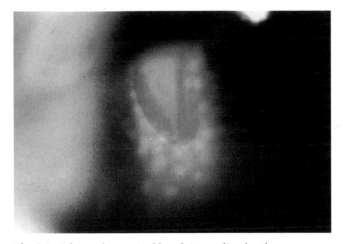

Fig. 9.3 A horseshoe retinal break immediately after argon green laser photocoagulation shows three rows of chorioretinal lesions immediately surrounding the edge of the tear.

difficult to obtain because peripheral cuneiform lenticular opacities are frequently present, preventing adequate visualiza-tion through a slit-lamp delivery system. Laser delivery through a binocular indirect ophthalmoscope may prove more effective. Failing this, transconjunctival cryopexy may offer an adequate alternative form of treatment, surrounding the anterior border of peripheral breaks.

Retinal tears may also cause vitreous hemorrhage, at times making it difficult to visualize the borders of the tear through a Goldmann lens via slit-lamp laser delivery. Again, laser delivery through an indirect ophthalmoscope or retinal cryopexy may be the treatment of choice because visualization of the tear with indirect ophthalmoscopy often proves much more acceptable. In cases where frank retinal detachment surrounds the retinal break, laser photocoagulation is contraindicated. Cryopexy with scleral buckling becomes the treatment of choice.

If at all possible, laser photocoagulation should be used rather than cryopexy for the treatment of retinal tears. Firstly, a subconjunctival injection of Lidocaine frequently has to be given before extensive cryopexy to minimize ocular discomfort. This procedure, coupled with the conjunctival applications by the cryoprobe itself, causes much more of an inflammatory conjunctival and uveitic reaction than laser photocoagulation. Secondly, retinal cryopexy produces a breakdown in the blood-retinal barrier with a lysis of RPE cells from the RPE. The liberation of peripheral RPE cells may result in their deposition posteriorly into the macular area with resulting metamorphopsia. In addition, extensive cryopexy, unlike extensive laser application, may increase the incidence of proliferative vitreoretinopathy (PVR). Lastly, a firm adhesion of the neurosensory retina to the pigment epithelium has been reported to occur within a matter of days with laser applications as contrasted to a week to 10 days for cryopexy as indicated by Lincoff and associates.

Lattice Degeneration

Lattice degeneration occurs in 8% to 10% of the population as shown in a study by Straatsma and coworkers (9). Karlin and Curtin (5) indicated lattice (Fig. 9.4) to be the most dangerous of all the peripheral chorioretinal degenerations. Approximately 35% of retinal detachments are associated with lattice degeneration according to Byer (10). The treatment of lattice degeneration remains controversial. Most surgeons would agree that if lattice degeneration without retinal breaks is discovered as an incidental finding in an asymptomatic eye, no treatment is necessary. The lattice should be "drawn but not quartered."

The controversy occurs in whether to treat lattice degeneration in which retinal tears are found within the area of the lattice. Two types of retinal tears can occur within the area of the lattice. Small, round retinal holes can be found anywhere in the involved area. Horseshoe retinal tears are seen at the ends of the lattice or at the posterior edge with the lattice located in the anterior flap (Fig. 9.5). Karlin and Curtin (5) have demonstrated that horseshoe breaks in areas of lattice are much more dangerous than small, round holes because the flap frequently exhibits vitreoretinal traction, which may lead to a retinal detachment. Most vitreoretinal surgeons would use laser to treat lattice with horseshoe retinal tears.

The controversy arises when one discovers lattice with small, round holes in an asymptomatic eye. Some retinal surgeons would treat all cases of lattice with small holes. Others would only treat lattice with holes located in the superior quadrants because superior tears are potentially more dangerous than inferior tears in leading to a retinal detachment. Lastly, other surgeons would only treat lattice with small holes if the location was in either the superior temporal or inferior temporal quadrants because the macula is more threatened than if the holes are located in the nasal quadrants.

All surgeons would agree that there are definite indications for the laser treatment of lattice degeneration

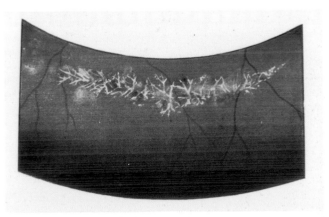

Fig. 9.4 Lattice degeneration shows the typical arborization of obliterated and sheathed retinal vessels.

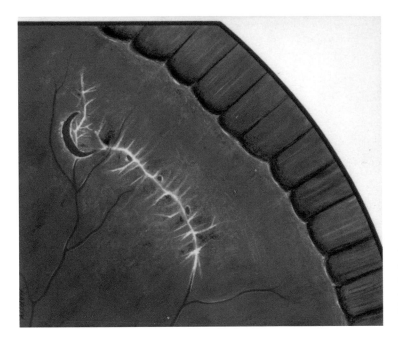

Fig. 9.5 Lattice degeneration exhibits the typical horseshoe retinal break located at the end or at the posterior edge of the lattice. Note that the lattice is located in the anterior flap. Small, round holes may be located anywhere within the area of lattice.

harboring any type of retinal break. If the patient sustained a retinal detachment in one eye and retinal tears were discovered in the fellow eye, laser photocoagulation should be performed, regardless of whether the breaks occurred in the area of lattice or independent of it. If retinal tears were discovered in an eye shortly to undergo cataract surgery, the eye should be treated with laser at least 2 weeks prior to anticipated cataract surgery. Similarly, if retinal breaks occur in an eye following cataract surgery, these breaks should be treated. Likewise, if retinal detachment occurred following cataract surgery in one eye, the fellow eye harboring retinal breaks should be treated. Laser therapy is also indicated in eyes having retinal breaks in which there is a strong familial history of retinal detachment or in which those eyes exhibit very high myopia. Retinal tears found in pseudophakic or aphakic eyes as well as in cases of Wagner's disease should also be treated.

Two to three rows of concentric laser burns of 500- to 1000-μm size should be placed contiguously completely surrounding the edge of normal retina adjacent to the area of lattice degeneration harboring retinal holes.

Risk Factors in Considering Treatment of Retinal Breaks

Many parameters have to be evaluated before determining whether to treat a retinal break. As stated previously, horseshoe retinal tears with elevated flaps signify much vitreoretinal traction and should be treated by laser photocoagulation before retinal detachment has a chance to develop. The small, round aphakic or pseudophakic tear occurring in the retinal periphery is much less likely to exhibit vitreous traction and is thus less dangerous. This is especially true when a freely floating operculum is seen overlying the atrophic hole. The fact that an operculum is present indicates that the vitreous traction no longer exists along the borders of the small hole because the vitreoretinal traction has succeeded in pulling a piece of retina into the vitreous cavity. It is important to remember to be semantically correct in noting that *tears have flaps* and *holes have opercula*. The tears with flaps are dangerous. Both retinal holes and horseshoe tears associated with elevated flaps should always be treated with laser if associated with symptoms of persistent photopsia. Flashes of light signify vitreoretinal traction on the retinal photoreceptors. Schepens has pointed out that photopsia limited to a single quadrant is much more ominous than flashes occurring 360°.

Lastly, this author believes that all retinal breaks occurring in eyes scheduled to have future YAG laser capsulotomy, miotic therapy for glaucoma, and any subsequent intraoperative procedure such as cataract surgery, should have prophylactic laser photocoagulation in an attempt to lessen the possibility of rhegmatogenous retinal detachment.

Selection of the Appropriate Laser and Contact Lens

The question is frequently asked about which laser to use to achieve maximum results. It should be emphasized that those lasers should be used that produce maximum heat absorption by the pigment of the RPE. The four lasers currently used with great effectiveness are argon blue-green, argon green, krypton, and the diode laser.

The argon and krypton lasers are gaseous, operating in the visual end of the spectrum, and require water cooling. The diode laser is a solid semiconductor laser, operating in the low infrared end of the spectrum, and is more compact because water cooling is not necessary. The argon green laser, operating at 514 nm, has become the laser of choice because maximum energy absorption occurs at the RPE level. The argon blue green laser, operating at 488 nm, is also absorbed by the RPE. However, argon blue-green is also absorbed by the vitreous. This feature may lead to vitreous contraction from heat produced in the vitreous cavity, with the possible development of PVR, which may result in a traction retinal detachment. Xanthophyll macula pigment together with xanthochrome lens pigment may also act as heat sinks when argon blue light is used. Blue light has been shown to be phototoxic to the retina and especially to its macular area. In fact, a study conducted within the Retina Society and Macula Society has shown that the phototoxic effect of argon blue may have resulted in less light sensitivity to some ophthalmologists constantly using the argon blue laser over many years' duration. The argon blue laser has therefore been largely replaced by argon green.

The gaseous krypton red laser, operating at 647.1 nm, and the solid-state semiconductor diode laser, operating at 810 nm, have a deeper absorption capability than the argon lasers. Not only is the maximum absorption at the RPE level, but Bruch's membrane and the inner layers of the choroid may frequently be involved. Thus, breaks in Bruch's membrane may occur, resulting in chorioretinal hemorrhage. In addition, retrobulbar anesthesia has to be given more frequently because more painful responses develop when administering krypton and diode laser therapy than when using the argon lasers. The main advantage in using the krypton red laser as well as the diode laser is better penetration through a cataractous lens as well as through vitreous hemorrhage.

Three corneal contact lenses are commonly being used to produce the necessary chorioretinal reaction in laser photocoagulation of the retina. The oldest is the Goldmann three-mirror lens (Figs. 9.6 and 9.7). It consists of a central lens for the posterior pole and three peripheral lenses set at various angles to cover the equatorial and peripheral areas of the fundus. Both the Rodenstock (Fig. 9.8) and the Mainster (Fig. 9.9) lenses provide larger fields than the Goldmann lens. They also have the dual advantages of minimizing "skip" areas as well as providing a safeguard for inadvertent laser applications to the macular area. The Rodenstock and Mainster lenses require a longer learning curve because they provide an inverted image of the retina, similar to the indirect ophthalmoscope. The Rodenstock lens also produces a larger

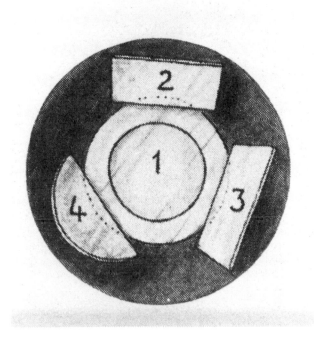

Fig. 9.6 The Goldmann three-mirror lens. The central mirror is used to view the optic disc and macular areas. The three peripheral mirrors have different inclinations to view the areas of the fundus from the posterior pole to the periphery.

lesion than that obtained with the Goldmann lens. For that reason, the micron size of the lesion must be adjusted downward when using the Rodenstock lens.

Laser Treatment Parameters for Retinal Breaks

Three variables must be controlled when administrating laser treatment for retinal breaks: size of lesion (in microns), time duration (in tenths of a second), and power setting (in watts). Usually 500- to 1000-μm size lesions are used contiguously in three concentric rows surrounding the tear. Time duration consists of 0.2 to 0.5 sec. The initial power setting starts at 150 to 200 mW and is adjusted upward in increments of 25 mW until a white lesion is obtained. If a cataract or slight vitreous hemorrhage is present preventing adequate lesions, turning the micron size down from 1000 to 500 will frequently produce the desired lesion because reducing the size of the lesion has the effect of increasing the power level. Increasing the time duration from 0.2 to 0.5 sec will also increase power output, holding micron size constant. It should also be remembered that in vitrectomized eyes having had a fluid gas exchange or in the silicone oil-filled eye, a lower wattage is frequently required because there is less heat absorption in the vitreous cavity with the gas-filled or silicone-filled eye. It should also be noted that while this

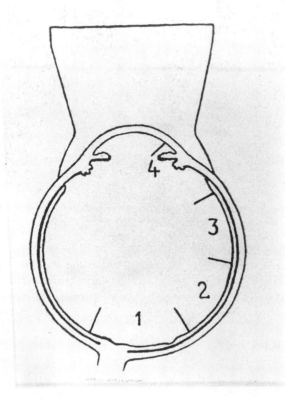

Fig. 9.7 An anteroposterior section of the eye indicates the anatomic areas of the retina seen with the various mirrors of the Goldmann lens as seen in Fig. 9.6.

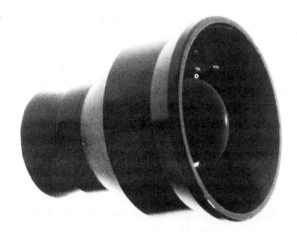

Fig. 9.8 The Rodenstock lens provides an inverted, larger field with a reduced magnification, as contrasted with the Goldmann lens.

author prefers the three concentric rows of lesions to be contiguous, some ophthalmologists prefer to create a honeycomb pattern to the lesions with 200-μm intervals of normal retina between the lesions.

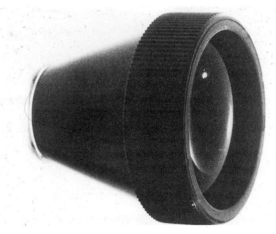

Fig. 9.9 The Mainster lens is similar to the Rodenstock lens in providing a greater field of view than the Goldmann lens. It also provides an inverted image similar to that seen with indirect ophthalmoscopy.

Laser Treatment in Retinal Detachment Surgery

Laser photocoagulation is infrequently used in typical cases of retinal detachment where scleral buckling procedures are used because subretinal fluid acts as an insulator preventing an adequate chorioretinal laser reaction. The chorioretinal adhesions are usually made via cryopexy or diathermy followed by the use of solid silicone or a silicone sponge as the buckling element. Drainage of subretinal fluid forms the third part of the procedure that is frequently performed.

Laser photocoagulation is often used as an adjunct following scleral buckling where residual subretinal fluid surrounding a retinal break fails to absorb. Penetration of laser energy through a thin layer of subretinal fluid in a flat retinal detachment can frequently produce a good chorioretinal adhesion, obviating the necessity of a subsequent intraoperative invasive procedure. The presence of postoperative fish-mouth retinal tears connecting into radial folds (Fig. 9.10) can be an ominous sign that may lead to the accumulation of subretinal fluid and re-detachment of the retina. Producing a good chorioretinal seal with laser burns surrounding the tear is an excellent way of preventing subsequent surgery. Lastly, laser photocoagulation can be used to wall off an area of subretinal fluid located anterior to the buckle. Although this does not eliminate the area of localized retinal detachment, it does contain the elevated retina in the periphery and may save the patient from a second surgical procedure.

The technique of pneumoretinopexy lends itself to laser photocoagulation in the postoperative period. Pneumoretinopexy is frequently considered in cases of localized superior retinal detachment harboring a superior retinal tear. Laser photocoagulation is applied postoperatively, completely surrounding the retinal tear through

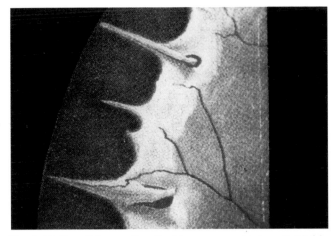

Fig. 9.10 Two fish-mouth retinal tears connect into radial folds at the ora serrata.

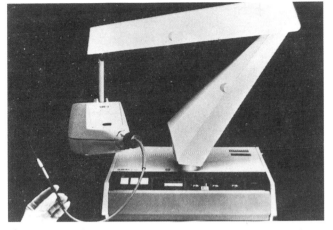

Fig. 9.11 Charles xenon arc endophotocoagulator shows the articulating arm that supports the xenon light source for the fiberoptic bundle to the handpiece.

the intravitreal gas bubble. The intravitreal gas bubble must, of course, flatten the retinal break against the RPE before laser photocoagulation can be applied. In all the above cases, laser photocoagulation consists of making three concentric rows of contiguous laser marks of moderate intensity, using 500- to 1000-μm size lesions completely surrounding the retinal break.

Endolaser Photocoagulation in Vitrectomy

The previous discussion of laser photocoagulation in retinal detachment surgery uses either slit-lamp or indirect ophthalmoscopic laser delivery systems to accomplish laser photocoagulation. Postoperative delivery of laser energy was also used. With the advent of endolaser photocoagulation, laser energy is applied during surgery, as an adjunct to pars plana vitrectomy procedures. The argon laser, operating in the visible spectrum, or the diode laser, operating in the low infrared end of the spectrum, is used.

Historical Background

Intraoperative laser endophotocoagulation has become a necessary tool in the armamentarium of the vitreous surgeon. During the course of a trans pars plana vitrectomy, vitreous hemorrhage may occur due to traction on a fibrovascular vitreoretinal membrane. Iatrogenic retinal tears may also develop. Before the advent of intravitreal photocoagulation, bipolar cautery or intravitreal diathermy were the instruments of choice in controlling hemorrhage.

Xenon Arc Endophotocoagulation

The development of the xenon arc endophotocoagulator by Charles (11,12) was the first application of an instrument using light to coagulate within the vitreous cavity during vitrectomy. It was used frequently in the late 1970s and early 1980s during vitrectomy procedures to coagulate hemorrhagic sites, treat retinal tears, or apply focal or panretinal photocoagulation (PRP) in selective cases of eyes with PDR. Charles' (11,12) portable xenon arc light coagulator (Fig. 9.11) was a system developed for transvitreal application of photocoagulation using a fiberoptic probe attached to a portable 500-W short xenon arc light source. The probe was sized to 20 gauge (0.89 mm diameter) and was 3.2 cm in length. The system was activated by a foot switch. The probe tip was positioned close to the retina during the vitrectomy operation.

Argon Laser Endophotocoagulation

In 1981, Fleischman and associates (13) as well as Peyman and coworkers (14) were the first to transmit argon laser energy through a portable fiberoptic pars plana endophotocoagulation system to produce chorioretinal lesions during a vitrectomy procedure. The argon laser was delivered through a 600-μm quartz fiber. The quartz fiber was coupled into a blunt needle sized to 20 gauge. The argon laser operated in the continuous mode. A safety filter shutter was introduced between the surgeon's binocular eyepiece and the lens objective (Fig. 9.12). The sclerotomy sites are sized so that the argon laser tip (Fig. 9.13) is interchangeable with either the vitrectomy cutter or the fiberoptic endoilluminator. Figure 9.14 shows the right fundus immediately after having received panretinal argon laser endophotocoagulation.

It has been shown that there are distinct advantages of substituting argon laser energy for xenon arc energy in cases where endophotocoagulation of the retina is indicated during a trans pars plana vitrectomy procedure. With xenon arc endophotocoagulation, the tip of the probe must be brought to within 0.5 mm of the target

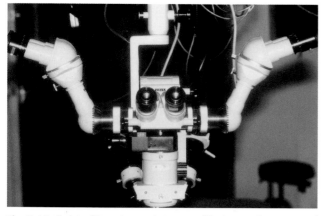

Fig. 9.12 Safety filter shutter interposed between the surgeon's binocular eyepiece and the lens objective. The filter is used while performing argon laser endophotocoagulation.

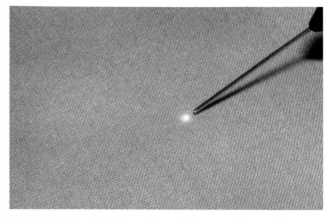

Fig. 9.13 Intravitreal laser tip used for argon laser endophotocoagulation.

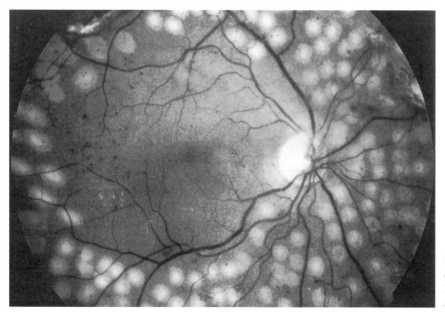

Fig. 9.14 Fundus of the right eye demonstrates panretinal argon laser photocoagulation immediately after treatment.

tissue. The risk of producing an iatrogenic retinal tear is therefore much greater than with the argon laser, which can effectively produce retinal photocoagulation even while operating in the midvitreous cavity. Variations in distance with the Charles endocoagulator can be no more than 0.33 mm. With the argon laser, variations of the distance between the probe and the retina within 1 mm do not produce dramatic changes. Also, the surgeon must wait between successive xenon arc applications so that the system can cool down and prevent probe failure. This increases the operative time in doing a PRP with the Charles xenon arc instrument. With argon laser endophotocoagulation, successive burns can be applied rapidly, thereby substantially shortening the treatment time. Thirdly, with the xenon arc delivery system, the probe must be fired in a fluid medium to dissipate the heat that is generated. A malfunction develops in cases where

a fluid/gas exchange has been performed. With the argon laser, the energy can also be delivered to the target tissue in the air-filled eye. Fourthly, light from the argon laser can be greatly attenuated by a yellow filter inserted in the microscope immediately below the surgeon's oculars. This filter provides full fundus visualization and protects the surgeon's eyes from potentially hazardous reflections. Contrasted to this, the Charles xenon arc coagulator uses white light that cannot be safely filtered without preventing fundus visualization.

Diode Laser Photocoagulation

The use of the diode laser, a solid-state laser operating in the low infrared end of the spectrum, as an alternative to the argon laser in performing endophotocoagulation during vitrectomy is discussed in Chapter 10.

Indications for Endophotocoagulation

Intravitreal laser photocoagulation is used at the time of vitreous surgery to control intravitreal hemorrhage, treat giant and posterior retinal breaks, coagulate retinal neovascularization, apply focal or panretinal laser photocoagulation, treat ciliary processes in eyes demonstrating neovascular glaucoma, and create pupillary enlargement in eyes with posterior synechiae, rubeosis irides, and miosis. Most of these conditions are found in vitrectomy performed in cases of PDR. Bovino and colleagues (15) have used laser photocoagulation to create an external sclerotomy for drainage of subretinal fluid. Endolaser photocoagulation is also performed surrounding a surgical retinotomy for endodrainage of subretinal fluid. It is also used to produce a good chorioretinal adhesion along the edges of a surgically created retinotomy to reattach a gliotic-contracted retina.

Posterior retinal breaks and macular holes are extremely difficult to treat by conventional scleral buckling procedures because accessibility to the tear with either the cryoprobe or diathermy tip is so difficult. Vitrectomy with focal laser endophotocoaglation coupled with a fluid/air exchange, with or without endodrainage of subretinal fluid, has emerged as the treatment of choice.

Laser endophotocoagulation has also become a necessary adjunct to the treatment of intraocular foreign body with and without accompanying retinal detachment.

Technique of Endolaser Photocoagulation

Producing endolaser photocoagulation in a phakic eye without a fluid/air exchange presents no difficulty, especially if the eye is widely dilated. The assistant indents the peripheral retina with a cotton-tipped applicator, which provides adequate visualization for laser treatment between the equatorial area and the ora serrata. With scleral depression, however, the power requirement usually is less than when performing coagulation posteriorly because the retina is closer to the tip of the probe. It is important to remember that unlike slit-lamp laser delivery, the distance of the laser exit port to the retina is not fixed during endolaser surgery.

The technique of endolaser photocoagulation consists of starting at a subthreshold milliwatt level and increasing the power until a white chorioretinal lesion is produced. The average milliwatt power will usually vary with each patient as a result of varying degrees of retinal pigmentation. Less power is required for a more heavily pigmented retina. One usually begins at 200 mW of energy power with a time duration of 0.2 to 0.5 sec and then increases the power by increments of 25 mW until the desired white lesion is obtained. The power levels frequently fall within 350 to 600 mW. Unlike exolaser delivery via a slit-lamp biomicroscopic approach, one does not dial in the micron size of the lesion. In endolaser photocoagulation, the size of the lesion depends on the proximity of the probe to the retinal target tissue. If the probe is held close to the retina, the lesion will be smaller and the power level, in milliwatts, will be less. If the probe is held father away from the retina, the size of the lesion will be larger. Also, the power level will be greater because the energy has to traverse a greater distance through the vitreous cavity to impact on the retinal target tissue.

A Landers −95 D lens must be used for retinal visualization in a phakic eye having had a fluid/air exchange. It is used to offset the high myopia induced in such an eye. In many cases, no contact lens is required when using endolaser in the air-filled aphakic eye.

The incidence of recurrent vitreous hemorrhage in PDR has been greatly reduced as a result of the use of argon laser endophotocoagulation during the course of the vitrectomy procedure. Liggett and coworkers (16) have shown the proportion of eyes requiring an additional surgical procedure to remove vitreous hemorrhage to be significantly lower in patients receiving laser endophotocoagulation.

The explanation for the beneficial effect of laser photocoagulation remains unclear. There are a number of reasons for the development of recurrent vitreous hemorrhage following vitrectomy in the diabetic eye. Renewed bleeding may occur from neovascularization of the disc and retina, fibrovascular epiretinal membranes, fibrovascular ingrowth at sclerotomy sites created during the vitrectomy operation, or from rubeosis irides. The majority of vitreoretinal surgeons would agree that in most instances, the exact source of the hemorrhage is rarely determined. Glaser and colleagues (17) have stated that a possible mechanism by which laser photocoagulation may induce vascular involution is the release of a chemical inhibitor by the damaged RPE cells. The effect of such an inhibitor might be potentiated by increased diffusion of this inhibitor in the fluid-filled vitreous cavity following vitrectomy.

Nd:YAG Laser Photocoagulation in Vitreous Surgery

The main advantage of using the neodymium:yttrium-aluminum-garnet (Nd:YAG) laser is that it is a painless and noninvasive procedure, performed on an outpatient basis. Its main use today has been in performing posterior lens capsulotomies following cataract extraction with intraocular lens implantation. A second indication is the creation of an iridectomy following an acute glaucoma attack. It has also been used in the anterior and midvitreous cavity, as will be discussed below. The Nd:YAG laser operates in the low infrared end of the spectrum. Its wavelength is 1.06 μm. The Nd:YAG laser produces optical breakdown through a physical effect resulting in

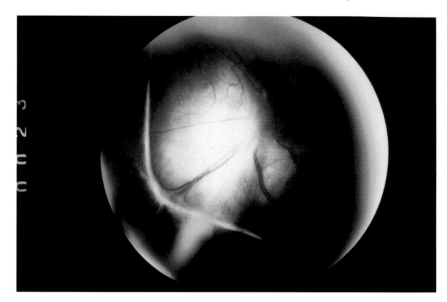

Fig. 9.15 An anterior traction retinal detachment due to trauma. Note an anteroposteriorly oriented traction membrane emanating from the optic disc as well as a more anteriorly placed limbus parallel vitreoretinal membrane.

explosive cutting, rather than creating a thermal change as seen with the argon, krypton, and diode lasers. The creation of a plasma shield acts as a barrier in attempting to prevent untoward results from the shock wave.

Remote acoustic effects produced by the Nd:YAG laser are responsible for chorioretinal burns if one attempts to cut a vitreoretinal or epiretinal membrane within 3 mm of the retina. The acoustic shock wave is also responsible for vitreous and intraretinal hemorrhage that may occur with the use of this wavelength.

Indications for Nd:YAG Laser Phototransection

Trauma

Vitreoretinal membranes frequently occur along the path of the wound of entrance and wound of exit as an intraocular foreign body or a sharp perforating object transverses the vitreous cavity.

Figure 9.15 shows the formation of a traction retinal detachment from a perforating injury. An anteroposteriorly oriented traction membrane as well as a more anteriorly placed limbus parallel vitreous membrane can be seen. A Nd:YAG laser using 3 mJ of energy level with three shots per burst for a total energy of 9 mJ succeeded in transecting the anteroposteriorly oriented vitreoretinal membrane as seen in Fig. 9.16. In Fig. 9.17, the distal part of this membrane is retracted onto the optic nerve, causing relaxation of the traction and reattachment of the previously detached anterior retina.

Proliferative Diabetic Retinopathy Causing Retinal Detachment

The elimination of vitreoretinal traction in a case of macular or extramacular diabetic traction retinal detachment

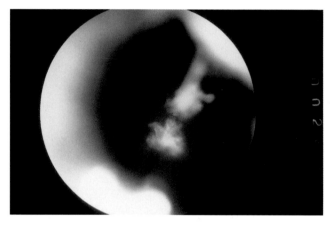

Fig. 9.16 Nd:YAG laser phototransection of the anteroposteriorly oriented traction membrane as shown in Fig. 9.15.

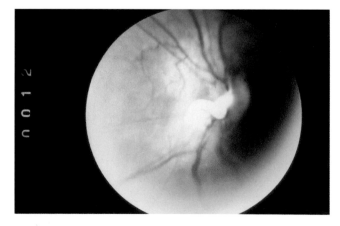

Fig. 9.17 The distal part of the anteroposteriorly oriented membrane shown in Fig. 9.16 is retracted back onto the optic nerve. This relieved traction on the anterior retina, resulting in reattachment of the entire retina.

can at times be accomplished through the transpupillary delivery of a Nd:YAG laser using a corneal contact lens. This can only be accomplished if a visible vitreoretinal membrane is seen in the mid or anterior vitreous cavity. The ocular media must be sufficiently clear with little cataract formation and little vitreous hemorrhage present.

Proliferative Vitreoretinopathy

Extensive cryopexy performed during the course of reattaching a retinal detachment can produce PVR with the subsequent formation of vitreoretinal membranes. In addition, massive vitreous hemorrhage may cause depolymerization of the collagen gel structure of the vitreous, with the formation of vitreoretinal adhesions. Occasionally, Nd:YAG laser photocoagulation can sever these membranes, resulting in the release of retinal traction and favoring the continued attachment of the retina.

Cystoid Macular Edema

Cystoid macular edema (CME) is a complication of cataract extraction, especially when an opening is created in the posterior lens capsule. Nd:YAG laser photocoagulation is a viable procedure in transecting a vitreous strand emanating from the edematous macula. In the rare case where the vitreous has been incarcerated in the corneoscleral incision following vitreous loss during cataract surgery, Nd:YAG laser therapy may be attempted. However, it has been the author's experience that this form of treatment gives rather poor results. In addition, because the cornea and iris are in proximity to the vitreous incarceration, the risk of producing corneal and iritic complications frequently makes Nd:YAG laser vitreolysis an unacceptable form of treatment.

Vitreous Opacities

The presence of vitreous opacities is usually not an indication for Nd:YAG laser treatment. Similarly, the occurrence of asteroid hyalosis almost never contributes to the loss of visual acuity, making Nd:YAG laser vitrectomy a virtually unnecessary procedure.

Technique of Nd:YAG Laser Capsulotomy

Although Nd:YAG laser vitreolysis can be performed without a contact lens, it is usually preferable to use such a lens. Figure 9.18 shows Peyman's (18) convex contact lenses of 12.5, 18.0 and 25.0 mm radii used for Nd:YAG laser vitreolysis. They are used when membranes are found to be present in the anterior and midvitreous locations. The advantages of a contact lens are that it helps focus the laser beam and helps to prevent untoward eye movement. Proparacaine hydrochloride 0.5% drops is

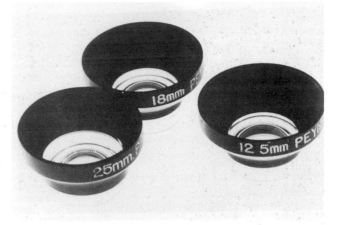

Fig. 9.18 The three Peyman convex lenses of 12.5, 18.0, and 25.0 mm radii used for Nd:YAG laser vitreolysis.

sufficent to produce topical anesthesia. The pupil is dilated with Mydfrin 2.5% and Mydriacyl 1%.

The procedure starts with 1 to 1.3 mJ of energy level and one pulse/burst. Then the millejoules as well as the pulses/burst are increased until the desired transection of the vitreoretinal membrane is achieved. It is important to remember that usually a greater energy level is required to cause transection of membranes within the vitreous cavity than to produce posterior lens capsulotomies.

Complications

For the most part, Nd:YAG laser vitrectomy is a safe, noninvasive surgical procedure. Postoperatively, a transient uveitis with a transient elevation of intraocular pressure may result. Vitritis may develop immediately following treatment if much debris forms in the vitreous cavity. This slowly clears. The limited use of Diamox tablets or Betoptic 0.5% drops usually effectively controls the pressure. Dilating the eye with Mydriacyl 1% or homatropine 2% coupled with temporary steroidal medication almost always results in resolution of the uveitis.

Cataract formation may result if one attempts to transect a membrane too anteriorly in the vitreous cavity. Iritis and keratitis can also result from using the Nd:YAG laser to cut a vitreous incarceration close to the iris or cornea. Vitreous hemorrhage can develop from Nd:YAG laser treatment in close proximity to retinal vessels or in areas harboring membranes with neovascularization.

Epiretinal membranes do not lend themselves to transection by the Nd:YAG laser. Jampol and colleagues (19) have demonstrated the production of chorioretinal lesions and retinal hemorrhages if the Nd:YAG laser is aimed at a target tissue within 3 mm of the retina. Figure 9.19 shows an epiretinal membrane lying within 3 mm of the retina in a case of PDR. Figure 9.20 indicates the presence of a chorioretinal lesion in addition to the transection of the membrane. Naturally, no diminution of central visual

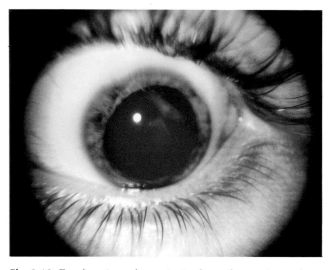

Fig. 9.19 Fundus view of an epiretinal membrane situated within 3 mm of the retina. (Courtesy of William Hagler, MD, Atlanta, GA.)

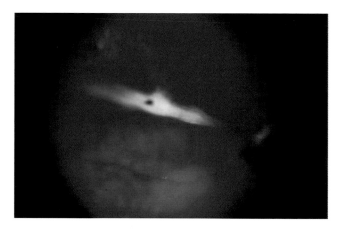

Fig. 9.20 Nd:YAG laser phototransection of the epiretinal membrane shown in Fig. 9.19. Note the occurrence of an acute chorioretinal lesion shown to the right, in addition to the cutting of the membrane. (Courtesy of William Hagler, MD, Atlanta, GA.)

acuity results if the chorioretinal lesion is located in the periphery. However, if the lesion was created in the macular area or overlying the disc, irreparable loss of central vision would result. Because most epiretinal membranes resulting from cases of PDR occur within the posterior pole, Nd:YAG laser transection of these membranes is contraindicated.

Retinal hemorrhage can also develop when focusing on a membrane located within 3 mm of the retinal surface. The acoustic shock wave is sufficiently strong to cause a rupture of the fine vascular walls of capillaries or neovascular vessels. Lastly, retinal tears and retinal detachment can occur when treating close to the retina as a result of faulty focusing or the forward movement of the patient.

Laser Treatment of Intraocular Tumors of the Posterior Segment

Solid Posterior Segment Tumors

Melanosarcoma of the choroid (malignant melanoma), retinoblastoma, and metastatic tumors to the choroid comprise the three most common solid intraocular tumors involving the posterior segment of the eye.

Melanosarcoma of the Choroid

Melanosarcoma of the choroid (malignant melanoma) is the most common malignant primary ocular tumor. The tumor usually presents in the late decades of life. Its most frequent occurrence is in the Caucasian population, especially in lightly pigmented individuals. It rarely presents itself in the African American race. The older Callender (20) classification is one of histopathologic cell type in which spindle cell A and B are found to be less malignant than the epithelioid and necrotic cell types. The more recent Collaborative Ocular Melanoma Study (COMS) has classified melanomas on the basis of the size of the lesion. Small melanomas are classified as those tumors measuring 3 mm or less in height; medium tumors comprise dimensions of 4 to 8 mm in height; large melanomas are those more than 8 mm in height. Consideration is also given to the width of the lesion in terms of basal diameter.

The ophthalmoscopic appearance of the lesion (Fig. 9.21) is characteristic, consisting of a dome-shaped, convex, solidly elevated choroidal lesion that may extend through the potential subretinal space, elevating the retina in a "collar button" fashion. Changes in the overlying retinal elevation consist of RPE changes, the appearance of drusen, and lipofuscin. Choroidal neovascularization, serous retinal detachment, and vitreous hemorrhage may be present.

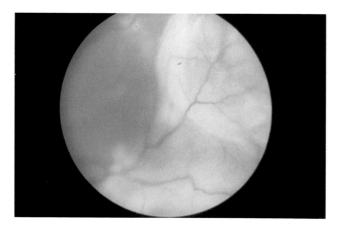

Fig. 9.21 Fundus photo of a choroidal malignant melanoma demonstrates a dome-shaped, collar button, convex, solidly elevated choroidal lesion.

The diagnosis of melanosarcoma of the choroid is usually made by the previous characteristic ophthalmoscopic appearance coupled with the following distinctive appearance of the ultrasonogram. A-scan ultrasound (Fig. 9.22) indicates a high initial spike with decreasing echoes as the sound waves penetrate deeper within the tumor. B-scan ultrasound (Fig. 9.23) demonstrates a solid mass with acoustic hollowing and orbital shadowing as the acoustic waves are absorbed by the tumor before reaching the orbit.

Historically, melanosarcoma of the choroid was treated by enucleation. However, small melanomas of the choroid were treated with multiple sessions of xenon arc photo-

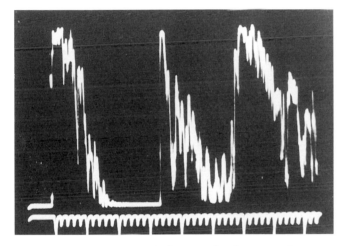

Fig. 9.22 A-scan ultrasound of a case of malignant melanoma of the choroid. Note a high initial spike with decreasing echoes as the sonic waves progress more posteriorly toward the orbital wall.

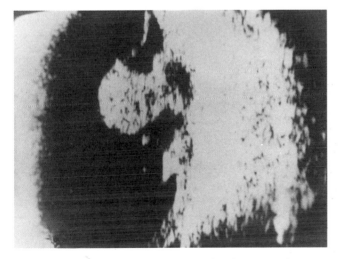

Fig. 9.23 B-scan ultrasound of a case of malignant melanoma of the choroid. Note the collar button appearance. Shadowing is present in the more posterior aspects of the orbit. Echo attenuation or "hollowing" is also seen at the posterior aspect of the tumor.

coagulation by Meyer-Schwickerath (21) or later, by laser photocoagulation. Unfortunately, frequent complications developed, including gliosis with preretinal fibrosis and macular pucker, traction retinal detachment, and retinal and vitreous hemorrhage. Unfortunately, laser photocoagulation could not always obliterate the tumor, resulting in recurrence of the malignant melanoma.

The treatment of malignant melanoma is currently in a state of flux, with no unanimity of opinion by experts concerning the best treatment for this condition. Fortunately, the COMS is addressing this dilemma. Specifically, this national prospective, multicentered clinical trial is trying to answer the following questions:

1. What is the place of enucleation as the treatment of choice? It appears that fewer eyes are currently being enucleated, especially those eyes harboring smaller tumors and possessing useful vision.
2. Does enucleation increase the risk of metastasis?
3. Does radiotherapy given before enucleation decrease the incidence of metastasis?
4. What method of radiation produces the optimal results?

Despite the fact that this randomized trial addresses the subject of enucleation versus radiation, there still are specific indications for the treatment of malignant melanoma by laser photocoagulation. Because of the following strict criteria, Shields (22) found that only 5% to 10% of melanomas are treated by laser therapy. Shields (23) states that small nasal malignant melanomas or temporal peripheral small melanomas located away from the macula and outside the superior temporal and inferior retinal arcades can be adequately treated with laser photocoagulation. The insertion of a radioactive plaque followed by laser photocoagulation frequently becomes the treatment of choice.

The following criteria govern whether laser therapy should be instituted. Laser therapy should only be considered if the melanoma is small, measuring less than 3 mm in height with a basal diameter less than 9 to 10 mm. Secondary serous detachment of the retina is a contraindication because a layer of fluid would tend to prevent adequate uptake of the laser energy by the underlying solid tumefaction. A third indication of laser treatment concerns the distance of the tumor from the posterior pole of the eye. Tumors lying within one disc diameter of the fovea or within one disc diameter of the optic nerve should not be photocoagulated because the radiation effect from the laser could cause a decrease in central visual acuity. However, if a posterior tumor is already causing a decrease in vision due to existing secondary retinal detachment, laser therapy may be considered, provided that adequate laser reaction can be placed completely surrounding the lesion without compromising the fovea or the optic nerve.

Argon and krypton lasers have been used for treatment in multiple sessions. The initial treatment is designed to disrupt the choroidal vascular supply to the tumor by applying 500-μm size lesions of long duration completely surrounding the tumor. Three rows of contiguous laser burns are made. A second application of laser burns is applied surrounding the melanoma 3 weeks later. Following this, contiguous laser applications are placed over the surface of the tumor. The treatment is repeated until the tumor together with its vascular supply is destroyed. The end point is reached when a flat or concave gliotic scar with pigmentation is obtained.

Unfortunately, laser treatment does not always obliterate a small malignant melanoma. Local radiation with iodine [125], cobalt [60], or ruthenium [106] plaques has largely replaced laser photocoagulation in treatment of small or moderately sized tumors of malignant melanoma. Large choroidal melanomas must, of course, be treated by enucleation. The COMS randomizes medium-size tumors to either enucleation or iodine [125] radiation plaque therapy. Large melanomas are randomized to enucleation or to external beam radiation before enucleation.

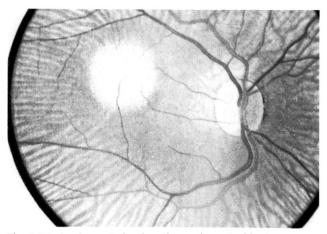

Fig. 9.24 A schematic fundus photo of a retinoblastoma.

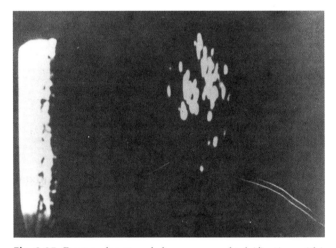

Fig. 9.25 B-scan ultrasound shows areas of calcification within a retinoblastoma as the decibel sensitivity is lowered.

Retinoblastoma

Retinoblastoma is the most common ocular tumor found in childhood. It is autosomal dominant with a 25% to 30% incidence of bilaterality. It occurs either as an isolated tumor or it may have a multicentric origin. Progression may occur toward the vitreous cavity (endophytic). It may also grow in the opposite direction through the choroid and sclera (exophytic). Leukocoria is the most common presenting sign. Strabismus is also very common because lack of adequate macular stimulation resulting from the leukocoric central opacity produces a turn in the affected eye. Proptosis, hyphema, and secondary glaucoma frequently signify local metastatic involvement. Invasion of the optic nerve with widespread systemic metastasis may follow.

The diagnosis of retinoblastoma is made on the ophthalmoscopic discovery of a white retinal mass (Fig. 9.24). Dilated tortuous retinal vessels may be present. Diagnosis is also made by B-scan ultrasonography demonstrating a solid mass with high-intensity reflection and orbital shadowing from the presence of tumor calcification. Figure 9.25 shows persistence of echoes from calcium deposits in the B-scan ultrasound of a case of retinoblastoma, in which the sensitivity in decibels had been markedly reduced.

The laser photocoagulation treatment protocol for retinoblastoma has been largely developed by Shields and colleagues (24) and Char (25). Laser criteria consist of a retinoblastoma measuring less than 4.5 mm in basal diameter and less than 2.5 mm in thickness. The tumor should be restricted to the neurosensory retina, located posterior to the equator, and situated at a distance from the fovea and optic disc.

Laser technique is designed to destroy the lesion by obliterating its feeding vessels. Laser applications are not made directly over the tumor. Double rows of contiguous laser burns of sufficient intensity are placed around the tumor to close off the vasculature supplying the tumor. The procedure may have to be repeated if there is evidence, demonstrated on fundus fluorescein angiography, that vascularity of the tumor is still present. The ophthalmic appearance of a depressed fundus scar demonstrating no angiographic leakage, is proof of adequate treatment.

Cryotherapy, radiotherapy, or enucleation become the treatments of choice if the tumor is larger than 4.5 mm in diameter or if laser photocoagulation fails to produce regression of the retinoblastoma. Cryotherapy is usually reserved for small, peripheral tumors that have not undergone metastasis.

Radiotherapy has been successful in the treatment of retinoblastoma. These tumors are highly radiosensitive. Treatment consists of either episcleral plaque therapy according to Shields and associates (26) or external beam radiation. The most common low-energy isotopes used as plaques today include iodine[125], cobalt[60], ruthenium[106], and iridium[192]. However, if the tumor is located in the parafoveal or juxtapapillary areas or if the tumor is very advanced with metastatic seedings, external beam radi-ation or chemotherapy become the treatments of choice. Enucle-ation becomes the treatment of choice for advan-ced large tumors that have produced massive loss of visual acuity without any chance of regaining useful central vision.

Metastatic Tumors

Breast carcinomas in women and lung carcinoma in men are the most common tumors metastasizing to the choroid. Malignant emboli reach the eye through the bloodstream by means of the short posterior ciliary arter-ies. Metastatic lesions can usually be found in the pos-terior region of the fundus. Ophthalmoscopically, these tumors (Fig. 9.26) are frequently seen growing along the plane of the choroid and retina with much less elevation than is found with melanoma or retinoblastoma. They present as placoid choroidal lesions and are frequently asymptomatic without requiring any direct treatment.

Localized laser photocoagulation is usually not indi-cated. Systemic chemotherapy comprises the treatment of choice. Gragoudas and Carroll (27) have advocated external proton beam radiation if the choroidal metas-tatic lesion involves the fovea or is located in the juxta-papillary areas where serious decreases in central visual acuity occur.

Vascular Posterior Segment Tumors

The following section discusses the most common vas-cular chorioretinal tumors. All of the tumors to be dis-cussed are rather uncommon. Von Hippel-Landau disease (retinal capillary hemangioma together with a sys-temic hemangioma), choroidal hemangioma, and retinal cavernous hemangioma will be presented.

Von Hippel-Lindau Disease

Ophthalmoscopically, this condition presents as an or-ange-red retinal capillary hemangioma with large, tortu-ous vessels traversing the tumor surface (Fig. 9.27). A feeder vessel can frequently be identified as well as a large drainage vessel. Retinal and vitreous hemorrhage, trac-tion retinal detachment, and secondary glaucoma may de-velop if the angioma is left untreated. Fundus fluorescein angiography reveals arteriovenous shunting over the sur-face of the tumor with leakage from both the tumor and its surrounding capillaries. Associated capillary heman-giomas may be found in the neurologic (cerebellum), gas-trointestinal (pancreas), and urinary (kidney) systems.

Argon laser photocoagulation is used to treat retinal capillary hemangioma. Initial treatment is directed at com-pletely surrounding the tumor with a good chorioretinal adhesion, using confluent 500-μm size burns. This will en-sure that the neurosensory retina becomes scarred down to the RPE. Following this, laser applications are made di-rectly over the surface of the tumor in subsequent sessions after waiting one to two weeks for a good chorioretinal scar surrounding the tumor. Once again, 500-μm size le-sions of long duration and in a contiguous pattern are applied over the lesion. Multiple treatment sessions are frequently required before one can document a slow re-gression of the angioma over a period of many months. The feeder vessel technique of attempting to close the feeding vessel with heavy intensity 500-μm size lesions

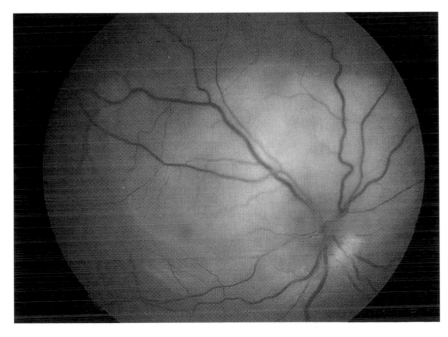

Fig. 9.26 Fundus photo of a metastatic tumor to the choroid. Note that growth occurs mainly in the plane of the choroid with relatively little elevation, as contrasted with malignant melanoma.

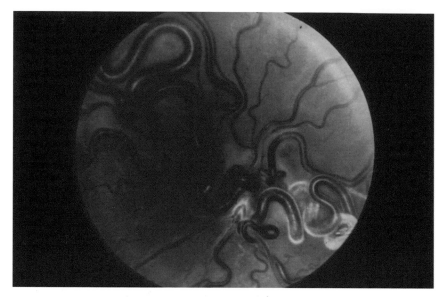

Fig. 9.27 Fundus photo of Von Hippel retinal capillary hemangioma. Note the large feeder and drainage vessels.

has infrequently resulted in successful obliteration of the tumor, even in cases of small tumors measuring less than 2.5 disc diameters.

Hemorrhagic complications may occur because of the extreme vascularity of the tumor. It is therefore important to remember to first surround the tumor with a good laser chorioretinal seal before working on the tumor itself. One should also treat with a sufficiently large micron size lesion so that the size of the laser burn is larger than the diameter of the vessel. If this is not adhered to, then the serious complication of a severe retinal or vitreous hemorrhage is possible. Lastly, the laser surgeon should always advise the patient, before laser therapy is begun, that although small retinal angiomas can readily be obliterated with laser photocoagulation, large tumors are frequently resistant to laser therapy and may result in vascular complications necessitating a pars plana vitrectomy.

Double or triple freeze-thaw cryopexy may also be successful in treating small peripheral retinal capillary hemangiomas or when a hazy vitreous prevents adequate laser photocoagulation.

Choroidal Hemangioma

Choroidal hemangioma frequently presents as a unilateral lesion located in the posterior pole. It may occur as an isolated choroidal tumor or may be associated with systemic findings such as in the Sturge-Weber syndrome in which facial and brain stem angiomas occur.

This benign choroidal tumor usually presents as a pink, slightly elevated fundus lesion (Fig. 9.28). No treatment is

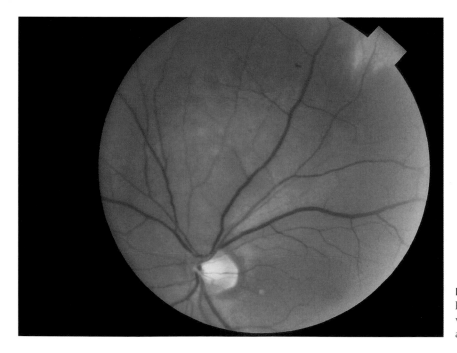

Fig. 9.28 Fundus photo of choroidal hemangioma. Note the slightly elevated lesion posteriorly located, just above the optic disc.

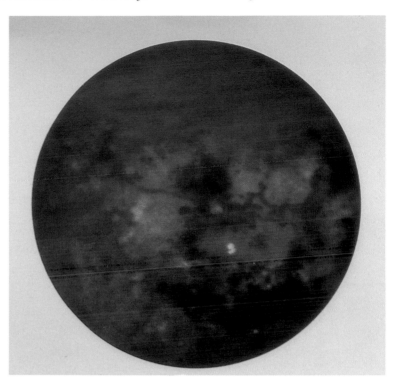

Fig. 9.29 Fundus photo of retinal cavernous hemangioma. Note the grapelike cluster of intraretinal blood-filled spaces together with retinal hemorrhage as part of the elevated vascular mass.

usually required because the tumors rarely enlarge and infrequently cause loss of central visual acuity. Diagnosis may be made by causing blanching of the tumor with digital pressure on the globe. Rarely, serous detachment of the overlying retina may develop with extravasation of fluid posteriorly involving the macular area. Documentation and monitoring of any progression should be made by serial fundus photography and fundus fluorescein angiography. Early filling of the large choroidal vessels is followed by staining of the tumor in the late stages of the fluorescein transit.

Gass (28) has treated choroidal hemangiomas using argon green or yellow dye laser photocoagulation if the secondary serous retinal detachment begins to involve the fovea. Argon laser photocoagulation over the surface of the tumor frequently results in resorption of the secondary serous detachment with preservation of central visual acuity.

Retinal Cavernous Hemangioma

This retinal hamartoma appears ophthalmoscopically as a grapelike cluster of intraretinal blood-filled spaces (Fig. 9.29). The tumors are usually unilateral and asymptomatic. However, retinal and vitreous hemorrhage may develop as a result of rupture of the thin-walled dilated blood vessels. Fundus fluorescein angiography demonstrates late venous filling but no leakage.

The tumor usually does not require treatment unless hemorrhage causes decrease in central visual acuity. Contiguous argon laser photocoagulation using 500-μm size lesions frequently results in successful destruction of the

cavernous hemangioma. Cryotherapy provides a successful alternative to laser photocoagulation.

References

1. Lincoff H, McLean JM, Nano H. Cryosurgical treatment of retinal detachment. Trans Am Acad Ophthalmol Otolaryngol 1964;68:412–432.
2. Meyer-Schwickerath G. Light coagulation. Translated by Drance SM. St Louis: CV Mosby, 1960, pp. 36–37.
3. Rutnin U, Schepens CL. Fundus appearance in normal eyes. IV. Retinal breaks and other findings. Am J Ophthalmol 1967;64:1063–1078.
4. Byer NE. Clinical study of retinal breaks. Trans Am Acad Ophthalmol Otolaryngol 1967;71:461–473.
5. Karlin DB, Curtin B. Peripheral chorioretinal lesions and axial length of the myopic eye. Am J Ophthalmol 1976;81: 625–635.
6. Javitt JC, Vitale S, Canner JK, et al. National outcomes of cataract extraction. I. Retinal detachment after inpatient surgery. Ophthalmology 1991;98:895–902.
7. Javitt JC, Tielsch JM, Canner JK, Kolb MN, Sommer A, Steinberg EP. National outcomes of cataract extraction. Increased risk of retinal complications associated with Nd:YAG laser capsulotomy. Ophthalmology 1992;99:1487–1498.
8. Lincoff H, O'Conner P, Block D, Nadel A, Kreissig I, Grinberg M. The cryosurgical adhesion: Part II. Trans Am Acad Ophthalmol Otolaryngol 1970;74:98–107.
9. Straatsma BR, Zeegen PD, Foos RY, Feeman SS, Shabo AL. Lattice degeneration of the retina. Trans Am Acad Ophthalmol Otolaryngol 1974;78:87–113.
10. Byer NE. Changes in prognosis of lattice degeneration of the retina. Trans Am Acad Ophthalmol Otolaryngol 1974;78: 114–125.
11. Charles S. Endophotocoagulation. Ophthalmol Times 1979; 4:68–69.

12. Charles S. Endophotocoagulation. Retina 1981;1:117–120.
13. Fleischman JA, Swartz M, Dixon JA. Argon laser endophotocoagulation. An intraoperative trans pars plana technique. Arch Ophthalmol 1981;99:1610–1612.
14. Peyman GA, Grisolano JM, Palacio MN. Intraocular photocoagulation with the argon-krypton laser. Arch Ophthalmol 1980;98:2062–2064.
15. Bovino JA, Marcus DF, Nelson PT. Argon laser choroidotomy for drainage of subretinal fluid. Arch Ophthalmol 1985;103:443–444.
16. Liggett PE, Lean JS, Barlow WE, Ryan SJ. Intraoperative argon endophotocoagulation for recurrent vitreous hemorrhage after vitrectomy for diabetic retinopathy. Am J Ophthalmol 1987;103:146–149.
17. Glaser BM, Campochiaro PA, Davis JL, Sato M. Retinal pigment epithelial cells release an inhibitor of neovascularization. Arch Ophthalmol 1985;103:1870–1875.
18. Peyman GA. Contact lenses for Nd:YAG application in the vitreous. Retina 1984;4:129–131.
19. Jampol LM, Goldberg MF, Jednock N. Retinal damage from a Q-switched YAG laser. Am J Ophthalmol 1983;96:326–329.
20. Callender GR. Malignant melanotic tumors of the eye: a study of histologic types in 111 cases. Trans Am Acad Ophthalmol Otolaryngol 1931;36:131–142.
21. Meyer-Schwickerath G. Photocoagulation of choroidal melanomas. Doc Ophthalmol 1980;50:57–61.
22. Shields JA. Diagnosis and management of intraocular tumors. St. Louis: CV Mosby, 1983, pp. 213–223.
23. Shields JA. The expanding role of laser photocoagulation for intraocular tumors. H. Christian Zweng Memorial Lecture, 1993. Retina (in press).
24. Shields JA, et al. The role of photocoagulation in the management of retinoblastoma. Arch Ophthalmol 1990;108:205–208.
25. Char DH. Current concepts in retinoblastoma. Ann Ophthalmol 1980;12:792–804.
26. Shields JA, et al. Episcleral plaque therapy for retinoblastoma. Ophthalmology 1989;96:530–537.
27. Gragoudas ES, Carroll JM. Multiple choroidal metastasis from bronchial carcinoid treated with photocoagulation and proton beam irradiation. Am J Ophthalmol 1979;87:299–304.
28. Gass JDM. Stereoscopic atlas of macular diseases—diagnosis and treatment, 3d ed. St Louis: CV Mosby, 1987.

10

Recent Laser Techniques in Vitreoretinal Surgery

David B. Karlin

Ophthalmology was the first specialty in medicine to use the laser as a clinical instrument to treat disease entities. Today, ophthalmic laser therapy comprises 50% to 60% of all medical laser procedures. Lasers were first used in ophthalmology to produce chorioretinal adhesions for retinal tears, before the development of a retinal detachment. A second use of ophthalmic lasers was in the treatment of leaking retinal vessels in cases of diabetic retinopathy, in an attempt to prevent the more advanced complications of vitreous hemorrhage, traction retinal detachment, and hemorrhagic glaucoma.

The first clinically successful use of light as a treatment modality was the development of the xenon arc photocoagulator (Fig. 10.1) by Meyer-Schwickerath (1). He used the rare gas xenon as the energy source to produce an intense beam of white light which, when focused, was able to produce a chorioretinal scar surrounding a retinal break. An external transpupillary approach was used. The xenon arc light coagulator was successfully used during the late 1950s and early 1960s to treat lid and adnexal lesions as well as retinal diseases and tumors.

Intravitreal endophotocoagulation using a 500-W, short xenon arc light source with a fiberoptic probe attached to the coagulator (Fig. 10.2) was developed by Charles (2,3) in the late 1970s. Xenon arc light photocoagulation via the transpupillary approach began to be supplanted in the mid and late 1960s by the ruby laser, developed by Campbell (4) and a team of physicists from the American Optical Company.

The first laser was a solid-state ruby laser. However, because of its lack of 100% reproducibility, it was replaced by the more dependable gaseous argon and krypton lasers.

The rationale for using lasers to treat chorioretinal disease is the laser's ability to produce a thermal reaction at the chorioretinal interface. This photocoagulation effect occurs as a result of both the argon and krypton lasers' transmissibility through the cornea, aqueous, lens, and vitreous to produce deposition of heat at the target tissue in the retinal pigment epithelial (RPE) layer.

Binocular Indirect Ophthalmoscope Laser Delivery System

In 1981, Mizuno (5) was the first to report on the use of argon laser photocoagulation transmitted through a binocular indirect ophthalmoscope (Fig. 10.3). This system was introduced as a commercially available instrument in the early 1980s. A separate helium-neon (HeNe) beam is transmitted down the same quartz optical fiber as is used for the argon laser. This separate HeNe beam serves as an aiming device. It can be greatly attenuated. Originally, only the argon laser was incorporated into the indirect ophthalmoscope. Today, indirect laser ophthalmoscopy can be performed using both the krypton and diode lasers. The method has been successfully used in cases of diabetic retinopathy, retinal vein occlusions, retinal tears and detachments, and retinopathy of prematurity.

Parameters in Laser Delivery Through an Indirect Ophthalmoscope

The parameter of spot size cannot be predetermined with laser delivery to the retina using an indirect binocular ophthalmoscope. With a slit-lamp delivery system, one can adjust the three parameters of laser output, duration of laser pulse, and laser spot size. The factors of power output in watts and the time interval in tenths of a second can be easily adjusted when using the indirect ophthalmoscope. However, the spot size cannot be predetermined because, unlike slit-lamp delivery where the distance of the patient's head and eye from the slit lamp is fixed, the working distance between the patient's eye and the ophthalmoscope mounted on the surgeon's head is variable.

Many factors contribute to the size of the retinal lesion when delivering laser energy through a binocular indirect ophthalmoscope. By increasing the condensing lens power from +20 to +30 diopters (D), the lesion will increase in size. The status of the patient's refractive error will also govern the size of the lesion. Myopes give smaller lesions than emmetropes. Hyperopes give larger lesions

197

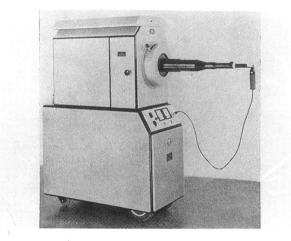

Fig. 10.1 Xenon arc light photocoagulator developed by Meyer-Schwickerath.

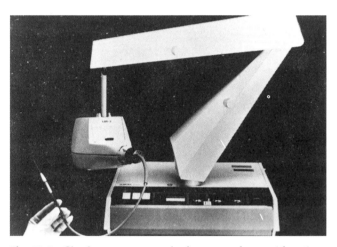

Fig. 10.2 Charles xenon arc endophotocoagulator with articulating arm used in vitrectomy surgery.

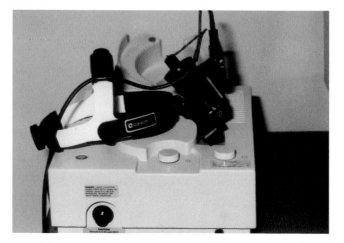

Fig. 10.3 Laser transmission through a binocular indirect ophthalmoscope.

than emmetropes. The surgeon's head movement relative to the patient's eye will also govern the spot size. If the laser focus is above the image plane, movement of the surgeon's head toward the patient creates a smaller lesion. Movement of the surgeon through the image plane and closer to the patient increases the size of the lesion.

The question of whether the eye is phakic or aphakic as well as whether an air bubble has been introduced into the vitreous cavity are two additional factors contributing to the size of the retinal lesion in laser delivery via an indirect ophthalmoscope. The eye becomes highly myopic in the phakic eye with intraocular air in the vitreous cavity. The spot size is reduced in such an eye as the surgeon holds the condensing lens further away from the patient's eye. The refractive power of the cornea is neutralized in an aphakic eye with intraocular air. Laser spots are very large in such eyes. Moving the +20 D lens closer to the patient's eye will reduce the size of the lesion.

In summary, spot size will increase when treating hyperopic eyes and decrease when laser is delivered to myopic retinas. With an air-filled phakic eye, the +20 D lens should be moved away from the patient to achieve a smaller spot size. In the air-filled aphakic eye, the lens should be moved closer to the patient's eye. Larger spot sizes can be obtained by increasing the power of the hand-held condensing lens.

Advantages of Indirect Laser Delivery

Perhaps the greatest advantage for indirect laser photocoagulation over slit-lamp delivery is the application of laser energy through a moderately sized gas bubble following trans pars plana vitrectomy surgery. Immediate postvitrectomy laser photocoagulation at the slit lamp is often difficult because of multiple light reflexes reflecting off the bubble. However, with indirect laser delivery, one can position the patient's head to move the bubble out of the path of the laser beam. Therefore, binocular indirect ophthalmoscopic laser delivery has frequently become the treatment of choice in cases of pneumatic retinopexy and giant retinal breaks flattened by air-fluid exchange.

There are many other advantages of performing laser photocoagulation via an indirect ophthalmoscopic delivery system following vitrectomy surgery. First, the eye is frequently chemotic and the cornea is, many times, edematous in the first few days following trans pars plana vitrectomy. Slit-lamp delivery of retinal photocoagulation using a corneal contact lens is therefore frequently impossible the first 2 to 3 days postoperatively. Second, the greater degree of fundus illumination via the indirect ophthalmoscope over that of the slit lamp provides more manageable photocoagulation in cases of lenticular opacification and miotic pupils. Third, there is a larger field of vision with the indirect ophthalmoscope allowing for photocoagulation up to the ora serrata. Fourth, a great advantage of laser delivery through the indirect scope is that photocoagulation is much easier when scleral depression is used in the retinal periphery. A corollary of this is that less power is required when performing laser photocoagulation with scleral depression. Two reasons may account for this phenomenon. Less distance has to be traversed through the vitreous cavity so that less laser energy is expended in the fluid vitreous. Scleral depression causes stretching of the vascular choroid. Less blood traversing the choroid will therefore prevent cooling of the retina and pigment epithelium during laser application.

There are other advantages of indirect laser delivery over slit-lamp delivery to the retina. Less chance of inadvertent laser photocoagulation of the macula occurs and fewer "skip" areas occur because a greater visual field allows better visualization of natural landmarks such as the macula and optic nerve. Additionally, many patients with advanced neurologic diseases and orthopedic problems cannot be properly seated and positioned in front of a slit lamp. For these people, indirect ophthalmoscopic delivery of laser energy provides an excellent alternative to slit-lamp laser photocoagulation. Binocular indirect laser photocoagulation has proven to be a good method of laser delivery in children with retinopathy of prematurity. The elimination of the corneal contact lens presents a great advantage in laser delivery through the binocular indirect ophthalmoscope. In recent cataract surgery, in recent suturing of corneal lacerations, and in laser application to young children, the ability to perform laser surgery without applying pressure on the cornea via the Goldmann or Rodenstock contact lens has made laser photocoagulation easier to perform.

Disadvantages of Indirect Laser Delivery

Naturally, as with all techniques, there are some disadvantages. In slit-lamp delivery, the patient's head is firmly held against both the forehead band and the chin rest. Because the laser is directed through the slit lamp, the distance is also fixed. In the binocular indirect laser delivery system, the laser is directed from the surgeon's head. Any movement of the physician's or the patient's head will vary distance and change the direction of the laser beam, perhaps causing laser photocoagulation in an area of the retina that was not intended to be treated. Similarly, any movement of the patient may also cause inaccurate photocoagulation. In addition, because the patient's head is not splinted with a contact lens when using the indirect scope, the patient's eye movement is possible, resulting in a potentially more dangerous situation.

Anesthesia and Technique

Topical proparacaine hydrochloride 0.5% is usually the only anesthetic required during retinal laser photocoagulation using a binocular indirect ophthalmoscope. This anesthetic reduces the blink reflex. Drying of the cornea is prevented by having the patient periodically close the eye. Occasionally, saline drops are required for additional corneal lubrication. A retrobulbar injection of lidocaine hydrochloride 2% will reduce the photophobia in patients with intense light sensitivity. The retrobulbar anesthetic also reduces ocular movement in patients who cannot fixate at one point. One disadvantage of a retrobulbar anesthetic is that the peripheral retina becomes difficult to visualize because the patient cannot move into the extreme positions of gaze. A cotton-tipped applicator applied by the surgeon to scleral tissue can usually bring the areas anterior to the equator into view.

It is also highly recommended that the patient's head be supported during treatment. Most frequently, it is best to have the patient lying down on a stretcher with the head in the supine position. If no stretcher is available, a reclining chair with a supporting head rest can be used as an alternative to prevent movement away from the laser source at a crucial point in laser therapy.

The most important consideration in applying laser photocoagulation through the indirect ophthalmoscope is that the surgeon be familiar with the technique of indirect ophthalmoscopy. A power setting of 200 mW with a time setting of 0.2 sec is initially used. The aiming beam is provided by either attenuating the argon laser beam or in some scopes by providing a separate HeNe aiming device. If neither the patient's head nor the surgeon's head moves, the size of the retinal lesion can be modified by turning a zoom lens mounted on the ophthalmoscope. Another way of increasing the size of the burn is to substitute a $+30$ D lens for a $+20$ D lens. The power setting is then turned up in increments of 25 mW until a moderately white retinal lesion is obtained. It must be remembered that power settings must be reduced when treating with scleral depression. If a choroidal hemorrhage is produced, moderate pressure should be applied to the eye, followed by three concentric, contiguous rows of laser around the hemorrhage, using reduced power.

Indications for Indirect Laser Photocoagulation

The most important indication for laser delivery through the binocular indirect ophthalmoscope is following pars plana vitrectomy surgery. This is especially true when air has been introduced into the vitreous cavity during the course of the vitrectomy procedure. Friberg and Eller (6) reported on the advantages of using laser photocoagulation via an indirect ophthalmoscope in cases of pneumatic retinopathy for retinal detachment. Indirect laser delivery is also preferable in cases where cataract opacification makes slit-lamp delivery difficult. Poor dilation of the pupil arising in cases of posterior synechiae following uveitis and in glaucoma patients using miotic therapy comprise another group of eyes where indirect laser delivery becomes the treatment of choice. The visualization of the retinal periphery is made easier with the indirect ophthalmoscope than with the slit lamp using the Goldmann triple-mirror or the Rodenstock lens. Therefore, cases of lattice degeneration harboring retinal breaks as well as peripheral neovascularization such as occurs in cases of sickle cell retinopathy are more efficiently treated with laser delivery through the indirect scope. Supplemental laser treatment in cases of giant retinal tears successfully reattached by an air-fluid exchange is also more easily performed by indirect laser delivery in the postoperative phase.

Complications of Indirect Laser Delivery

Inadvertent movement of the patient's or surgeon's head may cause deposition of laser energy in an area of the retina not intended to be coagulated. This is of small consequence when working in the retinal periphery or in the nasal quadrants. However, in administering laser burns in the temporal retina close to the macular area or in the juxtapapillary zone, an inaccurate laser application could result in macular dysfunction, optic neuritis, or even optic atrophy. For this reason, the practice model eye manufactured by MIRA of Waltham, Massachusetts is a useful method to be used before clinical treatment. The patient's eye can be stabilized by using a stretcher or a headrest for support. A retrobulbar anesthetic can also be used to avoid ocular motion.

Most other complications of indirect laser delivery are similar to those encountered in slit-lamp applications. Too much laser power can result in a retinal or choroidal hemorrhage. Firm digital pressure on the eye can frequently stop a hemorrhage from spreading. In addition, three rows of laser applications around the bleeding site should be performed using reduced energy, as a prophylactic approach to prevent a retinal detachment.

The Semiconductor Diode Laser

The first laser to be used for retinal photocoagulation following the introduction of the xenon arc photocoagulator was the ruby laser, introduced in the 1960s. The argon blue-green laser and the krypton red laser were the first continuous wave (CW) gaseous ion lasers introduced, respectively, in 1968 and 1972. The CW tunable organic dye laser was clinically accepted in 1981. The disadvantages of these gas ion lasers are that they require a high-voltage power supply, plumbing for water cooling, are bulky in size, not readily portable, and expensive to purchase. Many of these disadvantages have been corrected by the introduction of the solid-state semiconductor diode laser (Fig. 10.4).

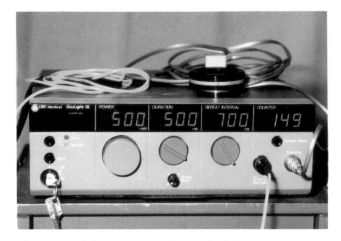

Fig. 10.4 Solid-state semiconductor diode laser.

Laser diodes are a special type of light-emitting diode. Laser diodes are made from semiconductor crystals of gallium arsenide (GaAs). "Doping" is the process of adding other atoms to the host semiconductor. The wavelength of the diode is a property of the semiconductor crystal. GaAs "doped" with aluminum (GaAlAs) is the most common semiconductor laser crystal. The diode laser operates in the low infrared region of the spectrum, between 780 and 850 nm. Light at 800 nm is easily transmitted through cornea, aqueous, lens, and vitreous to reach the retinal target tissue. Fortunately, there is little absorption by the xanthophyll in the macula. Unfortunately, only 25% of diode laser emission is absorbed by the RPE. Contrasted to this, there is 95% absorption by the RPE using the argon green laser operating at a wavelength of 514 nm. The result is that three to four times as much power is required with the diode laser than with the argon green laser to produce similar chorioretinal photocoagulation.

Puliafito and colleagues (7) were the first to clinically describe the chorioretinal lesions produced with a diode laser. Both endoscopic and transpupillary delivery systems were used. Histopathologic evaluation of retinal lesions showed no essential differences when the argon and krypton lasers, operating in the visible spectrum, were used or when the diode laser, operating in the low infrared region of the spectrum, was used.

The common diode laser operates at 810 nm. It has been used in the treatment of proliferative diabetic retinopathy (PDR), exudative diabetic maculopathy, panretinal photocoagulation (PRP), the treatment of retinal tears, and retinal vein occlusion. Its fiberoptic delivery system can be used as either an endophotocoagulator during vitreous surgery, or through a transpupillary slit-lamp delivery system. Greater power and longer exposure times are required with the solid-state diode laser than with the gaseous argon and krypton lasers. Power levels of 500 to 1200 mW and time intervals of 0.2 to 0.5 sec are frequently required. Pain is much more common with the red lasers of krypton and diode than with the argon blue-green and green lasers. One possible explanation is that there is less absorption of diode laser energy in the RPE, so that the energy is deposited deeper into the choroidal tissue. Thus, there may be more pain stimulation from receptors in the ciliary nerves. The increased power levels required to obtain a good laser reaction produce a more painful reaction when using the semiconductor diode laser. A retrobulbar anesthetic is therefore more frequently used with the diode laser than with argon.

Advantages of the Diode Laser

There are both technical and clinical advantages of using the semiconductor diode laser instead of the argon laser. The diode laser can operate off a standard 110-V line or can be battery driven. Therefore, no special 220-V electrical output is required. The diode laser is more compact and can be made portable. Its initial cost and its maintenance are much less than those of the argon laser. Expensive plumbing, as required with the argon laser, is unnecessary because water cooling is not required.

The clinical advantages of the diode laser over the argon laser are similar to those found with the krypton red laser. There is greater transmission of laser energy through cataractous lenses or slight vitreous hemorrhage and better laser penetration through macular edema and serous retinal detachment. There is less absorption of laser energy in areas of intraretinal hemorrhage than with the argon laser.

Disadvantages of the Diode Laser

As with other lasers, there still remain disadvantages with the use of the semiconductor diode laser. In the transpupillary delivery system, more pain is experienced by the patient. Higher power levels and longer time duration are required. The greater beam divergence with the diode laser results in less precise focusing than with the argon or the krypton lasers. As with the krypton laser, subretinal hemorrhage may be more common with the diode laser than with the argon laser. This also results from the fact that with the diode laser, there is less RPE absorption and deeper choroidal penetration.

New Advances in Laser Technology for Vitreoretinal Surgery

Historical Background

In the 1940s, Schepens and associates (8) devised the pioneering technique of scleral buckling as a means of reattaching the retina. Following this procedure, many eyes were salvaged that were formerly lost to retinal detachment. The success rate in detachment surgery increased dramatically. For the most part, scleral buckling is an extraocular procedure, the sclerotomy for drainage of subretinal fluid being the only invasive intraocular technique. In the 1960s, Lincoff and colleagues (9) demonstrated that the drainage of subretinal fluid was unnecessary in certain selected cases of retinal detachment.

Cibis (10) was the first to show in the 1960s that manipulations within the vitreous cavity could serve as an adjunct to the scleral buckling procedure in the more advanced and complicated forms of retinal detachment. He introduced the liquid silicone injection as an internal tamponade and devised microinstrumentation for manipulation within the vitreous cavity. Thus was born the age of vitreous surgery in a compartment of the eye that was formerly held to be inviolate. Shafer (11) used human eye bank vitreous as an implant within the vitreous cavity in the late 1950s. In the late 1960s and early 1970s, Machemer and coworkers (12) devised new techniques in vitrectomy surgery that have been adopted by vitreoretinal surgeons in the last two decades. Machemer and colleagues (12), O'Malley and Heintz (13), Douvas (14), Peyman and Dodich (15), and Klöti (16) devised the many mechanical cutters that served as prototypes for today's instruments used within the vitreous cavity.

In the 1960s, Karlin (17) and Purnell and associates (18), working independently, were the first investigators to use the radiation pressure effect of ultrasonic energy within the vitreous cavity to retrodisplace retinal tissue in cases of retinal detachment. Karlin (17) showed that the radiation pressure effect of ultrasound can retrodisplace retinal tissue in certain cases of retinal detachment. Best movement of retinal detachment occurred in those cases exhibiting retinal holes (rhegmatogenous detachments), whereas little movement was demonstrated in traction or nonrhegmatogenous detachments. Results indicated that therapeutic ultrasound may be a prognostic test for successful surgical reattachment of the detached retina. Karlin (19) also designed an ultrasonic probe for vitreous liquefaction (Fig. 10.5) in cases of massive vitreous hemorrhage with organized blood within the vitreous cavity. The probe was also used for experimental ultrasonic transection of vitreoretinal membranes created in the vitreous cavity of rabbit eyes. This was perhaps one of the first indications of the use of a nonmechanical cutter for transection of epiretinal membranes through the use of tractionless ultrasonic energy. Karlin (17) and Purnell and coworkers (18) demonstrated that ultrasound may also prove useful in treating giant retinal breaks, noninvasive external dissolution of vitreoretinal adhesions, and positioning air bubbles placed within the vitreous cavity.

The advent of ophthalmic laser surgery began in the late 1960s. Thus far, lasers have been clinically successful in vitreoretinal surgery via their photocoagulation effect. Today, many investigators are currently experimenting

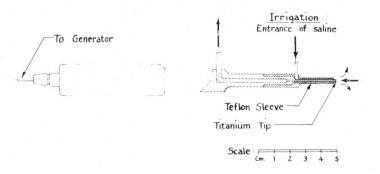

To Suction Pump
Exit of liquefied
blood clot and vitreous

To Generator

Irrigation
Entrance of saline

Teflon Sleeve

Titanium Tip

Scale:
Cm. 1 2 3 4 5

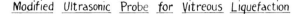

Modified Ultrasonic Probe for Vitreous Liquefaction

Fig. 10.5 Design of ultrasonic liquefaction transducer. (Reproduced by permission from Karlin [19].)

with various lasers at the animal level in an attempt to find a suitable laser to be used as a phototransector, or cutting instrument, within the vitreous cavity.

Lasers as Cutting Instruments Within the Vitreous Cavity

Laser surgery has been used successfully for over 30 years as a primary noninvasive procedure for the treatment of retinal tears. More recently, lasers have also been used as an invasive ancillary procedure in vitrectomy for the treatment of retinal holes as well as for their ability to coagulate retinal tissue. In both procedures, the argon, krypton, and diode lasers are used for their photocoagulation effect. At present, the use of lasers for phototransection (cutting) is at the verge of becoming a clinically applicable tool in the armamentarium of the vitreoretinal surgeon.

The primary advantage of using a laser for phototransection within the vitreous cavity is that it would eliminate the *traction* on retinal tissue that frequently occurs with the mechanical cutters, scissors, or pics used today. With the current mechanical cutters, vitreoretinal membranes have to be sucked into the open port of the instrument where they are severed by either the guillotine or oscillatory cutting action of the mechanical instrument. With the suction action, traction is transmitted to the fibrovascular membrane, frequently causing vitreous and retinal hemorrhage. In addition, distal traction on a vitreoretinal membrane may also cause retinal tears and retinal detachment. The alternate use of mechanical scissors and vitreoretinal pics used to dissect epiretinal membranes also have the potential complication of causing traction and may result in vitreous hemorrhage, retinal tears, and retinal detachment.

The following lasers designed for cutting within the vitreous cavity have the added advantage of providing tractionless surgery. These lasers, for the most part, operate in the infrared end of the spectrum, although one

of them, the excimer laser, functions at UV levels. The CO_2 laser, the sapphire-tipped neodymium: yttrium-aluminum-garnet (Nd:YAG) laser, the excimer laser, the erbium:YAG (Er:YAG) laser, the holmium:YAG (Ho:YAG) laser, and the picosecond neodymium: yttrium-lithium-fluoride (Nd:YLF) laser all have phototransection ability within the vitreous cavity. These lasers are discussed in the order of their historical appearance.

Carbon Dioxide (CO_2) Laser

Karlin and colleagues (20) and Miller and associates (21) were two of the earliest investigators to recognize the possibility of using the phototransection (cutting) ability of the CO_2 laser for intraocular ablation and tractionless segmentation of vitreoretinal membranes. Working independently, they used the cutting and coagulation ability of the CO_2 laser in the fabrication of CO_2 intravitreal probes to be used in trans pars plana vitrectomy procedures.

Shortly after the discovery of the CO_2 laser by Patel (22), coherent radiation in the infrared region of the spectrum drew the interest of the medical profession as a potential tool for a variety of surgical procedures. The CO_2 laser has its principal emission wavelength at 10.6 μm. It has been successfully used in dermatology (23), otolaryngology (24), gynecology (23), and burn surgery (25).

Ocular tissues are essentially opaque to CO_2 laser radiation. Fig. 10.6 shows the water extinction curves for the various lasers in wavelengths. In general, the extinction dimension is defined as the distance from the surface of water at which 90% of the incident laser radiation is absorbed. The extinction length is inversely proportional to the wavelength. Thus, the CO_2 laser produces almost all of its effect in the vicinity of the target tissue with little retrograde radiation extension.

The two most important lasers from an ophthalmologic clinical standpoint have been the argon and krypton

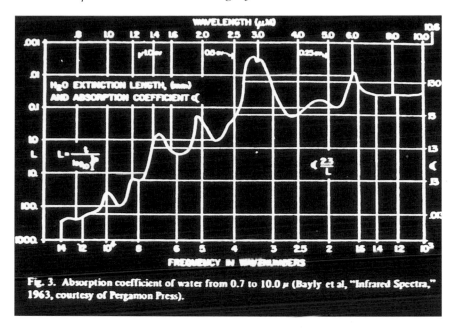

Fig. 10.6 Absorption coefficient of water at various wavelengths.

lasers. These lasers have emission wavelengths in the visible spectrum where ocular tissues and fluids are frequently transparent and not opaque, allowing penetration through the ocular media before depositing their energy at the retinal target tissue. The CO_2 laser is relatively opaque to ocular tissue, depositing its energy at the point of impact. The short penetration depth of the CO_2 laser was demonstrated by Bridges and associates (26) to be approximately one wavelength (10 μm). This means that the CO_2 laser's greatest effect will be at the first point of contact with ocular tissue and explains why little damage to neighboring tissue, and no damage to more distant tissue, are seen. For the application of ablating vitreoretinal membranes, the short penetration depth of the CO_2 laser is advantageous because little or no adverse effect would be produced in the underlying optic nerve or macular areas. In Fig. 10.7, Karlin shows the transection of the anterior hyaloid membrane of the vitreous with little retrograde extension of CO_2 laser energy.

Argon and krypton lasers are pigment dependent. Laser light emitted by these sources is absorbed by hemoglobin and by the pigment epithelium in the retina and choroid. Because of greater pigmentation in the macula, power levels that give a minimal lesion in the nonmacular area produce a moderately heavy lesion in the parafoveal area. Because of their pigment dependence, argon and krypton lasers produce almost no reaction in the albino or nonpigmented fundus. Karlin and associates (27) and Miller and associates (28) showed that chorioretinal lesions can be produced in white albino rabbit eyes with CO_2 laser radiation (Fig. 10.8). Thus, CO_2 laser photocoagulation is not pigment dependent. This is a definite advantage if the CO_2 laser is used to transect an avascular vitreoretinal frond during vitrectomy surgery.

One might speculate about the overall practicality of the CO_2 laser as an endophotocoagulator in vitrectomy, considering the acceptance of the argon, krypton, and diode laser endophotocoagulators. It has been shown that the CO_2 laser has the important dual potential advantages of cutting as well as coagulating, a function that the argon, krypton, and diode lasers cannot accomplish. The simultaneous ability of the CO_2 laser to photocoagulate and phototransect might offer improved results in clear media vitrectomy for PDR with massive fibrovascular membrane formation.

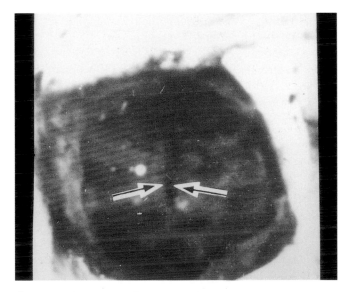

Fig. 10.7 Photograph of CO_2 laser phototransection through the anterior hyaloid membrane of the vitreous body, in a human eye bank eye. Distance between arrows indicates width of incision. (Reproduced by permission from Karlin et al. [20].)

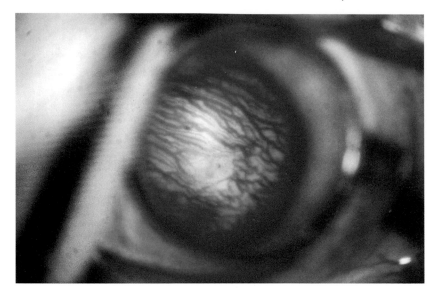

Figure 10.8 A chorioretinal lesion made in the albino rabbit eye shown immediately after CO$_2$ laser application; 0.4 W of energy level was used for 0.2 sec.

The dual effects of retinal photocoagulation and phototransection with the CO$_2$ laser require an invasive intravitreal approach because of the essentially complete absorption of CO$_2$ laser energy by all ocular tissue. Karlin and coworkers (20) demonstrated the great absorption of CO$_2$ laser energy by the vitreous body. However, it is necessary to make physical contact between the tip of the intravitreal CO$_2$ laser probe and the internal limiting membrane of the retina or the neovascular or avascular vitreoretinal membrane. At times, it is difficult to determine the exact point of contact of the tip to the target tissue. If the tip exerts too much pressure, an iatrogenic retinal tear may develop. If the probe does not closely approximate the retina or membrane, then much of the energy is absorbed by the intervening vitreous, which insulates the retina and prevents the production of an adequate chorioretinal lesion or a transection.

Karlin has shown in Fig. 10.9 a series of chorioretinal lesions made with a CO$_2$ laser in a rabbit's eye during the course of a vitrectomy procedure. Energy is held constant at 0.4 W. Time is variable with the lower lesions, seen from left to right, made at 0.125 sec, 0.25 sec, 0.50 sec, and 0.75 sec. The three lesions seen at the upper part of Fig. 10.9 were made at 1.0 sec, 2.0 sec, and 5.0 sec. Results indicated that CO$_2$ laser chorioretinal lesions made at lower power levels are indistinguishable from argon and krypton lesions. The last lesion made with 0.4 W for 5 sec demonstrates the intense laser radiation to be splayed out into the subretinal space.

Karlin has demonstrated two potentially adverse effects using a CO$_2$ laser. Bubble formation may occur within the vitreous cavity following the continuous application of CO$_2$ laser energy in both the production of chorioretinal lesions and the transection of vitreoretinal membranes during the course of a vitrectomy procedure (Fig. 10.10). It should be noted that only in rare cases does the presence of the bubbles interfere with the visual-

ization of the underlying retina. In addition, the bubbles dissolve within the vitreous cavity within a short period of time. Carbon deposition may occur within the chorioretinal lesion in those applications made with higher power levels (see Fig. 10.9). Future studies are necessary to determine what, if any, lasting effects may occur at these higher power levels.

Advantages of CO$_2$ Lasers

Table 10.1 summarizes the many advantages of substituting a CO$_2$ laser for the current argon, krypton, and diode lasers used in vitreous surgery. Perhaps the greatest advantage is the dual effect of photocoagulation and phototransection. This implies that when a neovascular vitreoretinal membrane is cut, the coagulation effect of the CO$_2$ laser will seal vessels, thus preventing retinal and

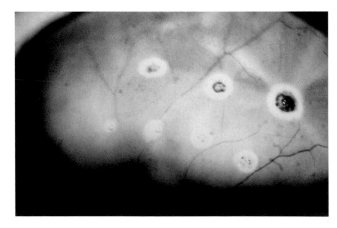

Fig. 10.9 Fundus photograph of a human eye bank eye shows a series of chorioretinal lesions using a CO$_2$ laser. Power levels were held constant at 0.4 W while time was varied from 0.125 to 5 sec. (Reproduced with permission from Karlin et al. [27].)

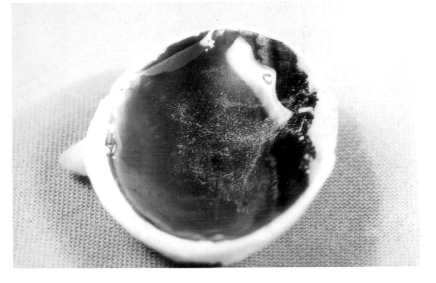

Fig. 10.10 Section of a rabbit eye demonstrates bubble formation in the vitreous cavity following continuous application of a CO_2 laser for photo-transection and photocoagulation during the course of a trans pars plana vitrectomy procedure.

vitreous hemorrhage. The CO_2 laser is not pigment dependent, which means that, unlike the argon laser, avascular membranes can be severed. Because ocular tissue is opaque to the CO_2 laser, almost all the energy is absorbed by the target tissue, with little retrograde extension to underlying or neighboring ocular tissue. It is well known that the preretinal membranes in the proliferative diabetic eye occur mainly overlying the macula and optic nerve. If one were to use argon laser in this area, one would certainly cause metamorphopsia, optic neuritis, or optic atrophy. However, with the almost complete absorption of energy in the target tissue by the CO_2 laser, this instrument provides an ideal surgical tool, preventing damage to these two most vital structures in the posterior segment of the eye.

Disadvantages of CO_2 Lasers

Despite the obvious advantages of the CO_2 laser, disadvantages are apparent (Table 10.2). CO_2 laser surgery implies contact or touch surgery. CO_2 energy cannot be

Table 10.1 Advantages of the Carbon Dioxide Laser

1. Dual effect of photocoagulation and phototransection via ablative surgery through tissue evaporation

2. Hemostasis and cutting under constant visible control

3. No pigment dependence; hence, cutting of avascular vitreoretinal membranes

4. High absorbency at the target tissue with minimal damage to neighboring ocular tissue

5. Micromanipulation
     High precision
     High control

6. Less postoperative pain because less edema or hemorrhage with photocoagulation

Table 10.2 Disadvantages of the Carbon Dioxide Laser

1. Nonfiberoptic delivery system

2. Direct contact with target tissue necessary

3. Carbonization at the end of the probe on the diamond window

4. Carbonization of the target tissue when using higher power

transmitted through the ocular media into the vitreous or at the chorioretinal interface. Carbon particles may be deposited on the diamond window of the probe, preventing adequate transmission of laser energy to the target tissue. If this situation occurs, the probe has to be removed from the vitreous cavity, the carbon removed from the enclosed diamond window with a Bard-Parker blade, and the probe reinserted into the vitreous cavity through the sclerotomy site.

The third and perhaps the greatest drawback to the use of the CO_2 laser in vitreous surgery is the inability to ef-

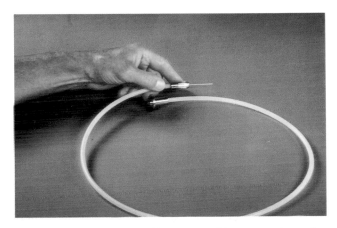

Fig. 10.11 Silver bromide fibers encased in a protective polyethelene sleeve used as the fiberoptic delivery system to transmit the CO_2 laser.

fectively transmit its energy through a fiberoptic delivery system. Karlin and colleagues (20), working at Bell Laboratories, attempted to transmit a CO_2 laser down 0.2 and 0.5 mm silver bromide fibers enclosed in a protective polyethelene covering and attached to a 20-gauge (0.89 mm) needle (Fig. 10.11). Although initial studies proved successful (Fig. 10.12), continuous use burned out the fibers and finally resulted in lack of CO_2 laser transmission. Because of inability to achieve fiberoptic delivery, one cannot miniaturize the CO_2 probe to a size that is compatible with the intravitreal mechanical cutters used today. Karlin and associates (29) patented an articulating arm delivery system for the CO_2 laser (Fig. 10.13), in which a series of quartz waveguide fibers propagate CO_2 laser energy to the probe. Their CO_2 laser, complete with a HeNe aiming beam, is shown in Figs. 14A and 14B.

Using this instrument, Karlin has produced chorioretinal lesions (see Fig. 10.8), transected vitreoretinal mem-

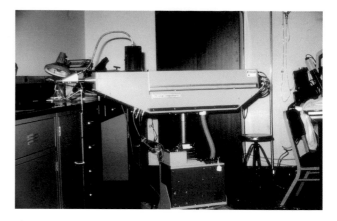

Fig. 10.14A   The CO_2 laser, as developed by Karlin in collaboration with Bell Laboratories, Murray Hill, NJ.

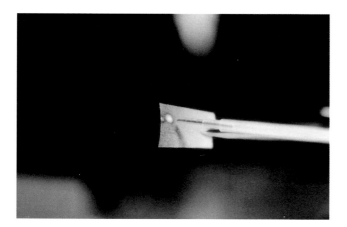

Fig. 10.12   The dual effect of photocoagulation and phototransection as a result of fiberoptic delivery of a CO_2 laser as shown in Fig. 10.11.

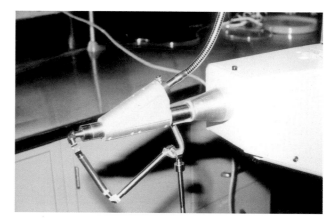

Fig. 10.14B   The distal end of the CO_2 laser instrument seen in Fig. 10.14A, and showing the articulating arm and the HeNe aiming beam.

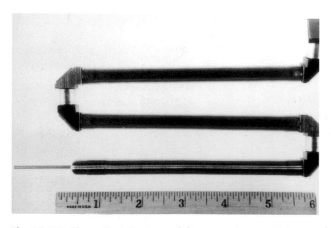

Fig. 10.13   The articulating arm delivery system used to transmit CO_2 laser radiation to ocular tissue. A series of quartz waveguide fibers propagate CO_2 laser energy to the probe.

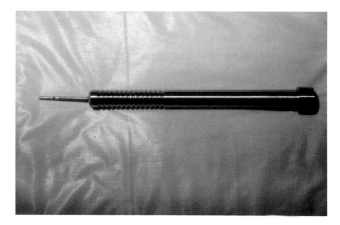

Fig. 10.15   The CO_2 laser handpiece measuring 2.5 mm in diameter and enclosed by the diamond window.

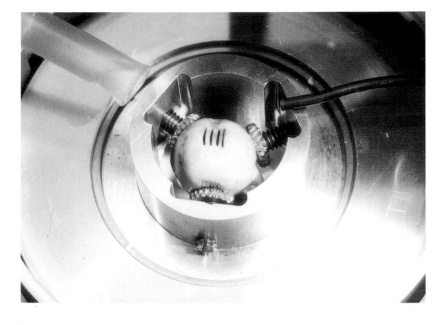

Fig. 10.16 Human eye bank eye mounted in holder. Four scleral incisions of approximately 0.5 cm in length have been produced by CO_2 laser phototransection. (Reproduced by permission from Karlin et al. [20].)

branes, and transected the anterior hyaloid membrane (see Fig. 10.7) in the experimental model rabbit eye. The tip of the handpiece is shown in Fig. 10.15. Karlin has also used this CO_2 laser instrument to create graded scleral incisions, as seen in Fig. 10.16. Histologic evaluation indicates sharp scleral cuts with increase in depth of penetration as the power level of the CO_2 laser is increased (Fig. 10.17). One notes little, if any, damage to neighboring scleral tissue as seen in the hemotoxylin and eosin stained scleral tissue. When one plots power in watts versus depth of penetration in millimeters (Fig. 10.18), one notes that it consistently required 2.75 W of energy level before the sclera was totally transected and choroidal tissue was entered. The implication is that the CO_2 laser may lend itself to the use of full ocular wall resection in the treatment of melanosarcoma of the choroid.

Harrington and Gregory (30) have reported on the use of hollow sapphire fibers for the delivery of CO_2 laser energy. Their new hollow waveguide is made of a single-crystal flexible sapphire tubing that has a low loss at 10.6 μm and can deliver near single-mode laser powers greater than 80 W. Harrington (30) believes that hollow sapphire fibers should be an excellent fiber delivery system for use in laser surgery. The smallest diameter fibers are sufficiently flexible to be useful in endoscopic procedures such as laser laparoscopy, bronchoscopy, and laser angioplasty of peripheral arteries. Karlin is, at present, collaborating with Harrington on the fiberoptic delivery system for the CO_2 laser in vitrectomy surgery.

Sapphire-Tipped Neodymium:YAG (Nd:YAG) Laser

The synthetic sapphire crystal is physically neutral to laser energy and does not alter laser transmission. Sapphire has great mechanical strength, low thermal conductivity, and a high melting point. All of these characteristics make sapphire a good conduit to transmit laser energy to the target tissue. Because of the optical properties and the geometric design, the exact shape and focal point of the beam can be determined by the design of the tips. The tips are placed in direct contact with the target tissue. Thus, the efficiency of laser delivery is increased without loss of energy via transmission across the vitreous cavity. The sapphire tip is coupled to either a Nd:YAG or an argon laser via a quartz fiber. Various sapphire designs have been fabricated, incorporating either narrow or broad tips (Fig. 10.19) and with either straight or curved configurations.

Federman (31) has performed transcleral laser photocoagulation of the retina using both the argon and Nd:YAG lasers. Karlin and Degan (32), working with Sharplan, have used the infrared sapphire-tipped CW

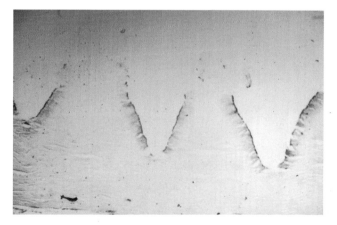

Fig. 10.17 Stained section of human eye bank eye showing same graded scleral incisions seen grossly in Fig. 10.16. Hematoxylin-eosin; ×10. (Reproduced by permission from Karlin et al. [20].)

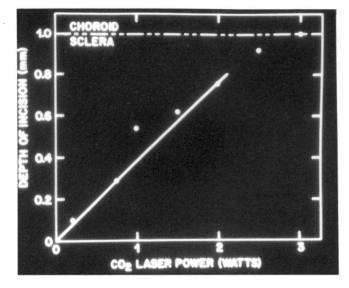

Fig. 10.18 Experimentally measured depth of incision in millimeters into scleral-chorioretinal coats of human eye bank eye as function of CO_2 laser power in watts. (Reproduced by permission from Karlin et al. [20].)

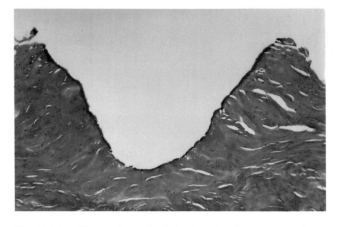

Fig. 10.20 Histopathologic slide of a scleral incision made with the sapphire-tipped Nd:YAG laser. Note the clean cut with little adverse effect on underlying scleral tissue. Hematoxylin-eosin; ×10.

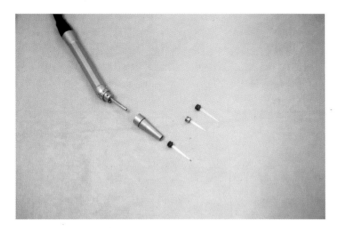

Fig. 10.19 Sapphire tips used with a CW Nd:YAG laser.

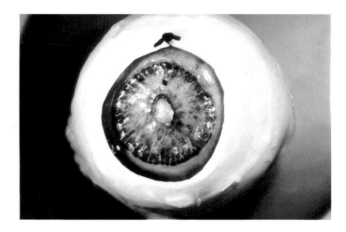

Fig. 10.21 An iridectomy made in the 12 o'clock meridian using the sapphire-tipped CW Nd:YAG laser.

Nd:YAG laser as a research surgical scalpel in both the posterior segment as well as in the anterior segment of the eye. Karlin created Nd:YAG retinal laser lesions as well as transections of vitreoretinal membranes. In addition, he created scleral (Fig. 10.20) and corneal incisions as well as iridectomies (Fig. 10.21).

The transcleral chorioretinal lesions made with the contact Nd:YAG sapphire tips are avascular and have strong adhesive qualities. The 1064-nm infrared wavelength of the Nd:YAG laser has a deeper tissue penetration than the 514-nm visible spectrum wavelength of the argon laser. Therefore, the sapphire-tipped Nd:YAG contact laser may prove clinically advantageous as a phototransector of both avascular and vascular vitreoretinal membranes. Federman (31) has shown that an endolaser scalpel for transvitreal surgery is capable of creating a retinotomy

in cases of retinal detachment with advanced proliferative vitreoretinopathy. Furthermore, sapphire-tipped Nd:YAG laser probes used in endophotocoagulation create lesions that appear to have immediate adhesive properties.

Advantages of the Sapphire Laser

The main advantage of the contact sapphire-tipped Nd:YAG laser scalpel is that it uses an efficient quartz fiberoptic delivery system. This is a distinct advantage over the CO_2 laser where the more cumbersome articulating arm delivery system is used. The contact laser scalpel using Nd:YAG energy operates as a cutter as well as a coagulator, thereby providing hemostasis. Like the CO_2 laser, it may also have applications to full eye wall resections in cases of melanosarcoma of the choroid. It may also be used as a contact delivery system for interstitial hypothermia in the treatment of ocular tumors. In animal studies, embedding contact laser probes in pancreatic and esophageal tumors and irradiating the tissue at a constant temperature for a specific period of time has resulted in a high percentage of death of tumor cells. This application may be found useful in the future treatment of ocular tumors.

Disadvantages of the Sapphire Laser

Certain problems associated with the use of the sapphire-tipped Nd:YAG laser in ophthalmic applications will have to be addressed before this laser becomes a clinically acceptable instrument. Like the CO_2 laser, the sapphire-tipped Nd:YAG laser uses a contact mode approach that ensures greater efficiency through less loss of energy because it does not have to be propagated through the vitreous fluid to reach the target tissue. However, it has thus far been difficult to obtan 100% reproducibility of lesions because it is difficult to determine at what point the tip engages ocular tissue. Fatigue sets in with repeated use of the sapphire tip, decreasing the efficiency of laser energy transmission and requiring a change to another sapphire tip. Karlin and Degan (32) found, as with the CO_2 laser, carbon deposition on the sapphire tip with repeated use of the instrument. A slight amount of carbon acts as a heat sink and enhances transmission of laser energy to the target tissue. With more carbon accumulation, the tip becomes insulated and prevents laser propagation to the target tissue. The contact sapphire-tipped Nd:YAG laser could easily become a clinically acceptable instrument if the above problems could be rectified.

Excimer Laser

The excimer (excited dimer) laser is composed of a rare gas, such as argon, combined with a halogen, such as fluorine, and operates in the UV end of the spectrum. Excimer lasers are photoablative in that they break up the intramolecular bonds of tissue. This UV laser has provided a well-controlled, highly precise method for corneal sculpting and cutting. Its use for cutting in vitreoretinal surgery has been advocated by some investigators.

Although there are many excimer lasers, they can be grouped into three, according to wavelength. The argon fluoride (ArF) laser, operating at a wavelength of 193 nm, is used for corneal contouring. Unfortunately for the vitreoretinal surgeon, it is not possible to transmit this laser down a fiberoptic delivery system. Hence, probes using 193-nm wavelength cannot be miniaturized to sizes compatible with other instruments already in use in vitreoretinal surgery. The xenon chloride (XeCl) laser, operating at a wavelength of 308 nm, is the best excimer laser used for vitreoretinal membrane transection. The 308-nm excimer laser has captured the imagination of the cardio-

vascular surgeons where it has been used in laser angioplasty to remove atheromatous plaques following balloon angioplasty (Fig. 10.22). Pellin and colleagues (33) have shown in experimental animal research that the XeCl laser, operating at a wavelength of 308 nm, is capable of transecting the fibrovascular vitreoretinal membranes occurring in cases of PDR. Furthermore, the 308-nm wavelength is capable of fiberoptic delivery. Using a red HeNe aiming beam, the 308-nm excimer laser has successfully cut vitreoretinal membranes produced in the experimental rabbit eye.

The problem with using UV light as an energy source to effect cutting within the vitreous cavity is the possibility of producing mutagenic changes in ocular tissue, potentially leading to carcinoma. The lower excimer wave length of 193 nm has been found by Trentacoste and coworkers (34) to be essentially free of mutagenicity. As the wavelength increases through the gamet of excimer lasers, the chance of mutagenicity increases. Krypton fluoride (KrF) at 248 nm has the highest possibility of mutagenic changes. The XeCl laser, operating at 308 nm, falls midway between the possible carcinogenic effect of the KrF laser of 248 nm and the almost nonexistent mutagenic possibility using excimer at 193 nm. Marshall and Slincy (35) have also shown retinal and lenticular changes using the excimer laser operating at a wavelength of 308 nm. Because of the above potentially hazardous complications, the use of the excimer laser as a cutting tool within the vitreous cavity has largely been abandoned.

Erbium:YAG (Er:YAG) Laser

Figure 10.6 shows the absorption coefficient of water for various wavelengths. One can see that the Er:YAG laser, operating at 2.94 µm in the mid infrared region, offers the best chance of cutting vitreoretinal membranes with the least chance of damage to neighboring ocular tissue. The reason for this laser offering the greatest promise is that at 2.94 µm, there is almost complete absorption of laser energy in water or vitreous with little transmission in a retrograde manner. Thus, there would be relatively little adverse effect on the underlying optic disc and macula while transecting epiretinal membranes overlying the macula (Fig. 10.23) and obliterating fronds emanating from the optic disc (Fig. 10.24).

Puliafito, Margolis, and colleagues (36) have shown that a pulsed Er:YAG laser, operating via an intraocular fiberoptic delivery system, allows almost tractionless cutting of vitreoretinal membranes created experimentally in rabbit eyes.

The Er:YAG laser, operating at 2.94 µm, is the most strongly absorbed by water of any of the lasers operating in the infrared, visible, or UV regions. Its absorption length is only 1 µm. Peyman and Katoh (37) were among the first to describe the effects of the Er:YAG laser on var-

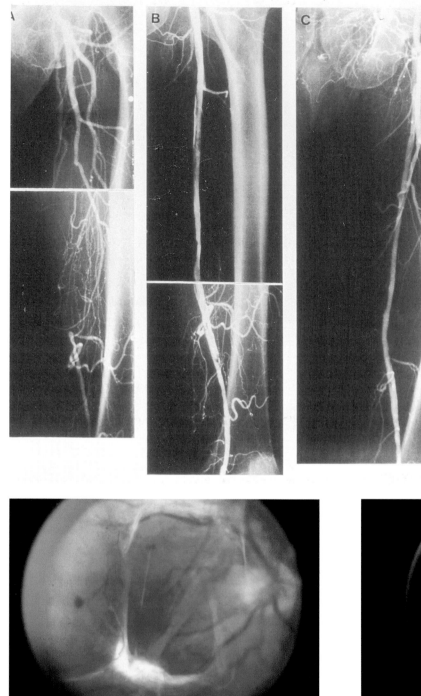

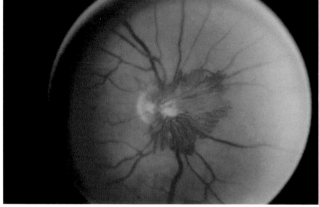

Fig. 10.22 A, Photo shows complete occlusion of the superior femoral artery. B, Immediately after balloon and excimer laser treatment. C, One year later, demonstrating patency of the artery. (Courtesy of Timothy Sanborn, MD, Cornell Medical School, New York, NY.)

Fig. 10.23 Three epiretinal membranes overlying the macular area as they run from the superior temporal to the inferior temporal vascular arcades in a case of PDR.

Fig. 10.24 Fundus photo depicting advanced neovascularization of the optic disc (NVD) with a fibrovascular frond emanating from the disc in a case of PDR.

ious ocular tissues. However, Puliafito and associates (36) first described the use of the Er:YAG laser in cutting experimentally formed vitreous membranes created in rabbit eyes. The threshold energy for membrane ablation was 3.6 mJ/pulse using a pulsed Er:YAG laser. Energy levels for membrane cutting were between 3.6 and

14 mJ/pulse. Retinal damage thresholds were determined for positions of the tip 1000, 1500 and 2000 μm from the retina. Some retinal burns as well as retinal hemorrhage occurred, especially when the tip was oriented in a perpendicular rather than a tangential fashion to the retinal surface.

Ellsworth and associates (38) used an Er:YAG laser to produce full thickness retinotomies. D'Amico and colleagues (39) have recently used an Er:YAG laser to produce laser photothermal retinal ablation in enucleated rabbit eyes. Laser output was delivered by a high midinfrared-transmitting fluoride fiber connected to a delivery probe consisting of a sapphire rod 375 μm in diameter. Graded retinal lesions were produced in both an air and a fluid medium.

Disadvantages of the Er:YAG Laser

The difficulty with using the Er:YAG laser is similar to that encountered with the previously discussed lasers. The adequate development of a reliable fiberoptic delivery system still remains the chief barrier preventing the clinical application of these lasers as an alternate cutting tool to the mechanical vitreous cutters and scissors used today. Low hydroxyl-fused silica fibers are used as the fiberoptic delivery system to couple the energy from the Er:YAG laser into the tip of the probe. Unfortunately, there is high attenuation of the radiation, necessitating very short silica fibers as a conduction vehicle. Puliafito and colleagues (36) have been experimenting with zirconium fluoride (ZrF_4) glass fibers as an alternate to the silica fibers. ZrF_4 has extremely low attenuation at 2.9 μm. It is stable at high energy levels. However, ZrF_4 has two disadvantages. Although the fiber is stable at high energy levels when used in air, it gives a markedly attenuated output when placed in a fluid medium, such as the vitreous. Secondly, the ZrF_4 fiber is very brittle and subject to repeated replacement.

Marburg and Harrington (38) have been working for many years on a suitable fiberoptic delivery system for the Er:YAG laser. They have grown single-crystal sapphire fibers. Er:YAG laser pulses of 600 mJ were delivered through these fibers with no laser-induced damage. Marburg and Harrington (40) have shown that single-crystal oxide fibers offer many advantages over glass fibers for the transmission of near to mid infrared radiation. Sapphire fibers offer an extremely high melting temperature (2050°C), excellent chemical durability, good mechanical properties, are bioinert, and possess high laser damage thresholds. A 340-μm diameter single-crystal sapphire fiber was used to deliver 600-mJ pulses at 2.94 μm (Er:YAG) wavelength at a pulse repetition rate of 1 Hz. The fiber did not show any evidence of laser damage over the 10-min period during which the test was conducted. Karlin has recently been collaborating with Harrington at the Rutgers University Fiber Optic Materials Research Program in the use of the single-crystal sapphire fiber as the delivery vehicle for the Er:YAG laser in the use of this laser for vitreoretinal and anterior segment surgery (Fig. 10.25).

Intravitreal bubbles due to cavitational effects can occur with the use of the Er:YAG laser as well as with the CO_2

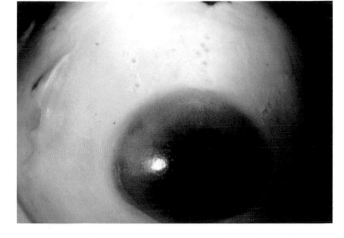

Fig. 10.25 Scleral incisions using an Er:YAG laser with a sapphire fiber delivery system. (Courtesy of Karlin and Harrington.)

laser. Unwanted deeper penetration of energy may occur as laser radiation is transmitted through the air medium of the bubble to more distal ocular tissue. Lin and associates (41) studied the formation of bubbles using an Er:YAG laser. They found a direct correlation between the size of bubbles and the amount of laser energy used. Changes in laser pulse delivery may serve to minimize these cavitational occurences.

Holmium:YAG (Ho:YAG) Laser

Infrared lasers provide perhaps the greatest possibility of any of the lasers in accomplishing tractionless cutting of vitreoretinal membranes. The holmium YAG (Ho:YAG) laser, operating at a wavelength of 2.12 μm, has been experimentally used by Puliafito (42) as an alternative to the Er:YAG laser because it may provide a more dependable delivery system to transmit its energy capability. The energy from a Ho:YAG laser is readily transmitted through flexible commercially available low hydroxyl-fused silica optical fibers with little power attenuation.

Borirakchanyavat and colleagues (42) inserted the silica fiber into a retinal shielding pic in some of their experimental work to prevent the underlying retina from being subjected to hemorrhage and retinal laser burns. The advantages of the Ho:YAG laser are that it is strongly absorbed by the target tissue (vitreoretinal or epiretinal membranes) and that it can be readily transmitted through a commercially available optical fiber.

The Ho:YAG laser is a solid-state pulsed laser. Membranes were successfully transected as close as 0.5 mm from the retinal surface without causing retinal injury while using the retinal shielding pic.

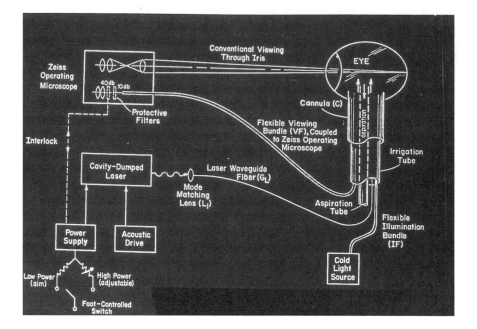

Fig. 10.26 Block diagram of multi-function vitrectomy probe shows laser fiberoptic delivery for phototransection and photocoagulation, irrigation and aspiration, and fiberoptic illumination and visualization.

Picosecond Neodyium:Yttrium Lythium Flouride (Nd:YLF) Laser

Because current nanosecond laser delivery may produce undesirable complications in the laser phototransection of vitreoretinal membranes as well as in laser sclerotomy for glaucoma, some investigators have turned to the picosecond ND:YLF laser as an example of a laser that may minimize damage to neighboring ocular tissue.

The Nd:YLF laser operates at 1053 nm, in the infrared region of the spectrum. Its main advantages comprise a high power with a short pulse and a high repetition rate. With the lasers previously discussed, retinal pathology may develop as a result of acoustic shock waves and cavitational phenomenon.

Some investigators feel that optical breakdown of epiretinal membranes with less effect on neighboring ocular tissue may be accomplished with much less energy by using lasers operating at the picosecond level rather than in the nanosecond range.

Summary

Present mechanical vitreous cutting instruments have undergone remarkable advancement in enabling the vitreoretinal surgeon to effectively cut vitreoretinal membranes. However, these cutters still present the distinct disadvantage of producing traction on epiretinal and subretinal membranes, sometimes resulting in massive retinal and vitreous hemorrhage, retinal tears, and retinal detachment. Even the use of finely designed microsurgical scissors and pics can exert traction on membranes located within the vitreous cavity.

It is evident that phototransection of vitreous membranes using one of the above mentioned infrared lasers offers the possibility of tractionless surgery within the vitreous cavity. Each of the five infrared lasers (CO_2, sapphire-tipped Nd:YAG, Er:YAG, Ho:YAG, and the picosecond Nd:YLF.) has distinct advantages and disadvantages over the other four. However, all of them are awaiting the implementation of a dependable fiberoptic delivery system before they can become part of the clinical armamentarium of vitreoretinal surgeons.

Figure 10.26 shows a block diagram depicting a laser with fiberoptic capability to accomplish the dual functions of photocoagulation and phototransection during the course of a vitrectomy procedure. By miniaturizing the laser portion of the probe to 0.2 to 0.5 mm, adequate room would be made available to incorporate fiberoptic visualization, suction of hemorrhagic vitreous, and reconstitution of intraocular pressure using a suitable irrigating fluid. Thus, future vitrectomy procedures may use a single sclerotomy site, wherein the various modalities are incorporated within a single instrument, instead of dividing the various functions into a three-sclerotomy procedure as is currently used today. True is the old saying that today's concepts frequently become tomorrow's realities.

References

1. Meyer-Schwickerath G. Light coagulation. Translated by Drance SM. St. Louis: CV Mosby, 1960.
2. Charles S. Endophotocoagulation. Ophthalmol Times 1979;4:68–69.
3. Charles S. Endophotocoagulation. Retina 1981;1:117–120.
4. Campbell C, Rittler M, Koester C. Laser photocoagulation of the retina. Trans Am Acad Ophthalmol Otolaryngol 1966;70:939–943.
5. Mizuno K. Binocular indirect argon laser photocoagulation. B J Ophthalmol 1981;65:425–428.
6. Friberg TR, Eller AW. Pneumatic repair of primary and secondary retinal detachments using a binocular indirect

ophthalmoscope laser delivery system. Ophthalmology 1988;95:187–193.

7. Puliafito CA, Deutsch TF, Boll J, et al. Semiconductor laser endophotocoagulation of the retina. Arch Ophthalmol 1987; 105:424–427.

8. Schepens CL, Okamura ID, Brockhurst RJ. The scleral buckling procedures. I. Surgical techniques and management. Arch Ophthalmol 1957;58:797–811.

9. Lincoff H, McLean JM, Nano H. Cryosurgical treatment of retinal detachment. Trans Am Acad Ophthalmol Otolaryngol 1964;68:412–432.

10. Cibis PA. Vitreoretinal pathology and surgery in retinal detachment. St. Louis: CV Mosby, 1965, pp. 199–248.

11. Shafer DM. The treatment of retinal detachment by vitreous implant. Trans Am Acad Ophthalmol Otolaryngol 1957; 61:194.

12. Machemer R, Buettner H, Norton E. Vitrectomy: a pars plana approach. Trans Am Acad Ophthalmol Otolaryngol 1971; 75:813–820.

13. O'Malley C, Heintz R. Vitrectomy via the pars plana: a new instrument system. Trans Pacific Coast Otol Ophth Soc 1972;53:121–134.

14. Douvas N. The cataract roto-extractor (a preliminary report). Trans Am Acad Ophthalmol Otolaryngol 1973;77:792.

15. Peyman G, Dodich N. Experimental vitrectomy. Instrumentation and surgical technique. Arch Ophthalmol 1971; 86:548–551.

16. Klöti R. Vitrektomie I ein neues Instrument für die hintere Vitrektomie. Graefes Arch Clin Exp Ophthalmol 1973; 187:161.

17. Karlin DB. Ultrasound in retinal detachment. A preliminary report. Arch Ophthalmol 1970;84:409–414.

18. Purnell EW, Sokollu A, Holasek E. The production of focal chorioretinitis by ultrasound. Am J Ophthalmol 1964; 58:953–957.

19. Karlin DB. Ultrasound in retinal detachment surgery. Trans Am Acad Ophthalmol Otolaryngol 1969;73:1061–1076.

20. Karlin DB, Patel CKN, Wood OR, Llovera I. CO_2 laser in vitreoretinal surgery: 1. Quantitative investigation of the effects of CO_2 laser radiation on ocular tissue. Ophthalmology 1979;86:290–298.

21. Miller JB, Smith MR, Boyer DS. Intraocular carbon dioxide laser photocautery. II. Preliminary report of clinical trials. Arch Ophthalmol 1979;97:2123–2127.

22. Patel CKN. Interpretation of CO_2 optical laser experiments. Phys Rev Lett 1964;12:588–590.

23. Kaplan I, Ger R. The carbon dioxide laser in clinical surgery. A preliminary report. ISRJ Med Sci 1973;9:79–83.

24. Andrews AH, Moss HW. Experiences with the carbon dioxide laser in the larynx. Ann Otol Rhinol Laryngol 1974;83:462–470.

25. Steller S, Ger R, Levine N, et al. Carbon dioxide laser for excision of burn eschars. Lancet 1971;1:945.

26. Bridges TJ, Strnad AR, Wood OR, Patel CKN, Karlin DB. Interaction of carbon dioxide laser radiation with ocular tissue. IEEE J of Quantum Electronics 1984;QE-20, No. 12:1449–1458.

27. Karlin DB, Jakobiec F, Harrison W, et al. Endophotocoagulation in vitrectomy with a carbon dioxide laser. Am J Ophthalmol 1986;101:445–450.

28. Miller JB, Smith MR, Pincus F, Stockert M. Intraocular carbon dioxide laser photocautery. I. Animal experimentation. Arch Ophthalmol 1979;97:2157–2162.

29. Karlin DB, Patel CKN, Wood O, Bridges T, Strnad R. Laser Surgical System Joint Patent held by Cornell University Medical College and Bell Telephone Laboratories. Awarded April 22, 1986.

30. Harrington JA, Gregory CC. Hollow sapphire fibers for the delivery of CO_2 laser energy. Opt Lett May 15, 1990; 15:541–543.

31. Federman JL. Round table forum: ophthalmic applications of lasers. Contemp Ophthalmic Forum 1986;4:No. 3.

32. Karlin DB, Degan J. The laser scalpel in ophthalmic surgery. Presented at the XVI Meeting, September 4–8, 1988, Club Jules Gonin, Bruges, Belgium.

33. Pellin MJ, Williams GA, Young CE, et al. Endoexcimer laser intraocular ablative photodecomposition. Am J Ophthalmol 1985;99:483–484.

34. Trentacoste J, Thompson K, Parrish RK, Hajek A, Berman MR, Ganjei P. Mutagenic potential of a 193 nm excimer laser on fibroblasts in tissue culture. Ophthalmology 1987; 94:125–129.

35. Marshall J, Sliney DH. Endoexcimer laser intraocular ablative photodecomposition. Am J Ophthalmol 1986;101: 130–131.

36. Margolis TI, Farnath DA, Destro M, Puliafito CA. Erbium-YAG laser surgery on experimental vitreous membranes. Arch Ophthalmol 1989;107:424–428.

37. Peyman GA, Katoh N. Effects of an erbium-YAG laser on ocular structures. Int Ophthalmol 1987;10:245–253.

38. Ellsworth LG, Kramer TR, Noecker RJ, Yarborough JM, Snyder RW. Retinotomy using Erbium:YAG laser equipped with a contact probe on human autopsy eyes. ARVO abstracts. Supplement to Invest Ophthalmol Vis Sci. Philadelphia: JB Lippincott, 1993:961.

39. D'Amico DJ, Moulton RS, Theodossiadis PG, Yarborough JM. Er:YAG laser photothermal retinal ablation in enucleated rabbit eyes. Am J Ophthalmol 1994;117:783–790.

40. Marberg G, Harrington J. Optical and mechanical properties of single crystal sapphire fibers. App Opt 1993; 32:3201–3209.

41. Lin CP, Stern D, Puliafito CP. High-speed photography of Er:YAG laser ablation in fluid. Implications for laser vitreous surgery. Invest Ophthalmol Vis Sci 1990;31;2546.

42. Borirakchanyavat S, Puliafito C, Kliman GH, Margolis TI, Galler EL. Holmium-YAG laser surgery on experimental vitreous membranes. Arch Ophthalmol 1991;109:1605–1609.

11

Lasers in Ophthalmic Plastic and Orbital Surgery

Albert Hornblass
Daniel J. Coden

Lasers are an integral part of most ophthalmologists' surgical armamentarium. In the past, most ophthalmic applications have been limited to the treatment of retinal vascular disease with the argon laser, and the discission of opacified posterior capsules with the neodymium:YAG (Nd:YAG) laser. Over the past several years, many oculoplastic and orbital applications of laser energy have been developed. The three types discussed in this chapter, CO_2, argon, and Nd:YAG have been used the most extensively to treat disorders of the ocular adnexa and orbit.

CO_2 Laser

The CO_2 laser, although unfamiliar to most ophthalmologists, is an extremely valuable tool in the treatment of eyelid and orbital disease. The laser's ability to cauterize as it cuts is advantageous when these vascular tissues are operated on.

The CO_2 laser, with an energy of 10,600 nm, operates in the infrared and, when focused to a very small beam, can be used to incise tissues. Its beam of energy can be defocused or broadened to vaporize tissues.

The CO_2 laser is invisible and, therefore, is used with a red, coaxial light beam generated by a helium-neon (HeNe) laser. This aiming beam allows accurate delivery of the CO_2 laser energy.

The CO_2 laser, unlike the argon laser, does not depend on the color of tissues, but instead is absorbed by water molecules, extracellular or intracellular. The CO_2 laser vaporizes cells at the tissue surface by flash boiling intracellular water at 100°C. Total absorption of the CO_2 laser energy occurs in 0.1 mm of soft tissue because it is composed of 80% to 90% water.

Lasers currently available have powers ranging from one to 100 W. For most ophthalmic applications, power less than 10 W is sufficient. The laser can be used as a single pulsed shot or as a continuous delivery of energy. The delivery system can be hand held or applied through an operating microscope (Fig. 11.1). One of the new technologies in CO_2 laser surgery is the superpulse laser, which is capable of delivering extremely high laser energy in millisecond pulses. Less total energy is delivered with a pulsed laser than with a continuous wave (CW) laser to accomplish the same task. By breaking up the impulse, less thermal damage is produced, which promises enhanced wound healing and less scarring. It should be noted, however, that the best hemostasis is obtained with a CW laser due to its wider zone of thermal injury.

The speed with which the laser is moved will affect the type of incision, coagulation, amount of charring, and thermal damage. If the laser is drawn across tissue too slowly, the penetration can be excessively deep and unwanted thermal damage occurs. Rapid movement will lead to an incision that is shallower than desired.

It is important that blood and fluid be kept out of the operative site as best as possible because these substances will absorb the CO_2 laser energy. The presence of these substances will greatly slow the rate at which an incision is produced.

Advantages of CO_2 Laser

A single pulse of the CO_2 laser will penetrate no more than 0.1 mm into soft tissue and, at the same time, cause only limited spread of thermal energy into the surrounding tissue. This allows precise delivery to the target tissue and minimizes the harm done to tissue surrounding the lesion.

Heat produced by the defocused CO_2 laser will predictably seal small vessels of less than 0.5-mm caliber. This gives the surgeon greater visibility during surgery, minimizes blood loss, and may make the patient feel more comfortable during the procedure. If bleeding should occur from larger blood vessels, they can frequently be heat sealed by grasping the end of the bleeding vessel with a pair of fine-tooth forceps and then, by defocusing the CO_2 laser beam, have their ends vaporized and welded shut with the CO_2 laser energy. Hornblass (1) has demonstrated the efficacy of using the CO_2 laser in high-risk patients with bleeding disorders. He was able to remove a subcutaneous lipoma from the brow of a patient with hemophilia and suggests that the CO_2 laser is similarly efficacious in patients who have thrombocytopenia or who are taking anticoagulants (Fig. 11.2).

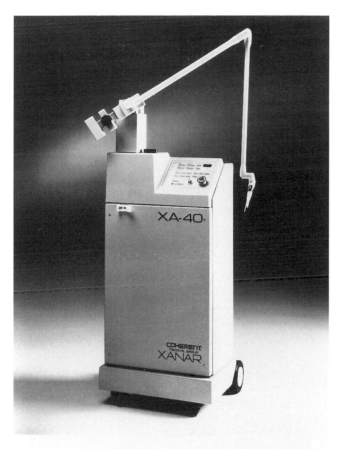

Coherent/Xanar XA-40 CO₂ Laser

Fig. 11.1 CO₂ laser system. Note articulated arm delivery system. Extension off the tip of the handpiece allows the surgeon to hold the tip at the proper distance from the tissue to be vaporized.

Just as the CO_2 laser seals small vascular channels, it also seals lymphatic vessels. This theoretically might convey an advantage when excising malignant tumors by reducing the risks of metastatic spread. This is also responsible for the minimal edema seen after CO_2 laser procedures.

Sensory nerve endings are sealed as they contact the CO_2 laser. In most bilaterally compared surgical cases, laser-treated sites are associated with less discomfort than the same procedure carried out with a scalpel (2).

The CO_2 laser offers an advantage in deep surgical cavities, such as orbital cases, in which the laser can be conveniently applied through an operating microscope, reaching areas that would otherwise be difficult to access.

Disadvantages of CO₂ Laser

Additional manual dexterity is necessary for the laser surgeon, at least initially, before this instrument can be used with the same degree of skill as obtained with traditional scalpel surgery. Because the laser beam is the only portion of the instrument that contacts tissue, the surgeon loses the normal tactile sensation of the scalpel blade contacting skin. Also, the bulky nature and limited articulation of the laser handpiece will require some practice to use effectively.

Strong evidence indicates that CO_2 laser incisions do not achieve the same tensile strength as scalpel-incised incisions until 3 weeks postoperatively (3,4). However, after this point, both types of wounds are indistinguishable from one another in cosmetic appearance and tensile strength. It is postulated that because of the quality of hemostasis obtained with the CO_2 laser, a normal fibrin clot, which forms after any injury, may not occur. This may delay the initiation of fibroblast migration across the wound and the subsequent collagen synthesis and development of tensile strength.

Safety Precautions

The CO_2 laser has a potential to ignite flammable substances, such as surgical drapes and clothing. One simple method to minimize this risk is to wet the surgical drapes surrounding the operative site with sterile water or saline before beginning the procedure. Surgical drapes are now available that are resistant to ignition from contact with the laser beam. All flammable materials should be removed from the operating room and all preoperative prepping agents containing alcohol must be excluded because they may be ignited if contact with the CO_2 laser beam occurs.

All patients, surgeons, and operating room personnel should use eye protection during CO_2 laser surgery (Fig. 11.3). Regular prescription glasses made from plastic or plastic goggles will prevent the beam from passing through and minimize the risk of ocular injury.

As the CO_2 laser vaporizes living tissue, a large amount of steam and smoke, called a laser plume, is generated. There is concern that this laser plume might contain viable microorganisms capable of infecting the surgeon and assistants or even other sites on the patient. The risk is greatest when cutaneous or mucous membrane lesions are vaporized at relatively low irradiances. It is, therefore, important that all operating room personnel have surgical masks capable of filtering out the smoke plume particles and that a smoke evacuator is used with the procedure.

The CO_2 laser has the ability to be reflected off shiny surfaces and it is important to use anodized or burnished tools that reduce reflected energy if the CO_2 laser beam should come in contact with an instrument. This is especially important in oculoplastic or orbital surgery because a reflected beam could be damaging to the globe. Although laser energy decreases inversely with the square of the distance, personnel without protective eyewear could be susceptible to keratitis. The reflected beam is also capable of causing cuts and burns to the surgical team if reflected.

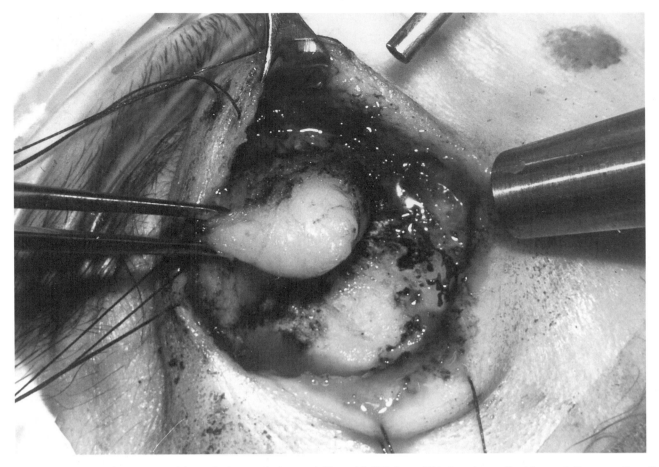

Fig. 11.2   Lipoma being excised from the brow of a hemophiliac with CO_2 laser. This laser's excellent hemostatic properties allow the surgeon to operate in a virtually bloodless field.

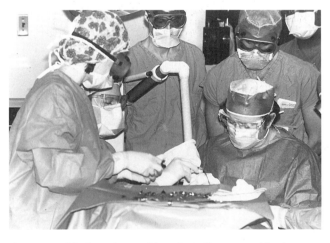

Fig. 11.3 CO_2 laser in use. Note that all personnel in the surgical suite, both surgeons and observers, are wearing protective goggles.

Plastic or methylmethacrylate eyeshields commonly used in oculoplastic and orbital surgery have the potential to become hot or even melt if prolonged contact with the CO_2 laser occurs. This could result in thermal conduction to the cornea with resulting injury. Because of these con-

siderations, many surgeons now use a buffed, stainless steel-type eye shield, which eliminates the possibility of thermal injury to the eye by reflecting the laser beam (5).

Oculoplastic and Orbital Applications of the CO_2 Laser

The CO_2 laser has been used successfully in many specialties. It has been used extensively in dermatology to treat many types of disorders, many of which may also involve the skin of the eyelids, such as adenoma sebaceum, neurofibroma, nevi, seborrheic keratoses, and port wine stains. More dermatologic examples follow.

This laser is especially useful for hemangiomatous lesions of the eyelids (Figs. 11.4 and 11.5), yielding excellent cosmetic results.

Beckman and colleagues (6) have used the CO_2 laser in the ablation of such lesions as papillomas and verruca and in the excision of a hemangioma, basal cell carcinoma, and a basal cell papilloma. They suggest the use of the CO_2 laser in any procedure that one might consider using electrocautery or cryotherapy. They note that the laser beam is convergent, which results in less of a necrotic zone than created by the divergent modalities of electrocautery and

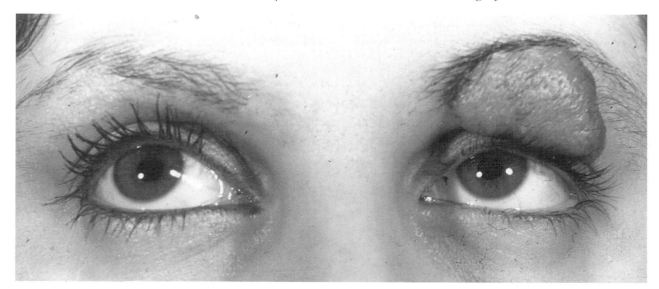

Fig. 11.4 Preoperative photograph of vascular lid tumor.

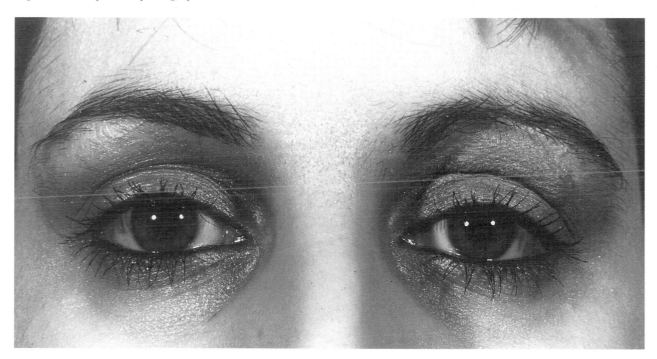

Fig. 11.5 The vascular lid tumor was easily excised with the CO_2 laser. The cosmetic result is excellent.

cryotherapy. They also report a successfully performed Ziegler procedure for minimal ectropion using the puckering effect of CW CO_2 emission.

The CO_2 laser is capable of creating flaps in a manner similar to a scalpel; however, Wesley and Bond (7) note that they avoid the application of the CO_2 laser to the skin or to areas on which a free graft may eventually be applied because vessels needed to nourish the graft are sealed.

Some surgeons have used the CO_2 laser to excise basal cell carcinomas. However, Wesley and Bond (7) have found the laser to be unacceptable for this purpose, due to the minimal surgical swath size of one millimeter, which

they have found to be excessive. For instance, when making additional surgical margins around an eyelid cancer to obtain a one-millimeter full-thickness specimen to be sent to pathology, 2 mm of lid margin must be destroyed: one millimeter of specimen and one millimeter of vaporized tissue by the laser.

Blepharoplasty

Baker and associates (8) reported their experience using the CO_2 laser in 40 patients undergoing blepharoplasties. For the skin incision, using a spot size of 0.1 mm, they found 6 W to be the optimal power setting. At lower power settings, the target tissues required significantly greater exposure to produce the incision. At higher power settings, the handpiece of the laser must be moved so rapidly to avoid damage to deeper structures that control of the incision direction and depth is compromised.

Technique

Upper lid blepharoplasty is performed in the following manner. The laser is set at 2 W in the single-pulse mode, at 0.05 sec/pulse. This is used to make small spot burns marking the proposed incision line every 5 mm. The laser is then set at 6 W of power in the CW mode and then is smoothly maneuvered to "connect the dots," cutting through skin and orbicularis muscle. The laser is then directed to the plane between the orbicularis muscle and orbital septum, and this tissue is cut by a side-to-side motion with firm tension maintained on the flap. Any intraoperative bleeding that does occur can most often be controlled by spot application to the bleeding site with the laser beam defocused. The operative field is usually bloodless because the laser cauterizes as it cuts. Orbital fat is clamped after the septum is divided transversely. This fat is then cut and cauterized using laser against the clamp. Lower lid blepharoplasty is carried out with the CO_2 laser in a similar fashion and the incisions are closed in the usual manner.

It was the impression of Baker and coworkers (8) report that the CO_2 laser incisions healed more slowly than scalpel incisions. They managed this by not removing skin sutures until the seventh or eighth day. They also noted that the final scar produced by the laser incision is one of slightly greater prominence, which related to thermal damage to the skin at the wound margins. They emphasized keeping the laser beam perpendicular to the skin to avoid undermining and to keep the beam well focused to produce a fine, sharp incision line.

Overly enthusiastic application of the laser may produce significant thermal damage to surrounding tissues. Baker and coworkers (8) report one case of ptosis produced by excessive application of the laser in an effort to deepen the lid fold, leading to a partial disinsertion of the levator aponeurosis.

David and Sanders (2) compared CO_2 laser blepharoplasty on one side with "cold steel" blepharoplasty on the other in 13 patients. They noted that a decreased operative time, on the average one third less, was noted in all 13 patients on the laser treated side. They also found bleeding to be considerably and consistently less on the laser side. Both bruising and swelling in the immediate postoperative period were less on the laser side, yet at 30 days they found the two sides to be indistinguishable. This differs with the patients in Baker's series who seemed to have more prominent scars with the CO_2 laser incision. How-

ever, Baker also noted the decreased operative time, lessened bleeding, and significant decreases in postoperative ecchymosis and swelling. He postulates that the sealing of lymphatics by the laser limits edema. He notes that postoperative pain is minimal or absent, which is attributed to laser cauterization of sensory nerves.

Xanthelasma

Xanthelasma palpebrarum represents deposits of fatty tissues in the periorbital area and may be associated with abnormal levels of cholesterol or triglycerides in the circulation, but may also occur as an inherited trait. The standard types of treatment available for this condition include surgical excision or treatment with a variety of caustic chemicals. Apfelberg and colleagues (9) have described the use of the CO_2 laser in the treatment of xanthelasma palpebrarum. They use a one-millimeter spot size with the power set between 4 and 9 W. Their initially focused beam vaporizes the overlying skin. Superficial defocused treatment, followed by gentle curettage with a small skin curette, removes residual pigment down to the upper dermis and occasionally to fascia overlying the orbicularis muscle. The wounds are not closed and are left to heal by epithelialization or secondary intention (Figs. 11.6 and 11.7).

In their series, all patients had satisfactory resolution of xanthelasma palpebrarum with excellent cosmetic effect and no recurrences. The skin is discolored initially, but fades and blends in 3 to 6 months. Pre- and posttreatment biopsies have demonstrated that the foam cells of cholesterol present initially are eradicated and that a normal epidermis over a fibrotic dermis replaces the original lesion. If the fatty material deposition extends to the ciliary margin, additional safety can be attained by infiltrating sterile saline under the treatment site. This absorbs CO_2 laser energy that might otherwise penetrate through to deeper vital structures.

Similar satisfactory results using the CO_2 laser to treat xanthelasma have been reported by Gladstone and associates (10).

Lymphangioma

A lymphangioma is a histologically benign but potentially aggressive tumor that usually occurs in young people. Lymphangiomas of the ocular adnexa, especially those in the orbit, are difficult to treat because the unencapsulated tumor freely interdigitates with normal orbital tissue, obliterating any potential surgical planes. Because of the hemorrhagic and friable nature of the tumor, conventional surgical techniques are frequently complicated by bleeding. Kennerdell and colleagues (11) reported data on 6 patients with orbital lymphangiomas where the CO_2 laser was used to remove the lesions subtotally by

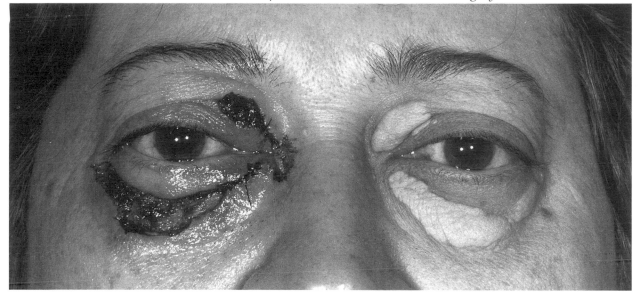

Fig. 11.6 Immediately postoperatively CO_2 laser vaporization of xanthelasma, right eye, with charred tissue left to heal by secondary intention. Preoperatively, the right eye appeared similar to the left eye as shown.

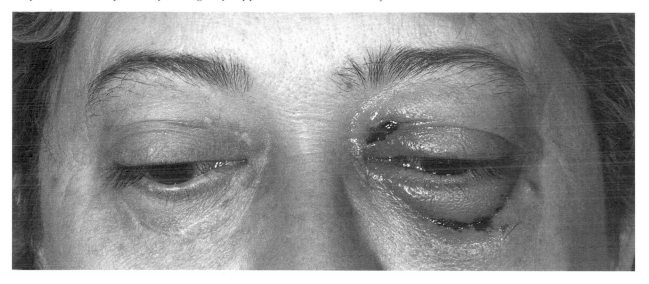

Fig. 11.7 Two months after vaporization of xanthelasma, right eye, with an excellent result. The left eye had been done 2 weeks previously and is beginning to granulate in.

controlled vaporization. The CO_2 laser was mounted on an operating microscope and was used first to cavitate the central portion of the tumor and then to vaporize the infolded sides. They used power settings ranging from 500 mW to 5 W for intraconal lesions and 8 to 15 W for eyelid lesions, depending on whether the tissue was cystic or solid. Their complications included 3 patients with dilated pupils postoperatively because of damage to the ciliary nerves and one case of corneal anesthesia, which led to recurrent corneal breakdown.

Chalazion

Chalazions are chronic lipogranulomas of the eyelids, secondary to the plugging of meibomian glands. They are most commonly treated with warm compresses, corticosteroid injections, or incision and drainage.

Wesley and Bond (7) have applied the CO_2 laser to chalazia extending through the conjunctival surface. The laser is directed to the center of the chalazion and the core carefully vaporized. Less anesthesia is required because a chalazion clamp application is unnecessary.

Korn (12) described good results using the CO_2 laser at 4 W in the CW mode and claims that contact lens wear can be resumed within an hour after surgery.

Syringoma

Syringoma of the face is a benign but cosmetically difficult condition. Each syringoma represents a collection of eccrine sweat glands and ducts and appears clinically as a small flesh-colored, one- to 3-mm papule that has a dome-shaped, smooth surface. Typically the post-pubertal woman presents with multiple papules located periorbitally or elsewhere on the face. Wheeland and coworkers (13) used the CO_2 laser to permit precise removal of the proliferating tissue with minimal injury to surrounding skin and an excellent cosmetic result. They used a defocused beam of 2 mm diameter with power set at 4 W to delivery 0.10- or 0.20-sec pulses of energy to each individual lesion and found that usually only two or three pulses were required to completely remove each lesion.

Apfelberg and colleagues (14) also have described the use of the CO_2 laser in treating syringomata. After initial unsuccessful trials with standard CW CO_2, they now report success with the CO_2 laser in the superpulse mode. After the epidermis is vaporized with the laser, a small white cyst is exposed. This cyst is evacuated with a 25-gauge needle and then a final defocused pulse of CO_2 laser accomplishes hemostasis if bleeding has been profuse.

Capillary Hemangiomas

Capillary hemangiomas are benign vascular tumors that usually appear within the first several months of life. The usual course is that of gradual enlargement followed by involution by the age of 4 to 5 years. Those appearing on the eyelids can lead to severe ptosis or induced astigmatism resulting in amblyopia if untreated.

The greatest utility of the CO_2 laser in ophthalmic plastic and orbital surgery appears to be procedures benefiting greatly from hemostasis. The CO_2 laser has been used effectively by Wesley and Bond (7) in vaporizing congenital capillary hemangiomas that have failed to resolve fully by the time the patient is a teenager or young adult. Their technique involves making a skin incision with a scalpel, retracting the edges of the skin, and then slowly vaporizing the hemangioma with the hand-held or microscope-mounted CO_2 laser.

Eruptive Vellus Hair Cysts

Vellus hair cysts are uncommon inherited lesions representing small collections of pilosebaceous structures typically distributed on the central face and periorbital areas. These well-encapsulated cystic structures may lead to much disfigurement. Huerter and Wheeland (15) described treating vellus hair cysts on the eyelids with the CO_2 laser. They use a defocused 2-mm beam and 3 W of power in 0.2-sec pulses. They do not curette the eyelid lesions as is done elsewhere on the face. There may be a temporary color change, usually in the form of hyperpigmentation, which resolves spontaneously in 4 to 6

months in most cases. They have had no recurrences of the cysts when treating with the CO_2 laser in this manner.

Meningioma

Meningiomas are invasive tumors that arise from arachnoidal villi and usually originate intracranially with secondary extension into the orbit. Surgical excision of this tumor is extremely difficult.

Takizawa and coworkers (16) reported the excision of an orbital meningioma using the CO_2 laser. The tumor tissue could not be removed by conventional methods, but the CO_2 laser scalpel allowed the surgeon to remove the tumor tissue adhering to the optic nerve and globe.

Exenterations

Wesley and Bond (7) have used the CO_2 laser to perform exenterations. Besides superior hemostasis, the CO_2 laser offers the advantage in cancer surgery of sealing vessels and lymphatics, possibly reducing hematogenous spread of tumors. After exenteration, they have applied the CO_2 laser to the bone in areas near possible tumor involvement because the CO_2 laser destroys cells, but does very little to remove bone. If bony involvement is suspected, the involved area is rongeured out and then the CO_2 laser is applied to the surrounding bone to obtain an extra margin of safety.

The CO_2 laser can be used in an exenterated orbit to stimulate granulation in areas of unhealed, exposed bone. Bailin and Wheeland (17) have described a method using a focused CO_2 laser beam of 0.1-mm diameter, 20 W of power and short pulses of 0.1 sec to create small holes in the outer table of the bone. When a small gridlike series of perforations have been created in an area of exposed cranial bone, granulation tissue will form through these small channels and epithelialization will occur.

Argon Laser

The argon laser is familiar to most ophthalmologists from its use in treating retinal vascular disease. It also has applications in oculoplastic surgery, which are discussed below.

Argon laser energy is created when a high-voltage electrical current is applied to the optical cavity containing argon gas. This laser light source is blue-green in color and has an emission spectrum between 488 and 514 nm. Besides the many ophthalmic applications familiar to the ophthalmologist, the argon laser has been used for years by dermatologists to treat vascular disorders and pigmented conditions of the skin and mucous membranes.

The emission spectrum for the argon laser has a distinct overlap with the absorption spectrum of hemoglobin and melanin. This leads to a relatively selective effect on these two types of tissues, although some scatter of energy occurs within skin and mucous membranes.

The argon laser, unlike the CO_2 laser, can be efficiently transmitted along fiberoptic cables without much energy loss. It is then delivered to the target tissue with a pencil-like handpiece.

The main usefulness of the argon laser in the treatment of cutaneous and mucous membrane disorders has been in the photocoagulation of vascular as well as pigmented lesions. Argon laser energy, when contacting melanin or hemoglobin in the skin, is converted into heat with resultant thermal injury to the cutaneous vasculature and pigment-containing cells. The greater the quantity of these pigments within the target tissue, the more superficial the effects will be because complete absorption of energy occurs nearer the skin surface, limiting penetration.

In general, the argon laser energy will penetrate to a depth of one to 2 mm before being completely absorbed by skin and mucous membranes. Therefore, the argon laser is not very useful in treating disorders where blood vessels are large or located in the deeper portions of the skin. Argon laser energy is scattered significantly in skin and mucous membranes, which can decrease the specificity of the interaction with the target chromophore and result in nonspecific thermal injury of the adjacent tissue. The thermal injury to the dermis may result in abnormal scar formation. Because of this scarring potential, a small test site within a larger treatment zone is treated, and then observed over a 6- to 12-week interval for possible abnormal scar formation or pigmentation that may compromise the final cosmetic result.

Safety Precautions

Several precautions should be taken when using the argon laser. The first is a simple posting on the laser operating room door that a laser is in use. Because the visible blue-green argon laser light can pass through glass without difficulty, there is a potential risk to outsiders. All external windows must be covered to prevent inadvertent injury to observers outside the operating room.

Because the argon blue-green laser is readily absorbed by the retinal pigment epithelium of the retina, there is a definite risk of injury if the laser is inadvertently fired at the patient, surgeon, or assistant. The laser energy can be focused by the patient's own lens onto the fovea, leading to irreversible damage to central vision. For this reason, during argon laser procedures, it is mandatory that the patient and all operating room personnel wear eye protection, which consists of simple plastic lenses or goggles of proper optical density that can be worn over or instead of prescription lenses. When working directly on the eyelids or the ciliary margin, eyeshields of either plastic or steel are used to reduce the risk of retinal injury.

Oculoplastic Applications of the Argon Laser

The argon laser has been used extensively in the treatment of numerous cutaneous and mucous membrane disorders and has been the mainstay of treatment for a variety of vascular conditions. The argon laser has been used to treat many skin disorders, some of which can affect the eyelids and periorbital area. These conditions include telangiectasias, senile (cherry) angioma, adenoma sebaceum, nevus of ota, cafe au lait spots, and pigmented seborrheic keratoses. Landthaler and coworkers (18) reported data on several patients who had xanthelasma of the eyelids successfully treated with the argon laser.

Port Wine Stains

Port wine stains are a subgroup of congenital vascular malformations, termed nevus flammeus, which most commonly involve the forehead, face, occiput, and nuchal regions, but can involve periorbital skin. Most of these lesions disappear in infancy; however, port wine stains persist into childhood or adulthood.

The argon laser has been used by many investigators in the treatment of port wine stains, as reviewed by Wisnicki (19). Most laser surgeons will perform a test treatment to an inconspicuous area of the stain before they begin actual therapy. The test site itself is broken up into four to six individual tests, each representing different combinations of time, beam diameter, and power. The immediate improvement, which is manifest as blanching, does not accurately represent the final degree of improvement that can be seen 3 to 6 months later.

Local anesthesia may be necessary for some patients, but it is important that non-epinephrine compounds be used. Epinephrine will lead to vasoconstriction and decrease the volume of the hemoglobin target and possibly be responsible for less than optimal improvement. The specific parameters used are decided after test patching. A spot size of 0.5 to 1 mm is used with power ranging from one to 5 W.

After an immediate blanching of treated skin, extensive epidermal and dermal necrosis occur by the third postoperative day. An eschar forms and falls off during the next week to 10 days. In 4 to 6 weeks, there is closure of the abnormal vessels, with recanalization with smaller vessels occurring in 2 to 4 months. This recanalization with smaller vessels combined with fibrosis lead to the desired lightening of the lesion. Lightening of angiomas following argon laser photocoagulation can continue for up to 18 months even though the greatest degree of improvement occurs in the first year postoperatively.

Cosman (20) and Apfelberg (21) reported separate large series with good to excellent results in 60% to 75% of patients. Noe and associates (22) have identified predictive criteria for the success of argon laser therapy. Clinical factors favoring a good result include patients greater than 37 years old and a purple-colored lesion. Undesirable results are associated with patients less than 17 years old or pink-colored lesions. Other important histologic criteria include the fraction of the dermis occupied by vessels and the percentage of vessels containing erythrocytes.

It has been suggested that chilling port wine stains immediately before argon laser therapy may improve results, and this has been shown clinically (23). This phenomenon has been attributed to a protective effect on the cutaneous appendages when exposed to thermal energy.

Chloasma

Chloasma, also known as the "mask of pregnancy," is a hyperpigmentation that occurs in the periorbital area after the use of oral contraceptives or following pregnancy. Argon laser may be beneficial in improving this hyperpigmentation. A series of small test sites is treated with different combinations of time and power. The patient is reexamined 6 weeks postoperatively to determine whether or not scarring or textural changes have occurred and to evaluate the degree of improvement in pigmentation. Once a satisfactory test result has been obtained, the treatment of the remainder of the pigmented lesion can proceed.

Capillary Hemangioma

Capillary hemangiomas are benign vascular tumors that usually appear within the first several months of life. These lesions are difficult to treat surgically due to their hemorrhagic tendency.

Gladstone and Beckman (24) reported the successful treatment of an upper lid capillary hemangioma using the argon laser. They used a one-mm spot size, 900 mW of power and one-sec exposure and found that smaller spot sizes led to rapid tissue destruction with too little hemostatic effect. Because penetration with the argon laser is limited, to treat the deeper parts of the tumor, it was necessary to remove coagulated tissue with a curet. The successful use of the argon laser in treating an upper eyelid capillary hemangioma has also been reported by Hobby (25). Selective absorption of the laser energy by the blood-filled tissue allows microablation of the lesion under ideal hemostatic conditions with minimal loss of normal lid tissue. This obviates the need for oculoplastic lid repair.

Phthiriasis Palpebrarum

The crab louse, *Phthirius pubis*, can infest the eyelashes. The mechanical removal of nits and parasites from the eyelashes is tedious and uncomfortable. Petrolatum ointment is effective in killing these parasites by smothering them but is ineffective against the nits. Awan (26) successfully treated phthiriasis palpebrarum in one session using an argon laser. The laser was set at a 200-μm spot size, 0.1-sec time, and 200 mW power and focused at the junction of the body and the head of each adult parasite, instantly killing it. The nits were treated in similar fashion. There were no recurrences and the only complication reported was the slicing of some eyelashes, which quickly grew to normal length.

Punctal Stenosis

Occlusion or stenosis of the lacrimal punctum is usually a congenital malformation but may result from inflammatory or traumatic lesions of the eyelids in the vicinity of punctal openings. Punctal stenosis is also associated with several dermatologic disorders or may be secondary to topical medications.

Awan (27) has described a punctoplasty procedure using the argon laser. After topical anesthesia is applied, the conjunctiva overlying the occluded punctum is marked with sterile mascara or dye. Using a 200-μm spot, 0.2-sec exposure time, and 1200 to 1500 mW of power, the painted area is treated. The initial central burn is followed by circles of burns around it, until a sufficiently large area has melted away. This forms a crater and creates an opening in the canalicular medial wall.

Blepharopigmentation

Blepharopigmentation involves the implantation of iron oxide pigment in the eyelid skin adjacent to the cilia for the purpose of eyelash enhancement (28). There has been no easy way to treat overcorrection or misplacement of pigment after it is applied.

Tanenbaum and colleagues (29) have described a method for removing unwanted pigmentation using the argon laser. Using a 50-μm spot size, 0.05-sec exposure and 300 to 800 mW of power, they focused the laser beam directly at the pigment. As the treatment progressed, a 2- to 3-mm incisional groove was created in the eyelid margin by the laser burns. This incisional groove healed by secondary intention leaving an almost imperceptible scar.

During the laser treatment, it is difficult to differentiate between the pigment itself and the tissue char produced by the laser. If the end point of the treatment is the partial dispersion of implanted pigment particles, residual pigment fades over several weeks following treatment.

Further studies are required to determine the optimal dosage of laser ablation treatment and to evaluate the long-term safety of this method, especially regarding the possibility of permanent loss of cilia.

Trichiasis

Trichiasis, misdirected cilia rubbing against the globe, is a difficult therapeutic challenge. Many treatments have been tried, each with advantages as well as drawbacks. Epilation is simple and quick, but the eyelashes quickly regrow. Electrolysis can be successful, but it is tedious to do and is uncomfortable for and poorly tolerated by the patient. Cryotherapy to the involved lid is effective but has the undesirable potential complications of visual loss, lid notching, corneal ulcer, symblepharon formation, xerosis, cellulitis, activation of herpes zoster, skin depigmentation and severe soft tissue reaction (30).

The use of the argon laser to treat trichiasis was first described by Berry (31). This technique was expanded on by Awan, who described success in a series of 11 patients (32). After tetracaine ointment is applied, the involved eyelid is rotated outward with the help of a sterile cotton-tipped applicator. With the laser set at a 50-μm spot size, 0.2-sec time, and 1000 to 1200 mW of power, the beam is focused at the root of each cilium. This initial shot of laser energy destroys the shaft of the eyelash at its root and creates a crater. The crater is then deepened to reach the follicle of the eyelash by increasing the spot size to 200 μm. A crater deep enough to destroy the follicles takes about a dozen applications. The follicles of eyelashes are 1.5 to 2.5 mm deep from the surface; hence, each crater must be about 2 mm deep to destroy the hair follicle effectively.

With this method, discomfort to the patient is minimal and there is no postoperative bleeding. Because of the accuracy of the laser beam, normal follicles and meibomian glands are not destroyed.

Bartley and associates (33) compared epilation, electrolysis, cryotherapy, and argon laser thermal ablation in removing eyelashes in rabbits and studied their histologic effects. Epilation was followed by total regrowth of eyelashes within 2 weeks. Electrolysis showed focal destruction of follicles with variable regrowth. Cryotherapy resulted in moderate to severe eyelid scarring with minimal regrowth. Argon laser thermal ablation produced focal necrosis and variable follicle destruction.

Nd:YAG Laser

The Nd:YAG laser was introduced to ophthalmology by Aron-Rosa and colleagues, who demonstrated its use in posterior capsulotomies (34). Daikuzono and Joffe (35) developed synthetic sapphire contact probes for the Nd:YAG laser in 1985.

The Nd:YAG laser is a near infrared laser light source of 1060 nm. This wavelength is absorbed by protein, unlike the CO_2 laser, which is absorbed by water, or the argon, which is absorbed by chromophores of the skin. Because of this protein absorption, the Nd:YAG laser scatters significantly as it impacts tissue and causes a diffuse thermal effect. As a consequence, the Nd:YAG laser is imprecise and leads to a zone of destruction much larger than is clinically apparent. It is, however, extremely effective in providing hemostasis.

The laser energy is delivered through a pencil-sized handpiece connected to a fiberoptic cable. The sapphire tip allows the surgeon to make contact with tissue, giving the same tactile clues found with the more familiar scalpel (Figs. 11.8 and 11.9).

Dickson and coworkers (36) compared the tensile strength of wounds created with the Nd:YAG laser scalpel to that of conventional steel scalpels in pigs. They found

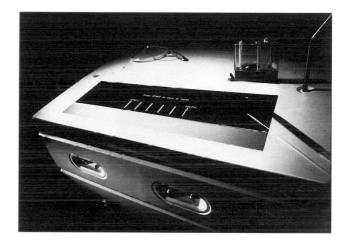

Fig. 11.8 Surface cutting YAG laser unit console.

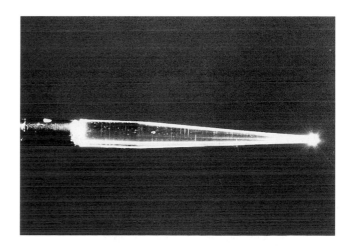

Fig. 11.9 Sapphire tip of surface cutting YAG laser. This tip, when inserted in the handpiece, gives the surgeon tactile sensation similar to the more familiar scalpel blade.

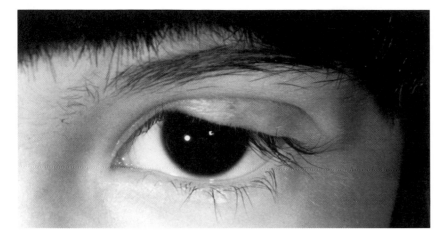

Fig. 11.10 Residual capillary hemangioma leading to a mechanical ptosis in an 8-year old girl.

that at 2 weeks, the tensile strength was greatest for wounds created with a steel scalpel. At 4 weeks, however, the tensile strength was similar in both groups.

Peyman and colleagues (37) described their experience with the contact Nd:YAG laser on rabbits. They were able to perform blepharoplasty without producing hemorrhage intraoperatively. No or minimal postoperative edema was observed and, after 3 weeks, the wound was healed with minimal scar formation. They note that, unlike the CO_2 laser, contact Nd:YAG laser energy does not cause tissue shrinkage, therefore allowing wound adaptation with minimal stress. They also studied the effect of the Nd:YAG laser on bone of the rabbit orbital rim and found that this could be penetrated easily.

The sapphire-tipped, surface contact YAG laser has also been used to excise vascular lid lesions with excellent hemostasis and cosmetic results (personal communications; Figs. 11.10 and 11.11).

Laser Dacryocystorhinostomy

Despite the high success rate of external dacryocystorhinostomies, which in most cases is 90%, in the last 4 years laser dacryocystorhinostomy has been introduced. The advantage for the laser dacryocystorhinostomy through an endonasal approach is elimination of cutaneous scar formation, reducing injury to adjacent medial canthal tendon structures and relatively minor morbidity (38). Another advantage is simplified secondary dacryocystorhinostomy repairs. The intranasal approach was originally described in 1983. However, because of poor instrumentation, it never really found success. Massaro and colleagues (39) and then later Gonnering and associates (40) described performance of intranasal dacryocystorhinostomy by either using the argon laser, the potassium-titanyl-phosphate (KTP): YAG laser or CO_2 laser.

Bleeding in a dacryocystorhinostomy can be a severe problem, sometimes even necessitating a transfusion. It also can make suture placement difficult and greatly slow the procedure. The incision of both periosteum and nasal mucosa can be carried out with the laser. This could potentially decrease intraoperative and postoperative bleeding, making the procedure both easier and safer. Hornblass has used the surface contact YAG laser to perform a dacryocystorhinostomy in a patient. The laser was used for the skin incision, to create the bony ostomy, as

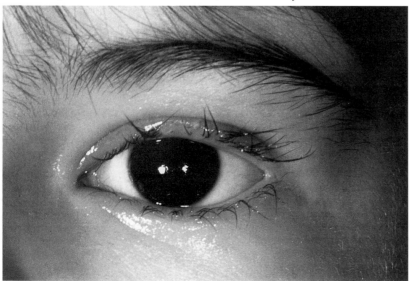

Fig. 11.11 The capillary hemangioma was excised using a sapphire tip, surface contact YAG laser. Bleeding was minimal and the cosmetic result is superb.

well as in creating lacrimal and nasal mucosal flaps. In comparison to conventional surgery, laser surgery gives rise to less intraoperative hemorrhage and postoperative edema, but leads to a more prominent scar.

Most recently, Woog and coworkers (38) described their experiences with an endonasal laser-assisted dacryocystorhinostomy technique using a Ho:YAG laser to achieve bone removal. Endoscopic sinus surgical instrumentation was used to obtain biopsy specimens of lacrimal sac mucosa.

Technique

Surgical technique described includes the use of various endonasal laser instrumentation and endoscopy. It can be performed under general or local anesthesia. Various companies have introduced the laser including Coherent Medical, which produces the Coherent versapuls Ho:YAG laser or the KTP laser. Laser settings are set anywhere between 0.5 to 1.0 J/pulse delivered at a rate of 5 to 10 pulses/sec. The pulse durations are 250 microsec. The power can range from 2.5 to 17 W. The laser energies are delivered through a 400 μm diameter quartz fiber.

The patient is anesthetized with a 4% cocaine solution inserted into the nose. One percent Xylocaine HCL with epinepherine 1:100,000 is injected submucosally in the middle turbinate and lateral nasal wall anterior to the attachment of the middle turbinate to relieve additional mucosal congestion. The lacrimal punctum is then dilated and a 20-gauge fiberoptic light probe is passed either through the punctum or canaliculus into the lacrimal sac. This light probe is important because it transilluminates the lateral nasal wall and assists in the localization of the lacrimal sac fossa. The YAG laser is directed into the area of transillumination along the lateral nasal wall. A one cm diameter area of mucosa is vaporized with the Ho:YAG laser or the KTP laser. Mucosal ablation is complete; the underlying bone can be removed with the laser, but it can also be removed with very small Rongeurs.

The lacrimal bone is removed in that fashion. A thicker bone on the maxilla constituting an anterior lacrimal crest may also be removed. If there are ethmoidal air cells, they can also be removed during this procedure. Once the medial wall of the lacrimal sac is exposed, it can be entered with angled endoscopic forceps and tissue can be removed. The lacrimal sac opening is enlarged to approximately 10 mm. An indication of the internal common punctum is extremely important and that is facilitated by simultaneous placement of probes to the superior and inferior canaliculus with visualization of a common point of entry in the lateral wall of the lacrimal sac. Several silicone tubes can be used. The silicone tube that we prefer is the Crawford tube. Dr. Woog has recommended a seflex lacrimal cap further developed by Dr. John Griffiths (41) to keep the silicone tubing in place. The tubes are placed into position and tied with nylon sutures.

The current success rate of endoscopic laser dacryocystorhinostomy is between 70% and 82%. Which laser one uses is not important as long as it functions well. Several lasers that have been used are the Nd:YAG laser, the Ho:YAG laser, the argon laser, and the CO_2 laser.

References

1. Hornblass A, Herschorn BJ. Carbon dioxide laser surgery in hemophilia. Am J Ophthalmol 1983;96:689.
2. David LM, Sanders G. CO_2 laser blepharoplasty: a comparison to cold steel and electrocautery. J Dermatol Surg Oncol 1987;13:110.
3. Cochrane JS, Beacon JP, Creasy GH, Russell RG. Wound healing after laser surgery: an experimental study. Br J Surg 1980;67:740.
4. Finsterbush A, Russo M, Ashur H. Healing and tensile strength of CO_2 laser incisions and scalpel wounds in rabbits. Plast Reconstr Surg 1982;70:360.
5. Wheeland RG, Bailin PL, Ratz JL, Schreffler DE. Use of scleral eye shields for periorbital laser surgery. J Dermatol Surg Oncol 1987;13:156.
6. Beckman H, Fuller TA, Boyman R, et al. Carbon dioxide laser surgery of the eye and adnexa. Ophthalmology 1980;87:990.
7. Wesley RE, Bond JB. Carbon dioxide laser in ophthalmic plastic and orbital surgery. Ophthalmic Surg 1985;16:631.
8. Baker SS, Muenzler WS, Small RG, Leonard JE. Carbon dioxide laser blepharoplasty. Ophthalmology 1984;91:238.
9. Apfelberg DB, Maser MR, Lash H, White DN. Treatment of xanthelasma palpebrarum with the carbon dioxide laser. J Dermatol Surg Oncol 1987;13:149.
10. Gladstone GJ, Beckman H, Elson LM. CO_2 Laser excision of xanthelasma lesions. Arch Ophthalmol 1985;103:440.
11. Kennerdell JS, Maroon JC, Garrity JA, Abla AA. Surgical management of orbital lymphangioma with the carbon dioxide laser. Am J Ophthalmol 1986;102:308.
12. Korn EL. Laser chalazion removal. Ophthalmic Surg 1988;19:428.
13. Wheeland RG, Bailin PL, Reynolds OD, et al. Carbon dioxide (CO_2) laser vaporization of multiple facial syringomas. J Dermatol Surg Oncol 1987;12:225.
14. Apfelberg DB, Maser MR, Lash H, et al. Superpulse CO_2 laser treatment of facial syringomata. Lasers Surg Med 1987;7:533.
15. Huerter CJ, Wheeland RG. Multiple eruptive cysts treated with carbon dioxide laser vaporization. J Dermatol Surg Oncol 1987;13:260.
16. Takizawa T, Yamazaki T, Miura N, et al. Laser surgery of basal, orbital and ventricular meningiomas which are difficult to extirpate by conventional methods. Neurol Med Chir 1980;20:729.
17. Bailin PL, Wheeland RG. Carbon dioxide (CO_2) laser perforation of exposed cranial bone to stimulate granulation tissue. Plast Reconst Surg 1985;75:898.
18. Landthaler M, Haina D, Waidelich W, Braun-Falco O. A three-year experience with the argon laser in dermatotherapy. J Dermatol Surg Oncol 1984;10:456.
19. Wisnicki JL. Hemangiomas and vascular malformations. Ann Plast Surg 1984;12:41.
20. Cosman B. Clinical experience in the laser therapy of port wine stains. Lasers Surg Med 1980;1:133.
21. Apfelberg DB. Argon laser treatment of port wine hemangiomas: summary of 10 years experience. In: Williams HB,

ed. Symposium on vascular malformations and melanotic lesions. St. Louis: CV Mosby, 1983:95–100.

22. Noe JM, Barsky SH, Geer DE, et al. Port wine stains and the response to argon laser therapy: successful treatment and the predictive role of color, age, and biopsy. Plast Reconstr Surg 1980;65:130.

23. Gilcrest BA, Rosen S, Hoe JM. Chilling port wine stains improves the response to argon laser therapy. Plast Reconstr Surg 1982;69:278.

24. Gladstone GJ, Beckman H. Argon laser treatment of an eyelid margin capillary hemangioma. Ophthalmic Surg 1983; 14:944.

25. Hobby LW. Further evaluation of the potential of the argon laser in the treatment of strawberry hemangiomas. Plast Reconstr Surg 1983;71:481.

26. Awan KJ. Argon laser phototherapy of phthiriasis palpebrarum. Ophthalmic Surg 1986;17:813.

27. Awan KJ. Laser punctoplasty for the treatment of punctal stenosis. Am J Ophthalmol 1985;100:341.

28. Angres GG. Angres permalid-liner method: a new surgical procedure. Ann Ophthalmol 1984;16:145.

29. Tanenbaum M, Karas S, McCord CD. Laser ablation of blepharopigmentation. Ophthalmic Plast Reconstr Surg 1988; 4:49.

30. Wood JR, Anderson RL. Complications of cryosurgery. Arch Ophthalmol 1981;99:400.

31. Berry J. Recurrent trichiasis: treatment with laser photocoagulation. Ophthalmic Surg 1979;10:36.

32. Awan KJ. Argon laser treatment of trichiasis. Ophthalmic Surg 1986;17:658.

33. Bartley GB, Bullock JD, Olsen TG, Lutz PD. An experimental study to compare methods of eyelash ablation. Ophthalmology 1987;94:1286.

34. Aron-Rosa DS, Gean-Jacques, Griesemann M, Thyzel R. Use of the neodymium-YAG laser to open the posterior capsule after lens implant surgery: a preliminary report. Am Intraocular Implant Soc J 1980;6:352.

35. Diakuzono N, Joffe SN. Artificial sapphire probe for contact photocoagulation and tissue vaporization with the neodymium-YAG laser. Med Instrum 1985;19:173.

36. Dickson JB, Flanagan JC, Federman JL. Contact neodymium-YAG laser: experimental studies and oculoplastic applications. Ophthalmic Plast Reconstr Surg 1989;5:17.

37. Peyman GA, Katoh N, Tawakol M, Khoobehi B, Federman J. Contact Nd:YAG laser for use in oculoplastic surgery. Jpn J Ophthalmol 1987;31:635.

38. Woog JJ, Metson R, Puliafito CA. Holmium:YAG endonasal laser dacryocystorhinostomy. Am J Ophthalmol 1993; 116:1–10.

39. Massaro BM, Gonnering RS, Harris GJ. Endonasal laser dacryocystorhinostomy. A new approach to nasolacrimal duct obstruction. Arch Ophthalmol 1990;108:1172.

40. Gonnering RS, Lyon DB, Fisher JC. Endoscopic laser assisted lacrimal surgery. Am J Ophthalmol 1991;111:152.

41. Griffiths JD. Nasal catheter used in dacryocystorhinostomy. Ophthalmic Plast Reconstr Surg 1991;7:177.

12

Medicolegal and Safety Aspects of Laser Surgery

Alfred E. Mamelok
David B. Karlin

Liability and Ophthalmic Lasers

Tort actions following the use of lasers in ophthalmology basically involve product liability related to the structure, function, and defects, if any, in the particular instrument being used and the skill or alleged lack of skill of the physician operating the instrument. Further consideration must be given to injury sustained by patients or laboratory personnel in the form of ocular damage caused by a reflected laser beam. Such a case involving the pulsed ruby laser was reported as early as 1968 (1). Protective goggles are now considered advisable when almost any type of laser is used today if the possibility of such damage exists. Generally, the operator behind the binocular microscope need not wear protective eyewear because a protective filter is provided. Laser caution signs on doors and locking of the latter can be helpful.

The concept of laser use in surgery has caught the public's imagination far more than expected. The term laser has acquired a type of magic often associated with science fiction. It is indeed true that the technologic advances of the past few years are astounding to the medical world. To the lay public, the capabilities of the laser have created myths and have led to expectations that are too great as well as inaccurate. An illustration of this commonly known to ophthalmologists is the use by the lay public of the term "laser" for phacoemulsification in initial cataract extraction. Currently, while there is promising work being done in the use of lasers to eliminate cataracts, it still has not received general acceptance at the date of this writing. When the lay public is led to expect what is often not possible to deliver, its frustration is fertile ground for liability action caused by negligence.

As in all surgery, the legal doctrine of informed consent can be of great value to the operating laser surgeon. If the patient is not to become a plaintiff, he or she must first be told in no uncertain terms that no promise for complete success can be made. Following this, any discouragement that such a declaration may engender can be counteracted by mentioning encouraging statistics for success. Complications must be mentioned and described. The fact that vision may become worse instead of improved following laser therapy, especially in the region of the macula, is a risk that the patient must be informed of and be willing to take. An attitude that "there's nothing to it" has to be avoided. Other surgical alternatives, including doing nothing, must be discussed. Written documentation of the above is essential.

There are special considerations in relating to liability when performing laser therapy. The first is that the practitioner must be able to show proper training and experience leading to proficiency in the use of the particular laser being used. New discoveries, alteration of instruments, and introduction of new instruments are constantly being made. Investigators for human studies must first obtain approval from the Institutional Review Boards (IRB) and then from the federal Food and Drug Administration (FDA) if the particular use of the laser in question is still investigational. This latter fact must be incorporated into the informed consent.

The initial decision as to whether a device constitutes a "significant risk" is made by the IRB, not the FDA. The latter can come in afterward and disagree with the IRB. If this occurs, the vulnerability of the investigator to malpractice action can be increased. Physician participation is mandatory in IRB and FDA panels. In choosing these physicians, conflict of interest must be avoided; financial disclosure, affiliations, and general activities must be revealed to avoid bias. The committee members, the institution, and the investigational team are all liable for any injuries produced.

Concerning product liability, the manufacturer can be held liable for mistakes in design, manufacture, testing, or failure to warn. If there is proof of misuse of a device or continued use of a device in the face of known or reasonably discoverable defect or wrong choice of a particular device, liability extends to the doctor using the device and the hospital housing the latter. The doctor must test the device being used and must not use it if it is known to be defective. Proper selection of the device with no misuse of the latter is necessary to avoid liability.

Safety Aspects and Hazards of Laser Surgery

The laser device must be properly serviced by adequately trained maintenance personnel, whether the device is located in the hospital or in the physician's office. All lasers are potentially hazardous because of deposition of thermal energy in the target tissue. Reflection of the laser beam with minimal loss of energy presents a formidable laser complication.

The use of lasers is relatively new in the world of law. This, coupled with the fact that many cases are settled without trial, accounts for a paucity of case reports.

The FDA requires manufacturers of laser instruments to report all injuries and accidents. Retinal injuries can occur from direct or reflected laser light. The laser surgeon should therefore never look directly into the path of either the treatment or aiming laser beam. Eyelid skin damage can develop from misdirected laser applications to lid lesions. In 1963, Campbell and associates (2) reported on the inadvertent macula photocoagulation complication in the eye.

Lobraico (3) has shown that the specialties that perform laser surgical procedures in areas close to vital structures, are the most prone to the development of complications. Thus, ophthalmology, the first specialty to use the laser for therapeutic applications, has one of the highest specialty rates of complications.

Retinal accidents occur when an uncooperative patient who has been instructed to look at a fixation light, focuses instead into the path of the laser beam. Thus, a retrobulbar anaesthetic is frequently given to patients in whom parafoveal laser photocoagulation is to be carried out.

All personnel observing a laser procedure should wear protective goggles to prevent direct or reflected laser light from striking the eye.

Laser injury to ocular tissue depends on the power, duration, and size of the laser lesion. In addition, lasers operating in the infrared and UV end of the spectrum are more dangerous than those in the visible spectrum, because these lasers cannot be visualized by the human eye. Therefore, it is imperative that a helium-neon beam is used coaxially as an aiming device when one uses lasers operating at wavelengths greater than 700 nm or less than 400 nm.

Safety Hazards with Various Lasers

Argon lasers are the most frequently used lasers in ophthalmology. The argon blue laser operates at a wavelength of 488 nm. The argon green laser operates at 514 nm. Both lasers perform in the visual end of the spectrum. Krypton and tunable dye lasers are other examples of laser energy that can clearly be perceived by the human eye. These lasers are selectively absorbed by red, orange, and yellow pigment. They have the capability of coagulating blood vessels, obliterating vascular tumors, and treating areas of telangiectasis. Used in cardiac surgery, the argon laser can incise and vaporize tissue at high-power levels. It serves as a heat source to a metal probe attached to the end of a fiber, as used to dissolve cholesterol plaques in angioplastic surgery. The hazard in laser angioplasty is perforation of the wall of the vessel.

The neodymium:ytrrium-aluminum-garnet (Nd:YAG) laser has a wavelength of 1064 nm and thus operates in the infrared region of the spectrum. This laser can also be delivered by a quartz fiber. The Nd:YAG laser has the capacity to penetrate 3 to 4 mm within the target tissue. Thus, immediate or delayed retinal hemorrhage may be an unwanted sequela from transecting an epiretinal membrane 3 to 4 mm from the surface of the retina in a patient with proliferative diabetic retinopathy.

The CO_2 laser, operating at a wavelength of 10,600 nm, is the most commonly used laser in general surgery today. It also operates in the infrared range. However, it is not generally used in the field of ophthalmology because it lacks fiberoptic delivery capability. Thus, the probe cannot be miniaturized for either intraocular endolaser treatment or for slit-lamp delivery. Its main use in eye surgery is in the area of oculoplastic orbital or lid reconstruction. The thermal energy of the CO_2 laser is rapidly absorbed by water, raising both the intracellular and extracellular water temperature to 100° Centigrade at the target tissue. At this boiling point, tissue explodes and vaporizes. The operative field in the immediate vicinity of the CO_2 laser must be kept moist to prevent explosive complications.

Hazards may occur if adequate precautions are not taken when using endotracheal anaesthesia during the course of a general anaesthetic used in an oculoplastic procedure. Thus, the thermal energy of the CO_2 laser produces vaporization, transection, and coagulation of ocular tissue. Destruction of bacteria will also occur at these high-power densities. If the CO_2 laser energy is not controlled, hemorrhage, scarring, and disruption of biologic tissue will occur.

The Physician's Role in the Safety Aspects of Laser Surgery

The attempt by some surgeons to complete the laser procedure in a relatively short period of time may lead to unnecessary risks. In such cases, increasing the power density above the accepted norms or failing to take the time to adhere to an adequate checklist prior to laser delivery may subject the patient to unnecessary hazards.

One must adhere to the basic principles of laser surgery. Unfamiliarity with the micron size of the lesion, laser time duration, and wattage to be used may result in an increase in power density and subsequent complications following laser delivery. Lobraico (3) states there is, on the average, a 6-foot zone surrounding the operative field, which has been identified as the nominal hazard zone. There is a real danger to anyone within that zone if a fiber fracture occurs or if a laser light leaks into the zone from a break in the equipment.

The unexperienced surgeon may apply too much laser to an area in an attempt to obtain the desired result. Thus, the novice vitreoretinal surgeon may place argon laser lesions in almost a contiguous manner instead of spacing them one lesion apart, creating loss of visual acuity and a decrease of visual field. The inexperienced oculoplastic surgeon may be overly cautious and move the CO_2 laser beam at a slower rate, providing deep burns with excessive carbon deposition.

Unfortunately, carbon serves as a heat conductor, increasing the temperature above 1000°C. Excessive necrosis, pain, and scarring may result. To avoid these complications, the laser surgeon should remove the carbon deposits from the tip of the probe.

Equipment Failure and Operating Room Safeguards

The manual provided by the laser company should be read thoroughly to acquaint the laser surgeon with the operative procedure and hazards associated with the instrument. The risks include a faulty shutter switch, leaks from a faulty laser head, broken fibers in the delivery system, the failure of a safety lock to shut down the equipment if the control panel registers a faulty reading, and the misalignment of the laser with its aiming beam. The laser should always be kept in the *standby* mode when not treating a patient. The system should be turned off by a key switch if the laser is left unattended. A hooded foot switch is mandatory to prevent unnecessary firing of the laser.

All mirrored surfaces should be eliminated from the path of the laser beam as well as in the vicinity of the laser room. This will minimize inadvertent reflected laser retinal burns to observing personnel in the operating suite. Volatile iodine surgical preps should be eliminated because iodine contact with the laser beam may result in smoke that may prove irritating to the mucous membranes of the patient as well as to the operating personnel.

Laser safety standards have to be established within the hospital. Quality control and peer review are necessary measures.

Conclusions

The basic problem of product and professional liability concerning lasers in ophthalmology does not differ from any other type of malpractice or product liability. With the increased use of multiple laser systems by ophthalmologists, there has been a marked increase of liability exposure in recent years.

The basic issues are not so much the concern with the laser itself and its therapeutic use, but the broader issues of liability involved in the handling of the case, such as diagnosis, timeliness of therapy, informed consent, and qualifications of the ophthalmologist using the laser. The difference, then, is added vulnerability by the necessity for precision and by the type of atmosphere created for the patient by the ophthalmologist. Forewarned is forearmed and if the clinician in these cases is careful enough to completely familiarize the patient with the positive and negative aspects of laser therapy, the liability in these cases can be markedly reduced.

In using a laser, the ophthalmologist directs an extremely powerful energy source into the target tissue within or surrounding the eye. Accidental exposure to anything other than the designated target tissue may result in potential complications, with the eye and the skin providing the two areas of the body exhibiting the greatest hazards. Exposure may be direct from the delivery device, or indirect in the form of specular or diffuse reflections from mirrored surfaces that may be present in the path of the laser beam.

Certain precautions must be taken when using laser energy in the operating room during surgery using general anaesthesia. The laser beam reacts with material that absorbs it, resulting in the production of heat. If flammable material is used, raising the heat to a critical temperature can produce the hazard of fire. To prevent such an occurrence, three precautions must be taken. First, a nonflammable anaesthetic must be used. Second, drapes and other flammable material must not be placed immediately adjacent to the target tissue. Third, moistening the drapes with saline or water around the operative site becomes a very good preventive measure.

In summary, a number of safety criteria must be in place to lessen medicolegal exposure and prevent complications from laser therapy. In many institutions, medical staff credentialling has occurred. Laser training courses and seminars should be made available. Many hospitals have their own certification procedures. In addition, the appointment of a laser safety officer can minimize hazards. A reliable laser safety policy frequently consists of education of the laser surgeon and staff personnel in the use of the laser, posting of warning signs outside of laser rooms, the wearing of goggles as a safety precaution for personnel, and familiarization with operating manuals and techniques by the laser surgeon for the various lasers used. Additional measures include instruction in anaesthetic safety when performing laser procedures under general anaesthesia, a fire and explosion safety policy, and documentation of laser use. Fewer risks of complications to the surgeon, the patient, and the operating personnel will occur if the above precautionary measures are rigidly enforced.

References

1. Curtin TL, Boyden DG. Reflected laser beam causing accidental burn of the retina. Am J Ophthalmol 1968;65:188–189.
2. Campbell CJ, Ritter MC, Koester CJ. The optical laser as a retinal coagulator: an evaluation. Trans Am Acad Ophthalmol Otolaryngol 1963;67:58–67.
3. Lobraico RV. Laser safety in health care facilities: an overview. Am Coll Surg Bull 1991;76:(8).

Index

ab externo/ab interno sclerostomy, 75
Abraham lens, 68f, 69
Absorption
  energy level diagram, 4f
  of light, 4
  spectrum, 2, 2f
Active medium of lasers, 4f, 4–5, 5f
Adult-onset diabetic retinopathy (type II), 92, 104
Age-related macular degeneration (AMD)
  atrophic "dry"/exudative "wet" forms, 112
  clinical features, 113–114
  diagnosis, 118–120
  fluorescein angiography, 114–117, 116f, 117f
  ophthalmoscopic signs, 113, 114f
  overview, 112
  pathology/pathogenesis, 112–113
  prognosis, 116
  treatment, 116–118, 120
Airy diffraction rings, 1, 2f
Albino fundus, CO_2 lasers and, 203, 204f
Alignment microscope, 35f
Alloplastic lamellar keratophakia, 50–51
Amplification of light, 4–5
Amsler grid, 131, 134
Anamorphic beam expansion devices, 33, 33f
Angioid streaks, 123–126, 125f
Angle closure glaucoma
  iridectomy, argon laser, 68–70
  iridectomy, argon peripheral, 68
  iridectomy, Nd:YAG laser, 69
  iridoplasty peripheral iris contraction, argon laser, 69–70
Anterior capsulotomy, 85, 86f
Anterior keratomileusis, laser
  complications, 53–54
  corneal leukoma, 53f
  historical aspects, 51–53, 52f, 54f
  operative technique, 52–53
  postoperative management, 53
Anticoagulants
  branch retinal vein occlusion and, 145
  central retinal vein occlusion and, 143
  CO_2 laser treatment and, 214

Aperture wheels, 34–35
Aphakic eye
  indirect laser delivery and, 198
  retinal tears and, 179, 182
  treatment, 72
Arcuate keratectomy, 60–62
Argon blue laser, 101, 183
Argon fluoride (ArF) laser, 31, 38, 42, 43f, 209
Argon green laser
  branch retinal vein occlusion, 148
  central retinal vein occlusion, 144
  central serous choroidopathy, 154
  Coats' disease and, 164
  juxtafoveal telangiectasis and, 158
  retinal breaks, 183
Argon-ion lasers
  Coherent 920, 13f
  emission spectrum, 3f
  energy level diagram, 11f
  fundamentals of, 11–12
  internal structure, 12f
Argon laser endophotocoagulation vitrectomy, 185–186, 186f
Argon laser iridectomy
  complications, 69
  patent, confirmation of, 68
  postoperative care, 68–69
  technique, 68–69, 68f
Argon laser iridoplasty peripheral iris contraction
  complications, 70
  technique, 69–70, 70f
Argon laser photocoagulation
  alternatives to, 102, 103–104
  binocular indirect ophthalmoscope, 197
  choroidal neovascularization, 122, 131–135, 133f, 134f, 135f
  diabetic retinopathy, 95, 96
  histoplasmosis, ocular, 122
  retinal capillary hemangioma, 193
Argon laser surgery
  blepharopigmentation, 222
  capillary hemangioma, 222
  chloasma, 222
  malignant melanoma, 191
  oculoplastic, 221–223
  phthiriasis palpebrarum, 222
  port wine stains, 221–222
  punctal stenosis, 222
  trichiasis, 223

Argon laser trabeculoplasty (ALT)
  complications, 72
  indications, 70
  technique, 70–72,
Argon lasers
  overview, 220–221
  safety precautions, 221, 228
Arteriovenous communication of the retina
  clinical features, 169–170, 170f
  fluorescein angiography, 170
  overview, 169
  pathology/pathogenesis, 169
  prognosis, 169
  treatment, 169
Aspirin
  branch retinal vein occlusion and, 145
  central retinal vein occlusion and, 145
  diabetic retinopathy, 95
Astigmatism
  laser anterior keratomileusis, 52
  noncentral refractive keratectomy, 56–57
Astigmatism wheel, 34, 35f
Atherosclerotic heart disease, 158
Atrophic "dry" age-related macular degeneration (AMD), 112
Autoplastic lamellar procedures, 50

"Bag of worms" configurations, 169
BBO (beta barium borate) nonlinear crystal, 21
Beam delivery system, excimer lasers, 32–36
Beam radius, defined, 6
Bell's phenomenon, 102
Benign vascular hamartomas, 164, 165, 168
Best's vitelliform dystrophy, 128
Beta barium borate (BBO) nonlinear crystal, 21
Bilateral juxtafoveal telangiectasis, 155, 158
Binocular indirect ophthalmoscope laser delivery. *See* Indirect binocular ophthalmoscope laser delivery
Blackbody radiation, 2, 3f
Bleeding disorders, CO_2 lasers and, 214

Blepharopigmentation, argon laser treatment, 222
Blepharoplasty, CO_2 laser treatment, 217–218
Blindness, causes of, 92, 93, 112, 121
Blood sugar levels, diabetic retinopathy and, 104
Branch retinal vein occlusion (BRVO)
  diagnosis and clinical course, 145
  fluorescein angiography, 145, 147f, 148f
  incidence, 144–145
  inferotemporal, 149f
  pathogenesis, 145, 147f
  treatment, 145, 148–149
Brightness of light, 3–4
Bruch's membrane
  age-related macular degeneration and, 112, 113
  breaks/perforation, 108, 121, 123
Bubble formation, CO_2 lasers and, 204, 205f

Candela MDL 2000 LaserTripter organic dye laser system, 16f
Candela SL 3000 Photocoagulator GaAs diode laser system, 20f
Candida albicans keratitis, 43f
Capillary hemangiomas
  argon laser treatment, 222
  clinical features, 165–166
  CO_2 laser treatment, 220
  fluorescein angiography, 166, 166f, 167f
  Ne:YAG laser treatment, 224f, 225f
  overview, 164–165
  pathology/pathogenesis, 165
  prognosis, 166
  treatment, 166–168
  von Hippel-Lindau disease and, 193–194
Capillary macular nonperfusion, 104, 104f
Capsulotomy. *See also* Nd:YAG laser capsulotomy
  anterior, 85, 86f
  dilated pupils, pre-operatively, 82
  posterior, 24f, 24–25, 187
Carbon deposition, CO_2 lasers and, 204, 205, 229
Carbon dioxide lasers. *See* CO_2 lasers
Cartwheel-shaped subretinal capillaries, 113, 115, 115f
Cataract laser surgery
  Nd:YAG lasers, impact on, 80
  opacification after, 24
  research, 85–88, 88f
Cavernous hemangiomas of the retina
  clinical features, 168
  fluorescein angiography, 169
  ophthalmoscopic signs, 195f
  overview, 168
  pathology/pathogenesis, 168
  prognosis, 169
  treatment, 169, 194
Central retinal vein occlusion (CRVO)
  electroretinography, 141–143, 144f
  fluorescein angiography, 141, 142f, 143f

macular edema and, 143, 144, 146f
medical conditions, associated, 140t–141t
neovascular glaucoma, 143–144
pathogenesis, 140t–141t, 140–141, 141f
treatment, 143–144
Central serous choroidopathy (CSC)
  clinical features, 152–153
  fluorescein angiography, 153, 153f, 154f
  laser treatment, 154
  pathology/pathogenesis, 152
  prognosis, 153–154
Chalazion, CO_2 laser treatment, 219
Charles xenon arc endophotocoagulator, 185f, 186, 198f
Children
  Coats' disease and, 162
  retinoblastoma, 192
Chloasma, argon laser treatment, 222
Chorioretinal lesions
  CO_2 lasers, 204, 204f
  Nd:YAG laser vitrectomy, 189–190
Choroid, melanosarcoma of, 190–192, 207
Choroidal hemangiomas, 194, 195f
Choroidal neovascularization (CNV)
  age-related macular degeneration and, 112–120
  angiography, morphology on, 115–116, 117f
  causes, 112–130
  central serous choroidopathy and, 153
  diabetic retinopathy and, 108, 109f
  histopathology, AMD and, 121
  idiopathic, 123
  laser treatment, 130–135, 133f, 134f, 135f
  management, 136f
  ophthalmoscopic signs, 113f
  prognosis, 116, 117f
  treatment, 116–118
Choroidal osteoma, 126, 131f, 132f
Choroidal rupture, 126, 130f
Choroideremia, 128
Choroiditis
  multifocal, 126, 127t, 128f
  serpiginous, 126, 129f
CO_2 laser surgery
  blepharoplasty, 217–218
  capillary hemangiomas, 220
  chalazion, 219
  eruptive vellus hair cysts, 220
  exenterations, 220
  lymphangioma, 218–219
  meningioma, 220
  syringoma, 220
  xanthelasma, 218, 219f
CO_2 lasers
  advantages, 203f, 205t, 214–215, 216f
  adverse effects, 204, 205f
  articulating arm delivery system, 206f
  Coherent/Xanar XA-40, 215f
  compared, argon/krypton lasers, 202–203
  disadvantages, 205–207, 206t, 215

energy level diagram, 10f
fiberoptic delivery system, 205–206, 206f
fundamentals of, 10–11
handpiece, 207f
internal structure, 10f
oculoplastic/orbital applications, 216–220, 217f
overview, 202–203, 214
safety precautions, 215–216, 228
Surgicenter 40 system, 11f
Coat's disease
  clinical features, 162f, 162–163
  fluorescein angiography, 163, 163f
  juxtafoveal telangiectasis and, 154
  laser treatment, 164
  overview, 161–162
  pathology/pathogenesis, 162
  prognosis, 164
Coherent 920 Argon laser photocoagulator, 13f
Coherent 7970 Nd:YAG Laser System, 17f
Coherent light, 2, 3
Coherent/Xanar XA-40 CO_2 laser, 215f
"Collar button" ophthalmoscopic sign, 190, 190f
Concentric resonator, 5f
Confocal parameter, defined, 7
Confocal resonator, 5f
Contact corneal lenses, 100–102
Contact Nd:YAG laser, 73
Continuous wave mode, laser operation, 7–8, 8f, 10
Corneal ablation, depth of, 25f
Corneal ectasia, 46
Corneal freezing, 51
Corneal fungal infections, 43, 45
Corneal laser surgery, 30–31. *See also* Photorefractive keratectomy
Corneal leukoma, 53f
Corneal opacities, removal, 45, 46f
Corneal sculpting/smoothing, 25, 44f, 45. *See also* Photorefractive keratectomy
Corneal trephination, 47, 47f, 49f, 50f
Cotton wool spots, 92
Cryopexy
  chorioretinal adhesions, 184
  retinal tears, 181
Cryotherapy
  arteriovenous communication of the retina, 171
  capillary hemangiomas and, 168
  cavernous hemangiomas of the retina, 169
  Coats' disease and, 164
  retinoblastoma, 192
Crystals, frequency-doubling/tripling, 21
Cyclocryotherapy (CCT), 73, 75
Cyclophotocoagulation, 73–75, 78
Cylindrical lens telescopes, 33
Cystoid macular edema (CME)
  branch retinal vein occlusion, 145
  fluorescein angiogram, 104f
  incidence, 81
  laser treatment, 173–174
  Nd:YAG laser capsulotomy, 85

Nd:YAG laser photocoagulation, 189
visual acuity and, 81, 104

D +60, +78, and +90 lenses, 99, 99f
Dacryocystorhinostomy, laser, 224–225
Diabetes mellitus, juxtafoveal telangiectasis and, 154, 155
Diabetic maculopathy, 104–105
Diabetic retinopathy
    classification, 92–94
    clinical trials, 94–95
    development, 92
    glycemic control and, 104
    laser diagnostic evaluation, 107
    laser photocoagulation, alternatives to, 103–104
    laser photocoagulation, complications, 107–109
    laser treatment guidelines, 101–104
    laser treatment indications, 95–96
    macular edema, modified grid laser for, 105–107
    maculopathy, 104–105
    management, 96–99, 98t
    panretinal laser photocoagulation, 99–101
    pregnancy and, 107
    subretinal neovascular membranes, detection, 109–110
Diabetic Retinopathy Study, 95
Diabetic Retinopathy Vitrectomy Study, 95
Diagnostics, optical, 25–27, 26f, 107
Diathermy
    capillary hemangiomas and, 168
    chorioretinal adhesions, 184
    Coats' disease and, 164
    retinal tears, 179
Diffuse macular edema
    diabetic retinopathy and, 104, 105
    modified grid laser, 105f, 105–107, 106f
Digital and ICG angiography, 118–120
Dilated pupils, pre-capsulotomy, 82
Dipyridamole (Persantine), 143
Directionality of light, 3
Disc, neovascularization of. *See* Neovascularization of the disc (NVD)
Disciform scarring, 114, 116, 126
Doping, defined, 200
Drainage sites, reopening failing, 73
Drusen, 112, 113
"Dumbbell" hemorrhage, 159
Dye laser systems. See Organic-dye lasers

Early Treatment Diabetic Retinopathy Study, 95
Early vitrectomy, 103
Ehlers-Danlos syndrome, 123
Einstein's E=hf formula, 4
Electromagnetic radiation, 1–2, 2f
Electron-hole recombination, defined, 19
Electroretinography, 141–143, 144f
Elschnig pearl formation, 81f
Emission spectrum, argon-ion laser, 3f
Endolaser photocoagulation, 96, 99

Endolaser photocoagulation vitrectomy
    complications, 189–190
    historical background, 185–186
    indications, 187
    Nd:YAG laser, 187–189
    technique, 187
Endophthalmitis, 80
Endophytic capillary hemangiomas, 165
Enucleation, 191, 192
Epikeratophakia, 50
Epikeratoplasty, laser, 54–55, 55f
Epikeratoplasty, laser-adjusted synthetic, 55–56, 56f
Epinephrine, contraindications to, 221
Erosions, recurrent, 45
Eruptive vellus hair cysts, CO_2 laser treatment, 220
Er:YAG lasers, 210–211, 211f
Excimer, defined, 12
Excimer lasers, 31f
    argon fluoride, 31
    beam delivery system, 32–36, 33f
    commercially available, 7f
    corneal surgical applications, 32f
    development, 30–31
    energy level diagram, 13f
    fundamentals of, 12–14
    internal structure, 14f
    laser subsystem, 32–33
    measurement subsystem, 35–36
    OnmiMed Excimer Laser Refractive Workstation, 14f
    optical subsystems, 33f, 33–35
    types/wavelengths, 13t
    vitreoretinal surgical applications, 209–210, 210f
Excitation of atoms, 4
"Excited dimer," 12, 209
Exenterations, CO_2 laser treatment, 220
Extinction dimension, defined, 202
Extracapsular cataract extraction, 80, 85
Extrafoveal choroidal neovascular membranes, 122
Extrinsic fluorescence, 26
Exudative "wet" age-related macular degeneration (AMD), 112
Eye protection, laser safety and, 215–216, 216f, 221, 228, 229

Facioscapulohumeral muscular dystrophy, 161
Fan-shaped subretinal capillaries, 115
Fiberoptic delivery system, CO_2 lasers, 205–206, 206f, 212f
Fibrillar haze formation, 39–40, 41, 46, 47f
Fibrotic scarring, diabetic laser photocoagulation, 108–109
5-D myope, 54f
Flammable materials, laser safety and, 215, 229
Flashlamp-pumped dye laser, 15
Fluorescein angiography, indocyanine green, 109–110, 118–120
Fluorescence, laser-induced (LIF), 26
Focal macular edema

diabetic retinopathy and, 104, 105
    resolution, 106
Food and Drug Administration (FDA), 227, 228
Foveal avascular zone (FAZ), 116, 117f
Foveal photocoagulation, 101, 108
Frequency-doubling crystal, 21
Frequency tripling, 21
Fundus flavimaculatus, 128
Fungal infections, corneal, 43, 45

G Laser 210 holmium laser, 75f
Gallium-aluminum-arsenide (GaAIAs) semi-conductor laser, 16, 20, 200
Gas lasers
    argon and other ions, 11–12
    carbon dioxide, 10–11
    fundamentals of, 8–14
    helium-neon, 9–10
Gaussian beams
    converging lens, effect of, 7f
    focusing, 6–7
    intensity profile, 33
    propagation, 6f
Geographic atrophy, RPE, 112
Glaucoma
    angle closure, 67–70
    anterior segment laser procedures, 72–78
    Nd:YAG laser iridectomy, 187
    open angle, 70–72
Glycemic control, diabetic retinopathy and, 104
Glycosylated hemoglobin, 104
Goldmann-Favre syndrome, 180
Goldmann lens, 69–70, 99, 100, 100f, 101, 179, 183f, 184f
Goniophotocoagulation, 73
Gonioscopy, 96
"Grape cluster" configurations, 162, 194, 195f
"Green" argon lasers, 144, 148, 154, 158, 164, 183
"Green" Nd:YAG lasers, 20, 22

Hallermann-Streiff syndrome, 152
Hamartomas, benign vascular, 164, 165, 198. *See also* Capillary hemangiomas; Cavernous hemangiomas of the retina
Harmonic generation, 20, 21
Haze formation, post-laser, 39–40, 41, 46, 47f
Helium-neon (HeNe) lasers, 9f, 9–10
Hemangiomas. *See* Capillary hemangiomas; Cavernous hemangiomas of the retina; Choroidal hemangiomas
Hemispheric (hemicentral) retinal vein occlusion (HRVO), 140, 149, 149f
Hemorrhagic PED, 114, 114f
HeNe lasers, 9f, 9–10
Hereditary dystrophies, CNV and, 128
"Histo spots," 121
Histoplasmosis, ocular, 121–123
Holmium (Ho) YAG lasers
    diode laser pumping, 18f

energy level diagram, 18f
fundamentals of, 17–18
sclerostomy, 75f, 75–77, 76f, 77f
Homoplastic lamellar procedures, 50
Horseshoe retinal break, 181f, 182, 182f
"Hot spots," 33, 115
Ho:YAG lasers, 17–18, 76–78, 211–212
Hruby non-contact lenses, 99
Hydroxyethylmethacrylate (HEMA)
    IOLs, 85
Hyperbaric oxygen, branch retinal
    vein occlusion and, 145
Hyperopia, correction of, 52
Hyperopia aperture wheel, 34, 34f
Hypertension, retinal arterial macroa-
    neurysms and, 158

Idiopathic central serous choroidopa-
    thy, 152–154
Idiopathic choroidal neovasculariza-
    tion, 123
Idiopathic juxtafoveal telangiectasis,
    154
Idiopathic polypoid choroidal vascu-
    lopathy, 130, 132f
Imaging, optical, 25–27, 26f
Incipient atrophy, RPE, 112
Incoherent light, 3, 3f
Indirect binocular ophthalmoscope
    laser delivery
    advantages, 198–199
    anesthesia and technique, 199
    apparatus, 198f
    disadvantages, 199
    indications, 199–200
    panretinal laser photocoagulation,
        99, 99f
    parameters in, 197–198
Indocyanine green fluorescein angiog-
    raphy, 109–110, 110f, 118–120,
    119f
Informed consent, 227
Injection process, defined, 19
Injury. *See* Trauma
"Ink blot" fluorescein angiographic
    pattern, 153
Intraocular lens (IOL)
    implantation, 24
    Nd:YAG capsulotomy and, 82, 84–85
Intraocular pressure (IOP), 84. *See also*
    Glaucoma
Intraocular tumors, posterior segment
    melanosarcoma of the choroid, 190f,
        190–192, 191f
    metastatic tumors, 193
    retinoblastoma, 192, 192f
    solid tumors, 190–193
    vascular, 193–195
Intraretinal microvascular abnormali-
    ties (IRMA), 92
Intrinsic fluorescence, 26
Ion lasers
    fundamentals of, 11–12
    major wavelengths of, 12t
Iridectomy
    after acute glaucoma attack, 187
    laser techniques, 67–69
Iridocapsular adhesions, lysis of, 85

Iris capture of posterior chamber IOLs,
    85
Iris neovascularization, 141
Ischemic central retinal vein occlusion,
    141, 142f
Isovolemic hemodilution, 143

Juvenile diabetic retinopathy (type I),
    92, 104
Juvenile retinoschisis, 180
Juxtafoveal telangiectasis
    clinical features, 155
    fluorescein angiography, 155, 157f,
        158f
    laser treatment, 158
    pathology/pathogenesis, 154–155
    prognosis, 158

"K-mirror" type beam rotator, 33
KDP (potassium dihydrogen phos-
    phate) nonlinear crystal, 21
Keratectomy. *See* also Photorefractive
    keratectomy; Phototherapeu-
    tic keratectomy
    arcuate, 60–61
    lamellar, 36–38, 43
    lamellar refractive, 50–51
    noncentral refractive, 56–57
    radial, 59f
    remodeling, post excimer-laser, 39,
        41
    transverse, 60f, 60–61, 61f, 62f
Keratitis, fungal, 43, 43f, 44f
Keratomileusis (KM), 50, 51–55, 55
Keratophakia (KF), 50–51
Keratoplasty, 43, 50–51
Krypton fluoride (KrF) laser, 209
Krypton laser photocoagulation
    advantages/disadvantages, 103
    choroidal neovascularization, 123,
        131–135, 133f
    diabetic retinopathy, 96
    histoplasmosis, ocular, 123
Krypton lasers
    central serous choroidopathy, 154
    malignant melanoma, 191
    retinal breaks, 183
KTP (potassium titanyl phosphate)
    lasers
    frequency-doubling crystals, 21f
    fundamentals of, 20–22
    Laserscope KTP/Nd:YAG XP Surgi-
        cal Laser System, 22f
    nonlinear crystals, 21f

Lacquer cracks, pathologic myopia
    and, 123
Lacrimal punctum, 222
Lamellar keratectomy, 36–38, 43
Lamellar refractive keratectomy, 50–51
Laser Doppler velocimeter (LDV), 107
Laser-induced fluorescence (LIF), 26
Laser photocoagulation
    capillary hemangiomas, 167–168
    cavernous hemangiomas of the
        retina, 169
    central serous choroidopathy, 154
    Coats' disease, 164
    complications, 108–109

diabetic retinopathy, 95–96
    macular edema, 105–107, 173
    malignant melanoma, 191–192
    modified grid, diffuse macular
        edema, 105–107
    radiation retinopathy, 173
    retinal detachment, 184–185
    retinal tears, 180–181
    retinoblastoma, 192
    vitrectomy, 185–190
Laser plume, defined, 215
Laser probes, 88f
Laser surgery, 30–31, 214. *See also* Ar-
    gon laser surgery; Cataract
    laser surgery; CO$_2$ laser
    surgery; Oculoplastic laser
    surgery; Photorefractive kera-
    tectomy; Phototherapeutic
    keratectomy; Vitreoretinal
    laser surgery
Laser(s). *See also* Argon lasers; CO$_2$
    lasers; Excimer lasers;
    Holmium (Ho) YAG lasers;
    Krypton lasers; Organic-dye
    lasers
    active medium of, 4f, 4–5, 5f
    delivery systems, excimer, 32–36
    delivery systems, fiberoptic, 205–206
    delivery systems, indirect, 99,
        197–200
    delivery systems, lenses and, 35
    delivery systems, slit-lamp, 22, 24f
    development, 1, 30
    Er:YAG, 211–212
    feedback control of, 27, 28f
    focusing gaussian beams, 6–7
    future applications, 25–28
    KTP (potassium titanyl phosphate),
        20–22
    liability issues, 227–229
    medical applications, selected, 22–25
    nature of light and, 1–4, 2f
    Ne:YAG, 223–225
    operating modes, 7–8, 8f
    optical resonators, 5–6
    output, 3f, 8f
    physics of, 4–7
    research, 87–88
    subsystems, 32–35
    surgical applications, 7–22, 8f
    terminology, illustrated, 4f
    types, commercially available, 7f
    water extinction curves, 204f
Laserscope KTP/Nd:YAG XP Surgical
    Laser System, 22f
"Late phase leakage of an undeter-
    mined source," 116
Lattice degeneration, 181f, 181–182,
    182f, 200
Legal aspects, ophthalmic lasers,
    227–229
Lens capsule, retroillumination, 82f
Lens(es). *See also* Goldmann lens;
    Mainster lens; Rodenstock
    lens; Yannuzzi lens
    Abraham, 70
    contact corneal, 99–101
    as delivery system component, 35
    Hruby non-contact, 99

noncontact corneal, 99
Peyman's, 189f
+60, +78, and +90 D, 99
Leukocoria, 166, 192
LIF (laser-induced fluorescence), 26
Light
brightness, 3–4
directionality, 3
as electromagnetic radiation, 1–2, 2f
monochromaticity, 2–3
properties of, 1–4, 2f
Light Amplification by Stimulated
Emission of Radiation. *See*
Laser(s)
Light amplifier. *See* Active medium of
lasers
"Light bulb" configurations, 162
Light-emitting diode keratoscope, 35,
36f
LiNbO₃ (lithium niobate) nonlinear
crystal, 21
Liquid lasers, organic dye, 14–15
Lithium niobate (LiNbO₃) nonlinear
crystal, 21
Longitudinal mode, 5
Lymphangioma, CO₂ laser treatment,
218–219
Lymphatic vessels, CO₂ lasers and, 215
Lymphatic vessels, sealing with CO₂
lasers, 220

Macroaneurysms
nonarterial, 175
retinal arterial, 158–161
Macular diseases
arteriovenous communications of
the retina, 169–171
capillary hemangiomas, 164–168
cavernous hemangiomas of the
retina, 168–169
Coat's disease, 161–164
idiopathic central serous
choroidopathy, 152–154
juxtafoveal telangiectasis, 154–158
radiation retinopathy, 171–173
retinal arterial macroaneurysms,
158–161
Macular edema. *See also* Cystoid macular edema (CME)
branch retinal vein occlusion, 145,
148
central retinal vein occlusion, 143,
144, 146f
diabetic retinopathy, 104f, 104–107
incidence, 93
management, 97–98
Macular pigmentary changes, 112. *See
also* Age-related macular degeneration (AMD)
Mainster lens, 100, 101, 183, 184f
Malignant melanoma, 190f, 190–192,
191f
Marfan's syndrome, 180
Mask of pregnancy, 222
Measurement subsystem, excimer
lasers, 35–36
Medical applications of lasers, 22–25
Medicolegal aspects, ophthalmic
lasers, 227–229

Melanosarcoma of the choroid,
190–192, 207
Meningioma, CO₂ laser treatment, 220
Metamorphopsia
capillary hemangiomas, 165
central serous choroidopathy, 152
exudative AMD, 113
Microaneurysms
diabetic retinopathy, 92, 96, 97f
macular edema, 105
Micropsia
capillary hemangiomas, 165
central serous choroidopathy, 152
exudative AMD, 113
Mode-locking laser operation, 7–8
Modes (of optical resonators), 5
Modified grid laser for diffuse macular
edema, 105f, 105–107, 106f
Molecular lasers, commercially available, 7f
Monochromaticity of light, 2–3
Multifocal choroiditis, 126, 127t, 128f
Myopia
laser anterior keratomileusis, 51, 52f,
55f
laser treatment, 25
pathologic, 123, 124f
retinal tears and, 179
Myopia aperture wheel, 34, 34f

Nanophthalamos, 69
Nd:YAG laser capsulotomy, 85, 86f,
189–190, 190f
Nd:YAG laser iridectomy, 69
Nd:YAG laser phacolysis probe, 88f
Nd:YAG laser phototransection,
188–189
Nd:YAG laser posterior capsulotomy,
187
complications, 83–85, 84f
contraindications, 81
impact on cataract surgery, 80
indications, 81, 81f
technique, 81–82, 82f, 83f
Nd:YAG laser transscleral cyclophotocoagulation (CPC), 73–75, 74f,
78
Nd:YAG laser zonulysis, 85
Nd:YAG lasers
applications, ophthalmic, 80
applications, potential clinical, 85
Coherent 7970 System, 17f
contact, 73
energy level diagram, 16f
fundamentals of, 15–17
green, 20, 22
internal structure, 17f
safety precautions, 228
sapphire-tipped, 207–209
vitreous surgery, 187–190
Neodymium YAG lasers. *See* Nd:YAG
lasers
Neovascular glaucoma, 96, 141, 149
Neovascularization, choroidal. *See*
Choroidal neovascularization
(CNV)
Neovascularization, idiopathic, 123
Neovascularization of the disc (NVD)
causes, 92

laser treatment, 102
ophthalmoscopic signs, 94f, 211
Neovascularization of the retina (NVE)
causes, 92, 145, 148–149
laser treatment, 102
ophthalmoscopic signs, 94f
Nevus flammeus, 221
Ne:YAG lasers, 223–225
Non-contact lenses, retinal photocoagulation, 99
Nonarterial macroaneurysms, laser
treatment, 173
Noncentral refractive keratectomy,
56–57
Noncontact Nd:YAG laser, 73
Nonlinear crystals, 21, 21f
Nonpigmented tissue, photocoagulation, 73, 203
Nonproliferative (background) diabetic retinopathy (BDR)
clinical course, 93
defined, 92
management, 97
ophthalmoscopic signs, 93f

Occult membranes, 113, 115
OCT (optical coherence tomography),
26
Ocular histoplasmosis, 121–123
Oculoplastic laser surgery, 214,
216–224
OnmiMed Excimer Laser Refractive
Workstation, 14f
Open angle glaucoma, 70–72
Operculum(a), 182
Ophthalmological applications of
lasers
liability/safety issues, 227–229
overview, 22–25
plastic and orbital surgery, 214
vitreoretinal surgery, 197, 202
Optic nerve, hemangiomas and, 164,
168
Optical coherence tomography (OCT),
26, 26f
Optical harmonics, 20–21
Optical imaging and diagnostics, laser,
25–27, 26f
Optical resonators, 5f, 5–6, 6f
Optical subsystems, excimer lasers,
33–35
Orbital laser surgery, 214
Organic-dye lasers
Candela MDL 2000 LaserTripter,
16f
CNV, 131–135
Coats' disease, 164
commercially available, 7f
energy level diagram, 14f
fundamentals of, 14–15
internal structure, 15f
juxtafoveal telangiectasis, 158
Oscillation, 1, 6

Paget's disease, 123, 125
Panretinal cryoablation, 103
Panretinal photocoagulation (PRP)
arteriovenous communication of the
retina, 171

complications, 108–109
contact corneal lenses, 99–101
defined, 22
diabetic retinopathy, 96
neovascular glaucoma, central retinal vein occlusion and, 143–144
non-contact lenses, 99
ophthalmoscopic signs, 23f
technique, 99–101
Paracentral scotoma, 107, 108
Pars plana vitrectomy
capillary hemangiomas, 168
endolaser photocoagulation, 185
indirect laser delivery, 198, 199
Pathologic myopia, 123, 124f
Peak (power) intensity, defined, 7
Penetrating keratoplasty
complications, 48–49
historical aspects, 47f, 47–48, 49f, 50f
indications, 43
operative technique, 48
Perforating injury. *See* Trauma
Peripheral iridectomy, 67, 68f
Peyman's lens, 189f
Phacolysis probe, Nd:YAG laser, 88f
Phakic eye, indirect laser delivery and, 198
Photoablation of the cornea. *See* Photorefractive keratectomy
Photocoagulation. *See* Laser photocoagulation; Retinal photocoagulation
Photodisruption of the posterior lens capsule. *See* Posterior capsulotomy
Photofrin, 26–27, 27f
Photomydriasis, 72
Photons, 2
Photopsia, retinal tears and, 182
Photorefractive keratectomy
clinical results, 37
contraindications, 36
development, 25, 30–31
excimer lasers, 31f, 31–36, 32f
histopathologic results, 37–42, 38f, 39f, 40f, 41f, 42
indications, 36
lamellar refractive keratectomy and keratoplasty, 50–51
laser applications of, 25, 25f
procedures, 36–37
Phototherapeutic keratectomy
clinical results, 37
complications, 46–47
contraindications, 36
corneal infections, 45
corneal opacity removal, 45, 46f
corneal smoothing, 45
excimer lasers, 31–36, 32f
histopathologic results, 37–42, 38f, 39f, 40f, 41f, 42
historical aspects, 43–44
indications, 36, 44–45
lamellar keratectomy and keratoplasty, 43
operative technique, 45
postoperative management, 45–46
procedures, 36–37

recurrent erosions, removal of, 45
Phototransection, Nd:YAG laser, 188–189
Phthiriasis palpebrarum, argon laser treatment, 222
Phthisis bulbae, 96
Physics, lasers and, 4–7
Picosecond Nd:YLF laser, 212
Pigment epithelial detachments (PEDs)
age-related macular degeneration, 112, 119f
central serous choroidopathy, 152
hemorrhagic, 113–114, 114f
Pigmented tissue, photocoagulation, 73, 203
Planar lamellar refractive keratoplasty (PLRK), 50
Plane parallel resonator, 5f
Plank's law, 2
Plasma, defined, 81
Plastic surgery, 214, 216–224
+60, +78, and +90 D lenses, 99, 100f
Pneumoretinopexy, 184, 198
Polymethylmethacrylate (PMMA) IOLs, 84
Population inversions
argon-ion lasers, 11
defined, 4
energy states, 5f
Port wine stains, argon laser treatment, 221–222
Posterior capsule opacification, 80, 81
Posterior capsulotomy, laser applications, 24f, 24–25, 187
Posterior keratomileusis, laser, 55–56
Posterior pole
hemorrhagic disorder of, 130
photocoagulation, 101
Posterior segment intraocular tumors, 190–195
Posterior uveal bleeding syndrome, 130
Potassium titanyl phosphate (KTP) lasers, 20–22
Potential acuity meter (PAM), 82
Pregnancy
chloasma, 222
diabetic retinopathy and, 104, 107
Prematurity, retinopathy of, 180
Preproliferative diabetic retinopathy (PPDR)
clinical course, 93
defined, 92
management, 97
ophthalmoscopic signs, 93f
Preretinal neovascularization, branch retinal vein occlusion and, 145, 148–149
Presumed ocular histoplasmosis syndrome (POHS), 121, 121f, 122f
Proliferative diabetic retinopathy (PDR)
clinical course, 93
defined, 92
management, 97–103, 106
Nd:YAG laser photocoagulation, 188–189
ophthalmoscopic signs, 92–93, 93f, 94f

retinal detachment, 180, 180f
retinal photocoagulation, 22
stages, 92
Proliferative vitreoretinopathy, Nd:YAG laser treatment, 189
Pseudophakic eye, retinal tears and, 179, 182
Pseudoxanthoma elasticum, 123
Pterygium removal, 44f
Pulse duration, defined, 31
Pulse-to-pulse energy level, defined, 31
Pulsed mode laser operation, 7–8, 8f
Pumping source of lasers, 4
Punctal stenosis, argon laser treatment, 222
Pupilloplasty, laser, 72
Pupils, dilated pre-capsulotomy, 82

Q-switched mode laser operation, 7–8, 8f

Radial keratectomy, 58f, 59f
Radial keratotomy, 25, 57–59
Radiation retinopathy
clinical features, 172, 172f
fluorescein angiography, 172f, 172–173
juxtafoveal telangiectasis and, 154
overview, 171
pathology/pathogenesis, 171–172
prognosis/treatment, 173
Radiation therapy, 192
Recurrent erosions, treatment of, 45
Refracting prisms, 33
Remodeling, post excimer-laser keratectomy, 39, 41
Retina. *See also* Capillary hemangiomas; Cavernous hemangiomas; Neovascularization of the retina (NVE); Vitreoretinal laser surgery
arteriovenous communications of, 169–171
Coat's disease, 154, 161–164
nonarterial macroaneurysms, 173
radiation retinopathy, 154, 171–173
Retinal arterial macroaneurysms
clinical features, 159
fluorescein angiography, 159, 160f, 161
laser treatment, 161
overview, 158–159
pathology/pathogenesis, 159
prognosis, 161
Retinal breaks
contact lens, selection of, 182–183
laser treatment, 182–184, 198
risk factors of treatment, 182
Retinal detachment
causes, 108
central serous choroidopathy, 152–153
incidence, 80
laser treatment, 184–185
Nd:YAG capsulotomy and, 83–84
proliferative diabetic retinopathy, 188–189
trauma, 188, 188f

Retinal edema, causes, 92
Retinal ischemia
  branch retinal vein occlusion, 148
  signs of, 92
Retinal photocoagulation. *See also* Diabetic retinopathy
  fundus view, 102f
  laser applications of, 22, 23f, 24, 24f, 197
  lenses for, 99–101
Retinal pigment epithelium (RPE)
  age-related macular degeneration, 112
  central serous choroidopathy, 152–153
  formation, 109
  tears, 114, 115f
Retinal tears
  fish-mouth, 185f
  formation, contributing factors, 179–180
  historical background, 179
  laser treatment, 180–181
Retinal vein occlusions
  branch (BRVO), 144–149
  central (CRVO), 140–144
  two-thirds, 150f
  types, 140
Retinitis pigmentosa
  central serous choroidopathy, 152
  Coats' disease, 161, 164
Retinoblastoma, 192, 192f
Retinopathy of prematurity, 180
Retrobulbar anesthesia
  disadvantages, 199
  indications, 101, 201, 228
Rodenstock lens, 99, 100–101, 101f, 108, 183, 184f
Rubella retinopathy, 126
Rubeosis irides, 96, 96f

Safety precautions
  argon lasers, 221
  CO$_2$ lasers, 215–216
  liability issues, 227–229
Sapphire-tipped Nd:YAG laser
  advantages/disadvantages, 209
  clinical applications, 208f, 208–209, 209f
  overview, 207–208
Sapphire-tipped Ne:YAG laser, 223f, 223–225
Scanning laser ophthalmoscope (SLO), 107, 109
Scatter laser therapy, branch retinal vein occlusion, 148
Scattering, optical tissue imaging, 26
Scleral buckling, 164, 168
Sclerostomy, holmium laser, 75–77
Scotoma, 152, 165
Semiconductor diode laser photocoagulation
  advantages/disadvantages, 103
  retinal breaks, 183
  vitrectomy, 186
Semiconductor diode lasers
  advantages/disadvantages, 201
  Candela SL 3000 Photocoagulator, 20f

development, 200–201
energy level diagram, 19f
fundamentals of, 18–20
glaucoma, 78–79
ICG as chromophore for uptake enhancement, 120
internal structure, 20f
solid-state, 200f
types/wavelengths, 19t
Senior-Loken syndrome, 161
Serpiginous choroiditis, 126, 129f
Sickle cell disease, 123, 154, 180
Slit-lamp laser delivery system, 22, 24f
"Smart lasers," 27
"Smokestack" fluorescein angiographic pattern, 153
Solid-state lasers
  fundamentals of, 15–22
  holmium (Ho) YAG, 17–18
  KTP lasers, 20–22
  neodymium (Nd) YAG, 15–17
  semiconductor diode, 18–20, 200f, 200–201
Spectral emittance of a blackbody, 3f
Spontaneous emission, 4f
Spot size, defined, 6
Steroids, AMD and, 118
Stickler's syndrome, 180
Stimulated emission of radiation, 4, 4f
Submacular fibrosis, 108
Subretinal neovascular membrane (SRN), 109f, 109–110, 110f, 127
Sufficient energy, defined, 31
Surgicenter 40 CO$_2$ laser system, 11f
Suture lysis, 73
Syringoma, CO$_2$ laser treatment, 220

Telangiectasis, juxtafoveal. *See* Juxtafoveal telangiectasis
TEM (transverse electromagnetic wave), 5
Thalassemia, 123
Tissue fluorescence, 26
"Top hat" intensity profile, 33
Trabeculectomy scleral flap suture lysis, 73
Traction, retinal tissue, 202
Transconjunctival cryopexy, retinal tears, 179
Transmission spectra, ocular chromophores, 23f
Transmittance, eye, 23f
Transpupillary argon laser ciliophotocoagulation, 72
Transscleral cyclophotocoagulation, 73–75, 78
Transverse electromagnetic wave (TEM), 5
Transverse keratectomy, 60f, 60–61, 61f, 62f
Transverse mode, 5, 6, 6f
Trauma
  Nd:YAG laser photocoagulation for, 188
  retinal detachment and, 180, 188f
Trichiasis, argon laser treatment, 223
Tumors, intraocular, 190–195
Turner's syndrome, 161

Two-thirds retinal vein occlusion, 150f

Ultrasonic liquefaction transducer, 202f
Ultrasonic phacoemulsification, 86
Unilateral juxtafoveal telangiectasis, 155, 158

Vascular posterior segment tumors, 193–195
Visual acuity
  age-related macular degeneration, 112
  arteriovenous communications of the retina, 170
  cystoid macular edema, 81, 104
Vitrectomy. *See also* Pars plana vitrectomy
  Diabetic Retinopathy Vitrectomy Study, 95
  early, 103
  endolaser photocoagulation, 185–190
Vitreolysis, cystoid macular edema, 173
Vitreoretinal laser surgery
  CO$_2$ lasers, 202–207
  cutting within the vitreous cavity, 202
  Er:YAG laser, 210–211
  excimer laser, 209–210
  historical background, 197, 201
  Holmium (Ho) YAG laser, 211–212
  picosecond Nd:YLF laser, 212
  sapphire-tipped Nd:YAG laser, 207–209
  tractionless, 202
Vitreous hemorrhage, 103f
  branch retinal vein occlusion, 145, 148
  vitrectomy procedure and, 187
Vitreous opacities, Nd:YAG laser treatment, 189
Vogt quadraspheric fundus lens, 100
Volk quadraspheric lens, 101
Von Hippel-Lindau disease, 164–165, 166, 193–194, 194f

Water, absorption coefficient at various wavelengths, 203f
Wyburn-Mason syndrome, 169, 170, 171f

Xanthelasma palpebrarum, 218, 219f
Xenon arc endophotocoagulation vitrectomy, 185, 185f
Xenon arc photocoagulation, 198f
  advantages/disadvantages, 103
  diabetic retinopathy, 95
  retinal tears, 179–180, 180f
Xenon chloride (XeCl) laser, 209

YAG (yttrium-aluminum-garnet), 15. *See also* Holmium (Ho) YAG lasers; Nd:YAG lasers
Yannuzzi lens, 100, 101

Zonulysis, Nd:YAG laser, 85